CHRONIC KIDNEY DISEASE AND RENAL TRANSPLANTATION

Edited by **Manisha Sahay**

Chronic Kidney Disease and Renal Transplantation
Edited by Manisha Sahay

Published by InTech
Janeza Trdine 9, 51000 Rijeka, Croatia

Publishing Process Manager Maja Kisic

Technical Editor Teodora Smiljanic

Cover Designer InTech Design Team

Additional hard copies can be obtained from orders@intechopen.com

Chronic Kidney Disease and Renal Transplantation, Edited by Manisha Sahay
p. cm.
ISBN 978-953-51-0003-4

For EU product safety concerns:
IN TECH d.o.o., Prolaz Marije Krucifikse Kozulić 3, 51000 Rijeka, Croatia,
info@intechopen.com or visit our website at intechopen.com.

Meet the editor

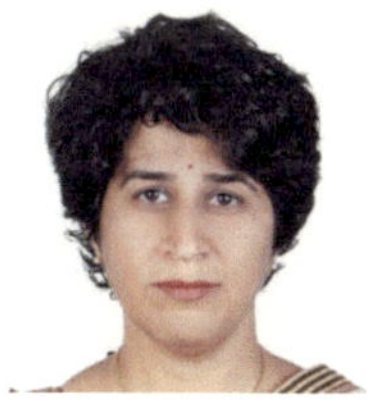

Dr Manisha Sahay is currently the Professor, and Head of the Department of Nephrology, Osmania General Hospital & Osmania Medical College, and Consultant Nephrologist at the Aditya Hospital, Hyderabad, Andhra Pradesh, India. She undertook her DNB in Nephrology in 2003 (under the National Board of Examinations, National Academy of Medical Sciences, India) in which she achieved first rank and a gold medal. She acquired her MD in 1998 from Osmania Medical College, Hyderabad, and MBBS from SMS Medical College, Jaipur, Rajasthan. She was a State topper in the 10th Board Examination and has, so far, been awarded 12 gold medals. She has also received the "Tanker – Young Investigator Award" of the Indian Society of Nephrology, and has many publications to her credit in both national and international journals. Dr Sahay is the Executive Committee Member of the Young Nephrologists' Committee of the International Society of Nephrology, and is also the Governing Body Member of the Indian Society of Nephrology. As well as having contributed to several textbooks, she is the reviewer for Indian and international journals, and is the Associate Editor of the *Journal of Academy of Medical Sciences* and Guest Editor for the *Indian Journal of Endocrinology and Metabolism-Renal Endocrinology*.

Contents

Preface

The first section deals with chronic kidney disease (CKD). CKD is assuming epidemic proportions. Metabolic bone disease is an important complication of CKD. Parathormone is an important uremic toxin and plays an important role in the pathogenesis of renal osteodystrophy and vascular calcification in chronic kidney disease. The role of elevated calcium and phosphorus product in the genesis of mineral bone disease is discussed. The presence of kidney disease, manifested by low glomerular filtration rates (GFR) and/or large amounts of protein in the urine, is independently associated with increased rates of cardiovascular disease (CVD). The severity of kidney disease is associated with graded increases in the risk of CVD and death. This is described in the chapter on cardiovascular diseases in CKD. Chronic kidney disease affects not only physical but also psychological health and well-being; this is highlighted in the chapter on social and psychological aspects of chronic kidney disease. Prevention of chronic kidney disease is the only solution to stem the increasing prevalence of CKD globally and hence emphasis should be on evolving screening methods for early detection, as is discussed in the chapter on screening for chronic kidney disease. The role of renin angiotensin system in the progression of renal diseases is stressed. The second section of the book includes chapters on renal transplantation that will be of use to the readers. I am sure this book will be a valuable addition to the reader's library.

Dr. Manisha Sahay
Department of Nephrology
Osmania General Hospital & Osmania Medical College
Hyderabad
India

Part 1

Chronic Kidney Disease

1

Screening for Chronic Kidney Disease

Ross Francis and David Johnson
Department of Nephrology
Princess Alexandra Hospital, Woolloongabba, Brisbane
Australia

1. Introduction

Chronic kidney disease (CKD), defined as reduced excretory kidney function (glomerular filtration rate (GFR) <60 mL/min/1.73m^2) or evidence of kidney damage (such as proteinuria) for a period of at least 3 months, is considered a major global public health problem (Levey, Atkins et al. 2007). The prevalence of CKD has been estimated at between 10-15% in industrialised countries and is increasing, likely as a result of population ageing and the increasing incidence of diabetes, vascular disease and obesity (Chadban, Briganti et al. 2003; Coresh, Astor et al. 2003; Coresh, Selvin et al. 2007; Stevens, O'Donoghue et al. 2007).
A definition and staging system for CKD was introduced in 2002 and has been widely accepted (Table 1) (K/DOQI 2002).

Stage	Description	GFR (ml/min/1.73m^2)
1	Kidney damage with normal or increased GFR	≥90
2	Kidney damage with mild reduction in GFR	60–89
3	Moderate reduction in GFR	30–59
4	Severe reduction in GFR	15–29
5	Kidney failure	<15 (or dialysis)

Table 1. National Kidney Foundation CKD classification (K/DOQI 2002)

More recent staging classification systems have attempted to improve CKD risk stratification by incorporating proteinuria (Table 2). Within the continuum of patients with CKD, there is a wide range of disease severities, from patients with an excellent long-term renal prognosis through to patients with end-stage kidney disease (ESKD) who require renal replacement therapy.
Many patients with CKD follow a predictable clinical course following disease initiation, with progressive renal dysfunction ultimately resulting in ESKD. Critically, CKD is clinically silent in up to 90% patients until it has reached an advanced stage (Chadban, Briganti et al. 2003; John, Webb et al. 2004; Nickolas, Frisch et al. 2004), and patients who reach ESKD without prior contact with nephrology services experience greater co-morbidity and poorer survival following initiation of renal replacement therapy (Roderick, Jones et al. 2002; Chan, Dall et al. 2007). There is therefore an opportunity to detect patients with asymptomatic CKD by screening, with the aim of applying therapies to ameliorate disease progression.

eGFR Stage	Albuminuria Stage (uACR value)		
	Normal (<2.5 mg/mmol [M], <3.5 mg/mmol [F])	Microalbuminuria (2.5-25 mg/mmol [M], 3.5-35 mg/mmol [F])	Macroalbuminuria (>25 mg/mmol [M], >35 mg/mmol [F])
1			
2			
3a			
3b			
4			
5			

* Risks of progressive CKD denoted as low (light grey), moderate (dark gray) and high (black).

Table 2. Modified CKD staging system recommended by the Caring for Australasians with Renal Insufficiency Early CKD Guidelines (Johnson and Toussaint 2011)

Apart from the risk of progression to ESKD, the presence of CKD is a potent risk factor for cardiovascular disease, such that individuals with ESKD have up to a 10- to 20-fold greater risk of cardiac death than age- and sex-matched controls without ESKD (Foley and Parfrey 1998). Moreover, as illustrated in Figure 1, people with earlier stages of CKD are up to 20 times more likely to die, predominantly from cardiovascular disease, than survive to the point of needing dialysis or kidney transplantation (Go, Chertow et al. 2004; Smith, Gullion

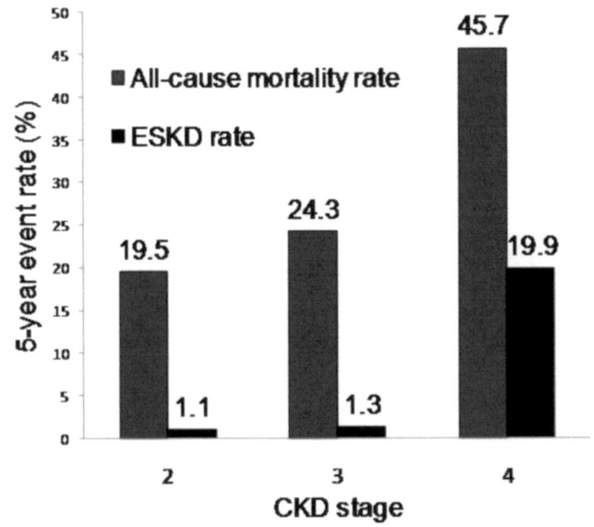

Fig. 1. Five-year event rates for all-cause mortality and end-stage kidney disease in CKD stages 2 to 4 (data derived from (Keith, Nichols et al. 2004)).

et al. 2004; Foley, Murray et al. 2005; Matsushita, van der Velde et al. 2010). As a result, a successful CKD screening programme would identify individuals who are likely to benefit from interventions to reduce heart disease risk.

Despite the theoretical benefits, screening for CKD remains controversial (Glassock and Winearls 2008; Grootendorst, Jager et al. 2009), and although several national and international organisations have made recommendations advocating routine screening for CKD, details regarding approaches to screening vary. This chapter will examine the role and cost-effectiveness of screening for CKD and make recommendations regarding the optimal screening strategy (i.e. who, how, when and what to screen).

2. Methods of screening

The presence of CKD can be readily identified using non-invasive investigations to estimate glomerular filtration rate and to detect proteinuria. Further information about future risk of progressive renal disease and ESKD can be obtained from monitoring blood pressure.

2.1 Proteinuria

Proteinuria is an early marker of kidney damage in many forms of renal disease, such as diabetic nephropathy and glomerulonephritis. Persistent proteinuria has a strong positive correlation with the subsequent development of ESKD. In a Japanese study of community mass screening, 193 of 107,192 subjects were identified as requiring RRT after 10 years of follow-up (Iseki, Iseki et al. 1996). Proteinuria was the strongest predictor of subsequent need for dialysis, with an adjusted odds ratio (OR) of 14.9 (95% confidence interval (CI) 10.9-20.2). Similarly, in a US study that followed 1832 subjects with type 2 diabetes for between 5-40 years, 25 reached ESKD (Humphrey, Ballard et al. 1989). The presence of proteinuria at the time diabetes was identified was the strongest risk factor for reaching ESKD (relative risk (RR) 12.1, CI 4.3-34).

There is also evidence from controlled trials that proteinuria is a risk factor for CKD progression. In the modification of diet in renal disease (MDRD) trial, there was a positive correlation between baseline proteinuria and the rate of decline in GFR (Peterson, Adler et al. 1995). This association was independent of other risk factors for decline in GFR such as blood pressure. Similarly, in a trial of 409 patients with type 1 diabetes, proteinuria was the strongest single risk factor for doubling of serum creatinine (Breyer, Bain et al. 1996).

The presence of proteinuria has also been shown to be an important independent predictor of subsequent cardiovascular disease, both in patients with diabetes and the general population (Mogensen 1984; Rossing, Hougaard et al. 1996; Hillege, Fidler et al. 2002; Romundstad, Holmen et al. 2003; Hallan, Astor et al. 2007).

Taken together, these observations strongly support the inclusion of proteinuria in CKD screening. The gold standard for assessing urinary protein excretion is a timed 24-hour urine collection. However, the difficulties of obtaining an accurately timed and complete urine collection and the inconvenience for the individual performing the collection reduce the utility of this test as a screening tool. Because the rate of creatinine excretion remains approximately stable over a 24-hour period, the creatinine concentration in a spot urine sample can be used as a control for urine concentration, allowing estimation of 24-hour urinary protein or albumin excretion from the urinary protein:creatinine ratio (uPCR) or albumin:creatinine ratio (uACR), respectively (Ginsberg, Chang et al. 1983). Alternatively, urine stick can be used to estimate urinary protein excretion (James, Bee et al. 1978; Allen,

Krauss et al. 1991; Higby, Suiter et al. 1995). However, meta-analysis of data extracted from the primary studies of proteinuria assessment indicate that urine stick testing has a sensitivity of 90% and specificity of 67%, compared to a sensitivity of 95% and specificity of 91% for protein:creatinine ratio (Craig, Barratt et al. 2002). For this reason, uPCR or uACR are the preferred modalities for CKD screening.

There is diurnal variation in urinary protein excretion, with the highest level of proteinuria in the afternoon and therefore where possible, spot urine testing for proteinuria should be performed on an early morning (first urinary void of day) sample. However, a number of studies have demonstrated that random urine samples are still acceptable if first void samples are impractical (Price, Newall et al. 2005; Cote, Brown et al. 2008; Witte, Lambers Heerspink et al. 2009). Importantly, transient increases in urinary protein excretion are seen in several circumstances other than CKD, including urine infection, febrile illness, heart failure and hyperglycaemia (Table 2). As a result, patients should only be labelled as having CKD if proteinuria persists for at least three months.

Urinary tract infection
High dietary protein intake
Congestive cardiac failure
Acute febrile illness
Heavy exercise within 24 hours
Menstruation or vaginal discharge
Drugs – e.g. non-steroidal anti-inflammatory drugs, ACE inhibitors, ARBs, calcineurin inhibitors

Table 2. Factors that may affect urinary protein excretion

2.2 Renal function

Glomerular filtration rate, or GFR, is determined by the total number of functional nephrons, and is considered the best overall measure of excretory kidney function. Furthermore, GFR is central to the current definition of CKD. Several equations have been derived that permit estimation of GFR from the serum concentration of renally-excreted endogenous molecules – typically creatinine. Creatinine is both filtered at the glomerulus and secreted in the proximal tubule, and therefore falls short of being a model molecule with which to assess GFR. This is particularly significant in patients with low GFRs, in whom tubular creatinine secretion contributes a greater proportion of total renal creatinine clearance. Nevertheless, several equations have been generated that allow estimation of GFR using serum creatinine levels. The first equation to be used widely in clinical practice was described in 1976 (Box 1) and estimates creatinine clearance (Cockcroft and Gault 1976). While useful for monitoring the clinical course of an individual patient or making dose adjustments of medications, the inclusion of body weight as a variable reduces the applicability of this formula for population screening.

More recent equations have been generated using data from large trials in which simultaneous data for serum creatinine and GFR measured by the renal clearance of radioactive isotopes, such as [^{51}Cr]-ethylenediaminetetraacetic acid, [^{125}I]-iothalamate or [^{99}Tcm]-diethylenetriaminepentaacetic acid, were available. At present, an equation generated using data from the modification of diet in renal disease trial (Box 2) is in widespread clinical use for GFR estimation (Levey, Bosch et al. 1999).

Creatinine clearance (ml/min) =

$$\frac{1.23 \times (140 - age\ (years))}{serum\ creatinine\ (\mu mol/L)}$$

$$\times\ 0.85\ (if\ female)$$

Box 1. Cockcroft and Gault equation

GFR (ml/min/1.73m^2) =

$$175 \times \left\{\frac{serum\ creatinine\ (\mu mol/L)}{1.004} \times 0.011312\right\}^{-1.154} \times (age\ in\ years)^{-0.203}$$

$$\times\ 0.742\ (if\ female)$$

$$\times\ 1.212\ (if\ black)$$

Box 2. Simplified modification of diet in renal disease (MDRD) formula

An advantage of the MDRD equation over the Cockcroft-Gault equation is that the former only requires knowledge of the serum creatinine, age and ethnicity. MDRD eGFR is currently reported automatically whenever a serum creatinine assay is requested in several countries including Australia and the UK. A significant problem with the MDRD equation is that the accuracy of the approximation to isotopic GFR varies with renal function. While it is acceptably accurate in patients with low GFR, it performs less well in patients with normal or near normal renal function (GFR >60ml/min/1.73m^2). The MDRD equation tends to underestimate GFR in patients with normal or near-normal renal function, which is of particular concern for the purpose of CKD screening, since this increases the probability of inappropriately labelling healthy individuals with CKD.

In an attempt to improve GFR estimation, a new creatinine-based eGFR equation was developed that includes a two-slope "spline" to improve accuracy in patients with good renal function (Levey, Stevens et al. 2009). Unlike the MDRD formula, which was developed from a population with CKD, the CKD-EPI formula was developed and validated in a large heterogeneous population with and without known CKD including subjects with diabetes, potential kidney donors and transplant recipients. Analyses using the CKD-EPI equation (Box 3) indicate that it is more accurate than the MDRD equation in individuals with a GFR >60ml/min/1.73m^2, and performs with equivalent accuracy to the MDRD equation when the GFR is <60 (Levey and Stevens 2010; Stevens, Claybon et al. 2011). Subsequent epidemiologic evaluations in North American (Matsushita K et al. 2010) and Australian general population studies (White, Polkinghorne et al. 2010) have shown that the CKD-EPI equation more appropriately categorises individuals with respect to long-term clinical risks of end-stage kidney disease, coronary heart disease, stroke and/or all-cause mortality than the MDRD equation. In particular, 1.9% of the AusDiab study population was re-classified as not having CKD and such re-classified individuals were predominantly younger women with a favourable cardiovascular risk profile and absence of significant albuminuria.

GFR (ml/min/1.73m²) =

$$141 \times \min\left(\frac{serum\ creatinine}{\kappa}, 1\right)^{\alpha} \times \max\left(\frac{serum\ creatinine}{\kappa}, 1\right)^{-1.209} \times 0.993^{age}$$

$$\times\ 1.018\ (if\ female)$$

$$\times\ 1.159\ (if\ black)$$

$$\kappa = 0.7\ , \alpha = \ -0.329\ if\ female$$

$$\kappa = 0.9\ , \alpha = \ -0.411\ if\ male$$

$$\min = \text{the minimum of } \frac{serum\ creatinine}{\kappa} \text{ or } 1$$

$$\max = \text{the maximum of } \frac{serum\ creatinine}{\kappa} \text{ or } 1$$

Box 3. Chronic Kidney Disease Epidemiology Collaboration (CKD-EPI) equation

Finally, equations are available that permit estimation of GFR from serum levels of an alternative renally-excreted endogenous molecule, cystatin C (Stevens, Coresh et al. 2006). Cystatin C is a 122-amino acid protein ubiquitously expressed in all nucleated cells that is freely filtered at the glomerulus, whereupon 99% of filtered cystatin C is reabsorbed and catabolised in the proximal tubule (Tenstad, Roald et al. 1996; Roald, Aukland et al. 2004). There is some evidence that cystatin C, like creatinine, is secreted in the proximal tubule. Early data suggest that estimated GFR based either on the serum level of cystatin C or the combination of cystatin C and creatinine may be more accurate than creatinine-only equations (Madero, Sarnak et al. 2006; Groesbeck, Kottgen et al. 2008; Kottgen, Selvin et al. 2008; Stevens, Coresh et al. 2008). At present, the relatively high cost of assaying cystatin C and the need for further validation of the potential benefits over creatinine as a filtration marker mean that this approach is not ready for use as a screening tool.

2.3 Hypertension

Systemic blood pressure is an important and modifiable risk factor for CKD progression (Haroun, Jaar et al. 2003). Furthermore, long-term population studies indicate that hypertension is a potent predictor of subsequent development of ESKD. For instance, in the Multiple Risk Factor Intervention Trial (MRFIT), a strong graded independent relationship between blood pressure and later ESKD development was observed (Klag, Whelton et al. 1996). The strength of the association between hypertension and ESKD risk was much greater for systolic blood pressure than diastolic blood pressure.

It remains unclear whether hypertension (other than accelerated or malignant hypertension) is causally related to, or a consequence of progressive renal impairment. Furthermore, no studies have specifically examined blood pressure as a screening tool for detecting patients with CKD. However, the strong epidemiological link between blood pressure and ESKD suggests that patients with hypertension should be monitored for the development of CKD.

3. Evidence of benefit from screening for CKD

There is little point in screening for a disease unless interventions are available that can improve outcomes following diagnosis. Unfortunately, there are no prospective randomised trials that have addressed whether screening for CKD leads to improvement in important outcomes such as progression of renal dysfunction or co-morbidity from cardiovascular disease. Despite this, there is an increasing evidence base to support a range of interventions in patients with CKD, providing indirect support for identifying these individuals at an earlier stage of disease. Specific therapies are available for a limited number of renal diseases, such as recombinant alpha-galactosidase in patients with Fabry disease. Immunosuppressive therapy can ameliorate disease progression in several immunologically-mediated renal diseases, such as lupus nephropathy. Importantly however, there are data to support the application of certain therapies in a broad range of patients with CKD, particularly blood pressure control and the use of HMG-CoA reductase inhibitors (statins).

3.1 Blood pressure lowering

Multiple studies have evaluated the impact of anti-hypertensive agents in patients with CKD. There is strong and consistent evidence from these data that antihypertensives, and in particular agents that inhibit the action of angiotensin II, reduce proteinuria (Gansevoort, Sluiter et al. 1995; Atkins, Briganti et al. 2005; Kunz, Friedrich et al. 2008; Parving, Persson et al. 2008), as well as the rate of progression of CKD (Peterson, Adler et al. 1995; Maschio, Alberti et al. 1996; Giatras, Lau et al. 1997; GISEN 1997; Jafar, Schmid et al. 2001; Strippoli, Bonifati et al. 2006). These data provide compelling support for blood pressure control in patients with CKD.

3.2 Lipid lowering

Until the recent publication of the SHARP trial (Baigent, Landray et al. 2011), there were no primary studies of lipid lowering in patients with CKD that were not on renal replacement therapy. Many patients with overt CKD were excluded from the early large trials showing a beneficial effect of statins on all cause mortality in both secondary and primary prevention studies (Wright, Flapan et al. 1994; Shepherd, Cobbe et al. 1995). Nevertheless, post-hoc analyses have identified many patients with modest renal impairment that were included in the trials. These data suggest that within these trials, similar benefits from statin use occurred in patients with or without modest renal impairment (Shepherd, Kastelein et al. 2008; Navaneethan, Nigwekar et al. 2009). In contrast, two randomised controlled trials specifically evaluating statin use in patients on dialysis found no evidence of improvement in mortality or cardiovascular endpoints, despite significant reductions in serum cholesterol levels (Wanner, Krane et al. 2005; Fellstrom, Jardine et al. 2009). The SHARP trial goes some way to bridge the gulf between these apparently contradictory findings. 9270 patients with CKD (serum creatinine >150 µmol/L in men or >130 µmol/L in women) were randomised to receive simvastatin plus ezetimibe or placebo (Baigent, Landray et al. 2011). The active treatment group experienced significantly fewer major atherosclerotic events (a composite endpoint of non-fatal myocardial infarction or coronary death, non-haemorrhagic stroke, or any arterial revascularisation procedure) – (RR 0.83, 95% CI 0.74–0.94; p=0.0021). There was no significant difference in mortality rate between the two groups. Overall, these data indicate that patients with CKD are likely to benefit from statin use.

4. Who should be screened for CKD?

Epidemiological studies indicate that many of the patients identified with CKD have a low probability of progressing to ESKD. As a result, most of the published guidelines on CKD screening have recommended targeted screening of groups considered to be at high risk of developing progressive CKD, such as individuals with diabetes or hypertension. This strategy will increase the cost-effectiveness of screening, at the expense of missing individuals who could benefit from CKD screening. For example, many individuals will have unrecognised risk factors for CKD – for example undiagnosed diabetes – and will therefore be omitted from targeted CKD screening. An 8 year follow-up of a cross sectional health survey (the HUNT II study) involving 65,604 people (70.6 % of all adults aged ≥20 years in Nord-Trøndelag County, Norway) found that screening people with hypertension, diabetes mellitus, or age >55 years was the most effective strategy to detect patients with CKD, such that 93.2% (95% CI 92.4-94.0%) of all CKD patients would be identified resulting in a number needed to screen of 8.7 (8.5 to 9.0). Nevertheless, the risk of end stage kidney disease among those detected was low (1.2% over 8 years) (Hallan, Dahl et al. 2006). Other strategies of targeting (e.g. only people with diabetes and hypertension) detected a lower percentage of CKD (44.2%) and were less effective. Another study reporting on the performance of similar screening strategies is the United States (US) Kidney Early Evaluation Program (KEEP), which targets individuals with diabetes, hypertension, or family history of diabetes or hypertension or CKD. Using this strategy, 7 people with diabetes or hypertension or with first degree relatives with diabetes, hypertension or kidney disease needed to be screened for one case of CKD to be found (Vassalotti, Li et al. 2009). An Australian report by Howard *et al.* using cost-effectiveness modelling outlined the potential effectiveness of screening and intensive management of the most important CKD risk factors - diabetes, hypertension and proteinuria (Howard, White et al. 2010). Cost-effectiveness was modelled in terms of the effect on overall mortality, on cardiovascular mortality and morbidity and on progression to ESKD and the report determined that a strategy based on screening of 50 to 69 year olds in general practice, plus intensive management of diabetes, hypertension and proteinuria, would be cost-effective. Similarly, a US cost-effectiveness study found that early detection of urine protein to slow progression of CKD and decrease mortality was not cost-effective unless selectively directed toward high-risk groups (older persons and persons with hypertension) (Boulware, Jaar et al. 2003). The CARI Guidelines recommend that patients should be screened with eGFR, urine albumin:creatinine ratio (uACR) and a BP measurement at least annually during routine primary health encounters if they have at least one of the CKD risk factors listed in Figure 2.

5. Conclusions

CKD is common, and can be readily detected using non-invasive assays. It causes considerable co-morbidity and premature mortality, and is frequently asymptomatic until disease has progressed to the point that there is little scope to modify disease progression or limit co-morbidity. At present, it is unclear whether screening for CKD has a beneficial effect on outcome. However, increasing evidence supports a range of interventions in patients with CKD, including blood pressure reduction, angiotensin-converting enzyme inhibition or angiotensin receptor blockade to reduce proteinuria and statin use to reduce cardiovascular events. Therefore, CKD fits many of the principles proposed by the WHO for population health screening programmes (Table 4). General population screening does not appear to be a cost-effective approach, and instead screening should be performed in individuals who have an elevated risk for CKD. An illustrative example of how a CKD screening programme may be organised is shown in Figure 2.

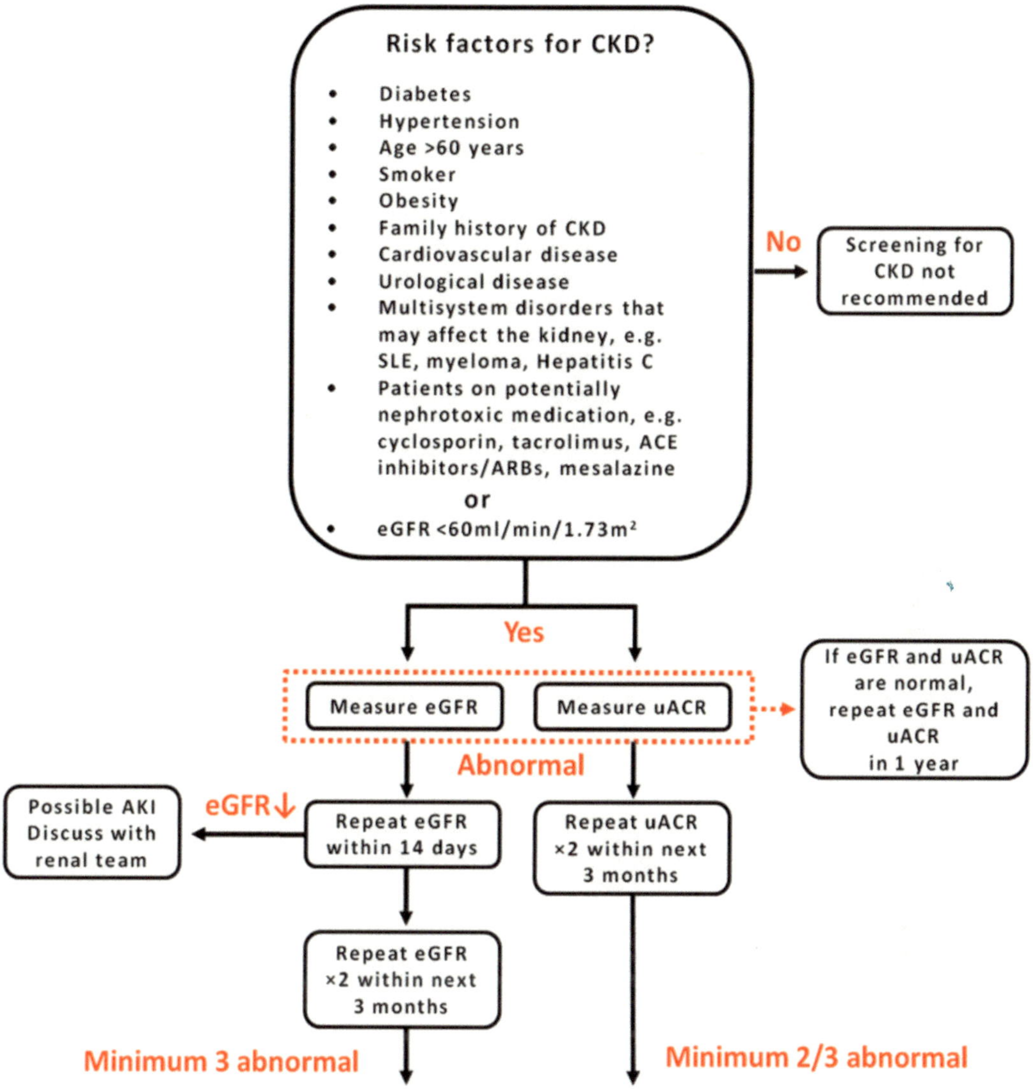

CKD stage	GFR (ml/min/1.73m²)
1	≥ 90
2	60-89
3	30-59
4	15-29
5	<15 (or on RRT)

Kidney damage Stage	uACR (g/mol)
Microalbuminuria	Men 2.5 – 25 Women 3.5 – 35
Macroalbuminuria	Men >25 Women >35

Combine CKD stage and kidney damage stage

Fig. 2. Recommended approach to screening for CKD

The condition should be an important health problem.
There should be a treatment for the condition.
Facilities for diagnosis and treatment should be available.
There should be a latent stage of the disease.
There should be a test or examination for the condition.
The test should be acceptable to the population.
The natural history of the disease should be adequately understood.
There should be an agreed policy on whom to treat.
The total cost of finding a case should be economically balanced in relation to medical expenditure as a whole.
Case-finding should be a continuous process, not just a "once and for all" project.

Table 4. World Health Organisation Principles of Screening (Jungner and Wilson 1968)

The clinical priorities in individuals detected to have CKD during screening will vary depending on the patient population. It is likely that many elderly patients with relatively poor excretory renal function (CKD stage 4-5) will be identified. However, many of these individuals are likely to have relatively stable renal function and to die either from alternative health issues or cardiovascular disease (O'Hare, Choi et al. 2007). In this population the principal benefit of CKD identification will be the potential to reduce the risk of cardiovascular complications. Younger patients with CKD are more likely to progress to ESKD, and the priorities will be both to ameliorate renal disease progression as well as to reduce cardiovascular co-morbidity (Menon, Wang et al. 2008).

6. Online resources

- National Kidney Foundation http://www.kidney.org/professionals/kdoqi/
- Kidney Disease Improving Global Outcomes (KDIGO) http://www.kdigo.org/
- Caring for Australians with Renal Impairment http://www.cari.org.au/
- UK Renal Association http://www.renal.org/home.aspx
- European Renal Association http://www.era-edta.org/
- UK NICE CKD guidelines http://www.nice.org.uk/CG73

7. References

Allen, J. K., E. A. Krauss, et al. (1991). "Dipstick analysis of urinary protein. A comparison of Chemstrip-9 and Multistix-10SG." *Arch Pathol Lab Med* 115(1): 34-37.

Atkins, R. C., E. M. Briganti, et al. (2005). "Proteinuria reduction and progression to renal failure in patients with type 2 diabetes mellitus and overt nephropathy." *Am J Kidney Dis* 45(2): 281-287.

Baigent, C., M. J. Landray, et al. (2011). "The effects of lowering LDL cholesterol with simvastatin plus ezetimibe in patients with chronic kidney disease (Study of Heart and Renal Protection): a randomised placebo-controlled trial." *Lancet*.

Boulware, L. E., B. G. Jaar, et al. (2003). "Screening for proteinuria in US adults: a cost-effectiveness analysis." *JAMA* 290(23): 3101-3114.

Breyer, J. A., R. P. Bain, et al. (1996). "Predictors of the progression of renal insufficiency in patients with insulin-dependent diabetes and overt diabetic nephropathy. The Collaborative Study Group." *Kidney Int* 50(5): 1651-1658.

Chadban, S. J., E. M. Briganti, et al. (2003). "Prevalence of kidney damage in Australian adults: The AusDiab kidney study." *J Am Soc Nephrol* 14(7 Suppl 2): S131-138.

Chan, M. R., A. T. Dall, et al. (2007). "Outcomes in patients with chronic kidney disease referred late to nephrologists: a meta-analysis." *Am J Med* 120(12): 1063-1070.

Cockcroft, D. W. and M. H. Gault (1976). "Prediction of creatinine clearance from serum creatinine." *Nephron* 16(1): 31-41.

Coresh, J., B. C. Astor, et al. (2003). "Prevalence of chronic kidney disease and decreased kidney function in the adult US population: Third National Health and Nutrition Examination Survey." *Am J Kidney Dis* 41(1): 1-12.

Coresh, J., E. Selvin, et al. (2007). "Prevalence of chronic kidney disease in the United States." *JAMA* 298(17): 2038-2047.

Cote, A. M., M. A. Brown, et al. (2008). "Diagnostic accuracy of urinary spot protein:creatinine ratio for proteinuria in hypertensive pregnant women: systematic review." *BMJ* 336(7651): 1003-1006.

Craig, J. C., A. Barratt, et al. (2002). "Feasibility study of the early detection and treatment of renal disease by mass screening." *Intern Med J* 32(1-2): 6-14.

Fellstrom, B. C., A. G. Jardine, et al. (2009). "Rosuvastatin and cardiovascular events in patients undergoing hemodialysis." *N Engl J Med* 360(14): 1395-1407.

Foley, R. N., A. M. Murray, et al. (2005). "Chronic kidney disease and the risk for cardiovascular disease, renal replacement, and death in the United States Medicare population, 1998 to 1999." *J Am Soc Nephrol* 16(2): 489-495.

Foley, R. N. and P. S. Parfrey (1998). "Cardiovascular disease and mortality in ESRD." *J Nephrol* 11(5): 239-245.

Gansevoort, R. T., W. J. Sluiter, et al. (1995). "Antiproteinuric effect of blood-pressure-lowering agents: a meta-analysis of comparative trials." *Nephrol Dial Transplant* 10(11): 1963-1974.

Giatras, I., J. Lau, et al. (1997). "Effect of angiotensin-converting enzyme inhibitors on the progression of nondiabetic renal disease: a meta-analysis of randomized trials. Angiotensin-Converting-Enzyme Inhibition and Progressive Renal Disease Study Group." *Ann Intern Med* 127(5): 337-345.

Ginsberg, J. M., B. S. Chang, et al. (1983). "Use of single voided urine samples to estimate quantitative proteinuria." *N Engl J Med* 309(25): 1543-1546.

GISEN (1997). "Randomised placebo-controlled trial of effect of ramipril on decline in glomerular filtration rate and risk of terminal renal failure in proteinuric, non-diabetic nephropathy. The GISEN Group (Gruppo Italiano di Studi Epidemiologici in Nefrologia)." *Lancet* 349(9069): 1857-1863.

Glassock, R. J. and C. Winearls (2008). "Screening for CKD with eGFR: doubts and dangers." *Clin J Am Soc Nephrol* 3(5): 1563-1568.

Go, A. S., G. M. Chertow, et al. (2004). "Chronic kidney disease and the risks of death, cardiovascular events, and hospitalization." *N Engl J Med* 351(13): 1296-1305.

Groesbeck, D., A. Kottgen, et al. (2008). "Age, gender, and race effects on cystatin C levels in US adolescents." *Clin J Am Soc Nephrol* 3(6): 1777-1785.

Grootendorst, D. C., K. J. Jager, et al. (2009). "Screening: why, when, and how." *Kidney Int* 76(7): 694-699.

Hallan, S., B. Astor, et al. (2007). "Association of kidney function and albuminuria with cardiovascular mortality in older vs younger individuals: The HUNT II Study." *Arch Intern Med* 167(22): 2490-2496.

Hallan, S. I., K. Dahl, et al. (2006). "Screening strategies for chronic kidney disease in the general population: follow-up of cross sectional health survey." *BMJ* 333(7577): 1047.

Haroun, M. K., B. G. Jaar, et al. (2003). "Risk factors for chronic kidney disease: a prospective study of 23,534 men and women in Washington County, Maryland." *J Am Soc Nephrol* 14(11): 2934-2941.

Higby, K., C. R. Suiter, et al. (1995). "A comparison between two screening methods for detection of microproteinuria." *Am J Obstet Gynecol* 173(4): 1111-1114.

Hillege, H. L., V. Fidler, et al. (2002). "Urinary albumin excretion predicts cardiovascular and noncardiovascular mortality in general population." *Circulation* 106(14): 1777-1782.

Howard, K., S. White, et al. (2010). "Cost-effectiveness of screening and optimal management for diabetes, hypertension, and chronic kidney disease: a modeled analysis." *Value Health* 13(2): 196-208.

Humphrey, L. L., D. J. Ballard, et al. (1989). "Chronic renal failure in non-insulin-dependent diabetes mellitus. A population-based study in Rochester, Minnesota." *Ann Intern Med* 111(10): 788-796.

Iseki, K., C. Iseki, et al. (1996). "Risk of developing end-stage renal disease in a cohort of mass screening." *Kidney Int* 49(3): 800-805.

Jafar, T. H., C. H. Schmid, et al. (2001). "Angiotensin-converting enzyme inhibitors and progression of nondiabetic renal disease. A meta-analysis of patient-level data." *Ann Intern Med* 135(2): 73-87.

James, G. P., D. E. Bee, et al. (1978). "Proteinuria: accuracy and precision of laboratory diagnosis by dip-stick analysis." *Clin Chem* 24(11): 1934-1939.

John, R., M. Webb, et al. (2004). "Unreferred chronic kidney disease: a longitudinal study." *Am J Kidney Dis* 43(5): 825-835.

Johnson, D. W. and N. Toussaint. (2011). "CARI Guidelines for early chronic kidney disease: Diagnosis, classification & staging of chronic kidney disease." from http://www.cari.org.au/DNT%20workshop%202011/5%20Classification%20Staging_Early%20CKD_DNT.pdf.

Jungner, G. and J. M. G. Wilson (1968). "Principles and practice of screening for disease." *WHO Public Health Papers* 22(11).

K/DOQI (2002). "K/DOQI clinical practice guidelines for chronic kidney disease: evaluation, classification, and stratification." *Am J Kidney Dis* 39(2 Suppl 1): S1-266.

Keith, D. S., G. A. Nichols, et al. (2004). "Longitudinal follow-up and outcomes among a population with chronic kidney disease in a large managed care organization." *Arch Intern Med* 164(6): 659-663.

Klag, M. J., P. K. Whelton, et al. (1996). "Blood pressure and end-stage renal disease in men." *N Engl J Med* 334(1): 13-18.

Kottgen, A., E. Selvin, et al. (2008). "Serum cystatin C in the United States: the Third National Health and Nutrition Examination Survey (NHANES III)." *Am J Kidney Dis* 51(3): 385-394.

Kunz, R., C. Friedrich, et al. (2008). "Meta-analysis: effect of monotherapy and combination therapy with inhibitors of the renin angiotensin system on proteinuria in renal disease." *Ann Intern Med* 148(1): 30-48.

Levey, A. S., R. Atkins, et al. (2007). "Chronic kidney disease as a global public health problem: approaches and initiatives - a position statement from Kidney Disease Improving Global Outcomes." *Kidney Int* 72(3): 247-259.

Levey, A. S., J. P. Bosch, et al. (1999). "A more accurate method to estimate glomerular filtration rate from serum creatinine: a new prediction equation. Modification of Diet in Renal Disease Study Group." *Ann Intern Med* 130(6): 461-470.

Levey, A. S. and L. A. Stevens (2010). "Estimating GFR using the CKD Epidemiology Collaboration (CKD-EPI) creatinine equation: more accurate GFR estimates, lower CKD prevalence estimates, and better risk predictions." *Am J Kidney Dis* 55(4): 622-627.

Levey, A. S., L. A. Stevens, et al. (2009). "A new equation to estimate glomerular filtration rate." *Ann Intern Med* 150(9): 604-612.

Madero, M., M. J. Sarnak, et al. (2006). "Serum cystatin C as a marker of glomerular filtration rate." *Curr Opin Nephrol Hypertens* 15(6): 610-616.

Maschio, G., D. Alberti, et al. (1996). "Effect of the angiotensin-converting-enzyme inhibitor benazepril on the progression of chronic renal insufficiency. The Angiotensin-Converting-Enzyme Inhibition in Progressive Renal Insufficiency Study Group." *N Engl J Med* 334(15): 939-945.

Matsushita, K., M. van der Velde, et al. (2010). "Association of estimated glomerular filtration rate and albuminuria with all-cause and cardiovascular mortality in general population cohorts: a collaborative meta-analysis." *Lancet* 375(9731): 2073-2081.

Menon, V., X. Wang, et al. (2008). "Long-term outcomes in nondiabetic chronic kidney disease." *Kidney Int* 73(11): 1310-1315.

Mogensen, C. E. (1984). "Microalbuminuria predicts clinical proteinuria and early mortality in maturity-onset diabetes." *N Engl J Med* 310(6): 356-360.

Navaneethan, S. D., S. U. Nigwekar, et al. (2009). "HMG CoA reductase inhibitors (statins) for dialysis patients." *Cochrane Database Syst Rev*(3): CD004289.

Nickolas, T. L., G. D. Frisch, et al. (2004). "Awareness of kidney disease in the US population: findings from the National Health and Nutrition Examination Survey (NHANES) 1999 to 2000." *Am J Kidney Dis* 44(2): 185-197.

O'Hare, A. M., A. I. Choi, et al. (2007). "Age affects outcomes in chronic kidney disease." *J Am Soc Nephrol* 18(10): 2758-2765.

Parving, H. H., F. Persson, et al. (2008). "Aliskiren combined with losartan in type 2 diabetes and nephropathy." *N Engl J Med* 358(23): 2433-2446.

Peterson, J. C., S. Adler, et al. (1995). "Blood pressure control, proteinuria, and the progression of renal disease. The Modification of Diet in Renal Disease Study." *Ann Intern Med* 123(10): 754-762.

Price, C. P., R. G. Newall, et al. (2005). "Use of protein:creatinine ratio measurements on random urine samples for prediction of significant proteinuria: a systematic review." *Clin Chem* 51(9): 1577-1586.

Roald, A. B., K. Aukland, et al. (2004). "Tubular absorption of filtered cystatin-C in the rat kidney." *Exp Physiol* 89(6): 701-707.

Roderick, P., C. Jones, et al. (2002). "Late referral for end-stage renal disease: a region-wide survey in the south west of England." *Nephrol Dial Transplant* 17(7): 1252-1259.

Romundstad, S., J. Holmen, et al. (2003). "Microalbuminuria and all-cause mortality in 2,089 apparently healthy individuals: a 4.4-year follow-up study. The Nord-Trondelag Health Study (HUNT), Norway." *Am J Kidney Dis* 42(3): 466-473.

Rossing, P., P. Hougaard, et al. (1996). "Predictors of mortality in insulin dependent diabetes: 10 year observational follow up study." *BMJ* 313(7060): 779-784.

Shepherd, J., S. M. Cobbe, et al. (1995). "Prevention of coronary heart disease with pravastatin in men with hypercholesterolemia. West of Scotland Coronary Prevention Study Group." *N Engl J Med* 333(20): 1301-1307.

Shepherd, J., J. J. Kastelein, et al. (2008). "Intensive lipid lowering with atorvastatin in patients with coronary heart disease and chronic kidney disease: the TNT (Treating to New Targets) study." *J Am Coll Cardiol* 51(15): 1448-1454.

Smith, D. H., C. M. Gullion, et al. (2004). "Cost of medical care for chronic kidney disease and comorbidity among enrollees in a large HMO population." *J Am Soc Nephrol* 15(5): 1300-1306.

Stevens, L. A., M. A. Claybon, et al. (2011). "Evaluation of the Chronic Kidney Disease Epidemiology Collaboration equation for estimating the glomerular filtration rate in multiple ethnicities." *Kidney Int* 79(5): 555-562.

Stevens, L. A., J. Coresh, et al. (2006). "Assessing kidney function--measured and estimated glomerular filtration rate." *N Engl J Med* 354(23): 2473-2483.

Stevens, L. A., J. Coresh, et al. (2008). "Estimating GFR using serum cystatin C alone and in combination with serum creatinine: a pooled analysis of 3,418 individuals with CKD." *Am J Kidney Dis* 51(3): 395-406.

Stevens, P. E., D. J. O'Donoghue, et al. (2007). "Chronic kidney disease management in the United Kingdom: NEOERICA project results." *Kidney Int* 72(1): 92-99.

Strippoli, G. F., C. Bonifati, et al. (2006). "Angiotensin converting enzyme inhibitors and angiotensin II receptor antagonists for preventing the progression of diabetic kidney disease." *Cochrane Database Syst Rev*(4): CD006257.

Tenstad, O., A. B. Roald, et al. (1996). "Renal handling of radiolabelled human cystatin C in the rat." *Scand J Clin Lab Invest* 56(5): 409-414.

Vassalotti, J. A., S. Li, et al. (2009). "Screening populations at increased risk of CKD: the Kidney Early Evaluation Program (KEEP) and the public health problem." *Am J Kidney Dis* 53(3 Suppl 3): S107-114.

Wanner, C., V. Krane, et al. (2005). "Atorvastatin in patients with type 2 diabetes mellitus undergoing hemodialysis." *N Engl J Med* 353(3): 238-248.

White, S. L., K. R. Polkinghorne, et al. (2010). "Comparison of the prevalence and mortality risk of CKD in Australia using the CKD Epidemiology Collaboration (CKD-EPI) and Modification of Diet in Renal Disease (MDRD) Study GFR estimating equations: the AusDiab (Australian Diabetes, Obesity and Lifestyle) Study." *Am J Kidney Dis* 55(4): 660-670.

Witte, E. C., H. J. Lambers Heerspink, et al. (2009). "First morning voids are more reliable than spot urine samples to assess microalbuminuria." *J Am Soc Nephrol* 20(2): 436-443.

Wright, R., A. Flapan, et al. (1994). "Randomised trial of cholesterol lowering in 4444 patients with coronary heart disease: the Scandinavian Simvastatin Survival Study (4S)." *The Lancet* 344(8939): 1765-1768.

2

The Role of Renin Angiotensin System Inhibitors in Renal Protection: Lessons from Clinical Trials

Ljuba Stojiljkovic
Department of Anesthesiology
Northwestern University, Feinberg School of Medicine
Chicago
U.S.A.

1. Introduction

The prevalence of chronic kidney disease (CKD) is on the rise, and it is estimated that more than 26 million Americans suffer from CKD[1]. The leading risk factors in the development of CKD are hypertension (HTN), diabetes mellitus (DM) and obesity. Because of the increasing prevalence of these risk factors as well as their frequent coexistence in the same patient, prevention strategies that would be able to decrease the progression of CKD to end stage renal disease (ESRD) are of paramount importance.

There is a growing body of evidence showing that the activation of the renin angiotensin aldosterone system (RAAS) plays an important role in the development of cardiovascular and renal disorders[2,3]. RAAS is one of the key players in human physiology, and under normal physiological conditions it regulates blood pressure homeostasis, water balance, renal function and cellular growth. RAAS consists of a cascade of peptide hormones, with the enzyme renin catalyzing the first step in a cascade leading to the production of angiotensin I (AngI) from a precursor angiotensinogen (Figure 1). The cleavage of angiotensinogen, catalyzed by renin, is the rate-limiting step in RAAS activation. AngI does not possess vasoconstricting abilities, and it is cleaved by angiotensin-converting enzyme (ACE) into active angiotensin II (AngII). AngII binds to angiotensin receptors and exerts powerful vasoconstricting abilities. AngII also activates aldosterone production, and regulates sodium and water reapsorption (Figure 1). The kidneys are one of the major targets for RAAS as evidenced by the robust expression of RAAS components and receptors in the kidney[4]. Renal effects of AngII include regulation of renal blood flow, glomerular filtration rate (GFR) and sodium and water balance[5]. Upregulation of renal RAAS has been linked to the development of CKD in both HTN and DM[4].

Hence, therapies that modulate RAAS have emerged as essential tools in decreasing the progression of CKD. Pharmacological inhibition of RAAS can be obtained via three different mechanisms: 1. Inhibition of conversion of AngI to active AngII via angiotensin I converting enzyme inhibitors (ACEI); 2. Selective inhibition of angiotensin receptor 1 (AR-1) via angiotensin receptor blockers (ARB); 3. Direct inhibition of AngI production via direct rennin inhibitors (DRI).

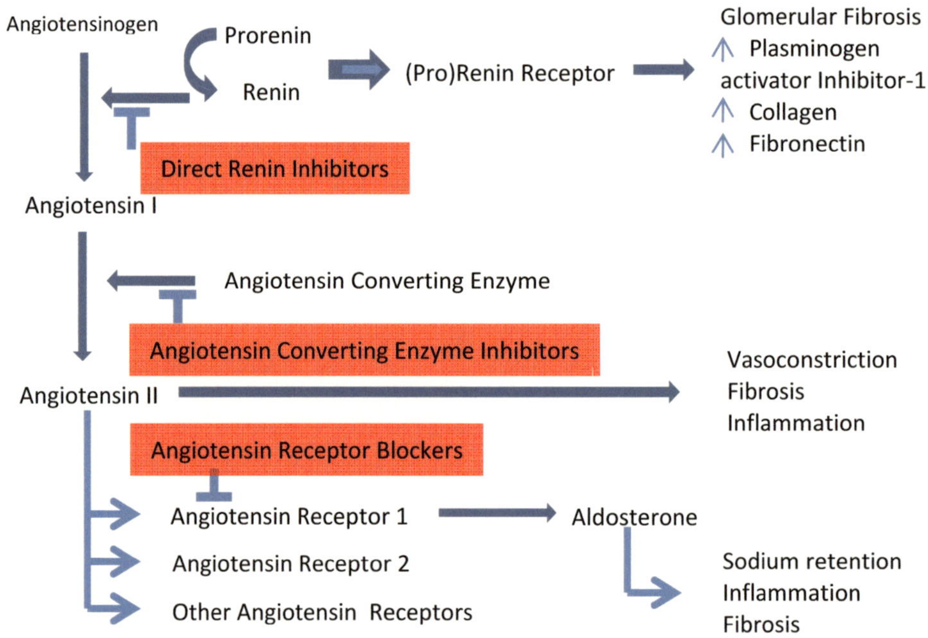

Fig. 1. Renin Angiotensin System Activation Cascade and its Effects on Target Tissues

In this chapter we will summarize the role of RAAS inhibitors on renal outcomes obtained from large clinical outcome trials. Clinical outcome trials have become an essential tool in evaluating treatment strategies and are now a cornerstone of evidence-based medicine. In addition, we will outline future RAAS modulation strategies that may become an important part of the clinical armamentarium for renal protection and prevention of CKD in the future.

2. ACEI in patients with type 1 diabetes mellitus and nephropathy

Patients with DM are more prone to cardiovascular and renal complications. Diabetic nephropathy is the leading cause of ESRD in developed countries [6-8]. Even small amount of albumin in the urine (microalbuminuria) strongly predicts the development of diabetic nephropathy[9]. Since RAAS plays one of the most important roles in renal physiology, several clinical studies have been conducted to evaluate the effect of ACEI on the progression of diabetic nephropathy[10-12]. The landmark study by Lewis et al. [1993], examined the effect of ACEI captopril on the progression of diabetic nephropathy in patients with type 1 diabetes mellitus (T1DM)[13]. The primary endpoint was defined as doubling the serum creatinine to at least 2 mg/dL. Treatment with captopril was associated with a 48% risk reduction for doubling the serum creatinine as compared to the placebo. The beneficial effects of ACEI on the progression of diabetic nephropathy were subsequently confirmed by the results of two large randomized clinical trials in the patients with T1DM[11,12]. The North American Microalbuminemia Study Group evaluated whether ACEI captopril reduces the progression of microalbuminuria to overt diabetic nephropathy in 409 normotensive patients with T1DM[11]. The primary outcome was the progression of microalbuminuria (defined as albumin excretion rate of 20-200 μg/min) to clinical proteinuria (defined as albumin excretion rate of > 200 μg/min, and at least 30% above the baseline). Over a median 3 year follow-up period, patients receiving captopril had a 67.8% risk reduction as compared to those receiving the placebo. According to the results of this clinical trial, for every 8 patients treated with captopril, the progression to proteinuria will be prevented in 1 patient in a 2-year period[11]. The EURODIAB controlled trial of lisinopril in insulin dependent diabetes (EUCLID) studied 530 normotensive T1DM patients either with little or no albuminuria (normoalbuminuria, albumin excretion rate < 20 μg/min) or with microabuminuria (albumin excretion rate > 20 μg/min)[12]. After a 2-year follow-up, the albumin excretion rate was 18.8% lower in patients who received lisinopril. When patients with normoalbuminuria and microalbuminuria were examined separately, the relative treatment difference was 49.7% in the microalbuminuric group and only 12.7% in the normoalbuminuric group. A stratified analysis of the normoalbuminuric group showed that most of the beneficial effect occurred in patients with albumin excretion rate >5 μg/min[12]. A meta-analysis of 12 clinical trials examining the effect of ACEI on T1DM confirmed the protective effect of ACEI on the progression of diabetic nephropathy in T1DM patients[14]. T1DM patients with higher urinary albumin excretion rates appear to achieve a greater benefit from RAAS blockade with ACEI[14].

A summary of the clinical trials on RAAS inhibition in T1DM patients with nephropathy is presented in Table 1.

Study	ACEI	Number of Patients	Renal Outcome	Risk Reduction (%)	Reference
Collaborative Study Group	Captopril	207	Doubling baseline creatinine	43	13
North American Microalbuminuria Study Group	Captopril	215	Progression to clinical proteinuria (AER > 200μg/min)	67.8	11
EUCLID	Lisinopril	530	Change in AER in all patients	18.8	12
			Change in AER in normoalbuminuric patients	12.7 (NS)	
			Change in AER in microalbuminuric patients	49.7	

ACEI: Angiotensin converting enzyme inhibitor; AER: Albumin Excretion Rate; NS: not significant

Table 1. Clinical Trials in Patients with Type 1 Diabetes Mellitus and Nephropathy

3. ACEI and ARB in type 2 diabetes mellitus and nephropathy

Nephropathy secondary to type 2 diabetes mellitus (T2DM) accounts for the majority of the increase in incidence and prevalence of renal failure in the last two decades. Healthcare costs for patients with ESRD are already reaching more than $18 billion per year in the United States and are on the rise. Since ACEIs have been shown to provide renal protection in patients with T1DM and microalbuminuric nephropathy[11-13], it was of paramount interest to examine whether ACEIs have similar effect in patients with T2DM. The MICRO-HOPE substudy of the HOPE trial examined the effect of ACEI ramipril on the development of nephropathy in 3,577 patients with type 2 diabetes mellitus (T2DM)[6,15]. Over a 4.5 year follow-up period, treatment with ramipril decreased the risk of development of overt nephropathy by 24%. However, in the follow-up analysis no change in the slope of serum creatinine rise or in the incidence of doubling serum cratinine was observed[15]. The Bergamo Nephrologic Diabetes Complication (BENEDICT) trial randomized 1,204 T2DM hypertensive patients with normal baseline renal function to receive ACEI trandolapril, calcum channel blocker verapamil or combination therapy (trandolapril plus verapamil). The primary endpoint was the development of persistent albuminuria. After a 3 year follow-up, patients who received trandolapril had a lower incidence of albuminuria, and the effect was not enhanced with the addition of verapamil[16]. The effect of verapamil alone was similar to that of the placebo[16]. Since the development of albuminuria is a major risk factor for the cardiovascular complications and death in this patient population, the authors concluded that in T2DM hypertensive patients with preserved renal function, ACEIs may be the treatment of choice[16]. In the subsequent BENEDICT-B trial they examined the effects of the addition of verapamil on trandolapril therapy in hypertensive T2DM petients with established microalbuminuria[17]. The BENEDICT-B trial showed that addition of verapamil did not improve albuminuria in T2DM patients with nephropathy. Conversely, the trandolapril treatment caused a reduction of albuminuria in 50% of the patients, and this reduction translated to a significantly lower rate of cardiovascular complications in these patients [17]. These results are in sharp contrast to the DIABHYCAR study, which failed to show the beneficial effect of ACEI ramipril on cardiovascular and renal outcomes in T2DM patients with established albuminuria[18]. The lack of an effect due to ACEIs in the DIABHCYAR study may be attributed to a mixed patient population; both normotensive and hypertensive T2DM patients with albuminuria were included in the study.

The renal protection effect of ARB in patients with T2DM was studied extensively in the early 2000s. Two studies, the Irbesartan in Patients with Diabetes and Microalbuminuria (IRMA-2) and the Diabetics Exposed to Telmisartan and Enalapril (DETAIL) study, examined the effect of ARB in T2DM patients with microalbuminuria, but without overt diabetic nephropathy[19,20]. In patients with T2DM the presence of microalbuminuria increases the risk of development of diabetic nephropathy (defined as albumin excretion rate > 200 μg per minute) by a factor of 10 to 20. The IRMA-2 study showed that treatment with irbesartan significantly reduces the rate of progression of microalbuminuria to overt diabetic nephropathy in patients with T2DM[19]. Furthermore, the study revealed that treatment with irbesartan was associated with significantly more common restoration of normoalbuminuria as compared to standard therapy[19]. All these effects were achieved independently of the systemic blood pressure. The DETAIL study compared renoprotective effects of ACEI enalapril and ARB telmisartan[20]. In this head-to-head comparison of these two classes of RAAS inhibitors, the authors showed that both enalapril and telmisartan were equally effective in preventing the progression of renal dysfunction, measured as a decline in the GFR[20]. Two other studies, the Reduction of Endpoints in NIDDM with Angiotensin II Antagonist Losartan (RENAAL) and the Irbesartan Diabetic Nephropathy Trial (IDNT) examined patients with T2DM, but with a higher rate albuminuria and established renal insufficiency [10,21]. In the RENAAL study, treatment with ARB losartan was associated with a 25% reduction of risk for doubling serum creatinine level and the risk of developing ESRD was reduced by 28%[21] Again, the favorable effect seemed to be independent of blood pressure effect. The IDNT compared the effect of ARB irbesartan and calcium-channel blocker amlodipine against the progression of nephropathy[10]. The primary endpoint was a composite of doubling the serum creatinine concentration, development of ESRD, renal transplantation and death. IDNT revealed that irbesartan decreased the relative risk of

reaching the primary end point by 20% when compared to the placebo and by 23% when compared to amlodipine. IDNT data showed that the renoprotective effect of irbesartan in patients with T2DM and overt nephropathy is due to the slowing of the progression of glomerulopathy[10]. The Incipient to Overt: Angiotensin II Blocker Telmisartan, Investigation on Type 2 Diabetic Nephropathy (INNOVATION) study examined the effect of ARB telmisartan in 527 normotensive and hypertensive T2DM Japanese patients with microalbuminuria[22-24]. After a follow-up of 52 weeks, transition to overt nephropathy was significantly lower with telmisartan[23,24]. In a trial comparing telmisartan versus losartan in T2DM patients with overt nephropathy (AMADEO) both agents reduced blood pressure, however telmisartan was more effective in reducing albuminuria as compared to losartan[25]. In the head to head comparison of ACEI ramipril and ARB telmisartan (ONTARGET) study, an increase in urinary albumin secretion was significantly lower in the telmisartan group as compared to ramipril[26,27].
A summary of the clinical trials in patients with T2DM and nephropathy is outlined in Table 2.

Study	ACEI or ARB	Number of Patients	Renal Outcome	Risk Reduction (%)	Reference
MICRO-HOPE	Ramipril (ACEI)	3,577	Overt nephropathy	24	6, 15
BENEDICT	Trandolapril (ACEI) with or without verapamil	1,204	Development of persistent albuminuria (>200 μg/min)	Delay of onset of albuminuria by factor 2.1	16
BENEDICT-B	Trandolapril (ACEI) vs. Trandolapril/Verapamil	281	Development of persistent albuminuria (UAE >200 μg/min)	NS (between trandolapril alone vs. trandolapril/verapamil)	17
DIABHYCAR	Ramipril (ACEI)	4,912	Combined incidence of cardiovascular death, non-fatal myocardial infarction, stroke, heart failure leading to hospital admission, and end stage renal failure	0.97 (NS)	18
IRMA-2	Irbesartan (ARB)	590	Development of persistent albuminuria (UAE >200 μg/min, or ≥ 30% from baseline)	HR 0.56 (150 mg group) HR 0.32 (300 mg group)	19
DETAIL	Telmisartan (ARB) vs. enalapril (ACEI)	250	Change in GFR	ARB not inferior to ACEI	20
RENAAL	Losartan	1,513	Composite of doubling serum creatinine, ESRD or death	25	21
IDNT	Irbesartan (ARB) vs. amlodipine	1,715	Doubling baseline serum creatinine, onset of ESRD, serum creatinine of 6mg/dL and death from any cause	20 (vs. placebo 23 (vs. amlodipine)	10
INNOVATION	Telmisartan (ARB)	527	Transition rate from incipient to overt nephropathy (UACR > 300 mg/g and increase ≥ 30% from baseline)	55	23,24
AMADEO	Telmisartan (ARB) vs. Losartan (ARB)	860	Change in UPC from baseline	Telmisartan superior to losartan (29.8% vs. 21.4% reduction)	25
ONTARGET	Ramipril (ACEI), Telmisartan (ARB) or both	25,620	Composite of dialysis, doubling of serum creatinine, and death	HR 1.00 (Ramipril vs Telmisartan) HR 1.09 Combination Therapy	27

ACEI: Angiotensin converting enzyme inhibitor; AER: Albumin Excretion Rate; GFR: Glomerular Filtration Rate; UACR: Urinary albumin-to-Creatinine ratio; UPC: Urinary Protein-to-Creatinine; HR: Hazard Ratio; NS: not significant

Table 2. Clinical Trials in Patients with Type 2 Diabetes and Nephropathy

As a result of the renoprotective effect of RAAS blockade in T1DM and T2DM patients with established albuminuria, the American Diabetes Asociation (ADA) recommends using ACEI and ARBs in diabetic patients with nephopathy[28]. Specifically, the ADA recommends ACEI in hypertensive T1DM patients with albuminuria and ACEI or ARB in hypertensive T2DM patients with albuminuria. In hypertensive T2DM patients with already established renal insufficiency, ARBs are recommended as a first line of treatment[28].
Even though ACEIs and ARBs have become a cornerstone of treatment of diabetic patients with established nephropathy (secondary prevention), it is still unclear whether RAAS blockade may be beneficial in preventing renal damage in diabetic patients without proteinuria. More recent clinical trials focused on the effect of ACEIs and ARBs on normotensive diabetic patients with normal renal function in order to examine whether early RAAS inhibition could prevent the development of renal disease in this patient population. It is estimated that about 20-30% of T1DM and T2DM patients develop nephropathy over the course of their illness[28]. The DIRECT program was established to investigate the effect of ARB candersartan in the development of diabetic retinopathy, and as a secondary outcome it addressed the effect of candersartan in the primary prevention of diabetic nephropathy (DIRECT-Renal)[29]. They included 3,326 T1DM and 1,905 T2DM patients, and after a follow up of 4.7 years, candersartan did not prevent microalbuminuria in normotensive patients with either T1DM or T2DM[29]. The Telmisartan Randomised Assessment Study in ACE Intolerant Subjects with Cardiovascular Disease (TRANSCEND) examined the effect of ARB telmisartan on cardiovascular outcomes in ACEI intolerant patients[26,30]. In this multicenter multinational study they included 5,926 diabetic patients with known cardiovascular disease, but without microalbuminuria. After 56 months follow-up, no important difference was found in the composite renal outcome (dialysis, doubling serum creatinine, changes in albuminuria and GFR) between patients treated with telmisartan versus placebo[30]. In the Renin - Angiotensin System Study (RASS), the authors examined whether a blockade of RAAS with either ACEI enalapril or ARB losartan prevents the development of structural glomerular changes consistent with the nephropathy in renal biopsy specimens of 285 normotensive T1DM patients with preserved GFR[31]. The results showed no significant difference in the progression of glomerular structural changes among the treatment groups[31].
Taken together, the present evidence does not support the use of ACEI or ARB in the primary prevention of diabetic nephropathy in patients with T1DM or T2DM.
A summary of the clinical trials in patients with DM and without HTN and nephropathy is presented in Table 3.

4. Direct renin inhibitor aliskiren and renal protection

The recent discovery of (pro)rennin receptor has added a new perspective to the RAAS physiology, and has opened new avenues for drug development and RAAS targeting[32]. It has became clear that both prorenin and renin can bind to (pro)renin receptors and activate intracellular signal transduction pathway, independent of angiotensin receptor activation[33,34]. Activation of the (pro)rennin receptor-mediated pathway results in glomerular fibrosis, due to upregulation of transforming growth factor β (TGF β) and increased synthesis of plasminogen activator inhibitor-1 and fibrotic glomerular matrix components, fibronectin and collagen I (Figure 1)[35].

Study	ARB	Number of Patients	Renal Outcome	Risk Reduction (%)	Reference
DIRECT-Renal	Candesartan (ARB)	3,326 T1DM 1,905 T2DM	Primary Prevention of Diabetic Nephropathy (secondary outcome)	NS over placebo	29
TRANSCEND	Telmisartan (ARB)	5,926	Composite renal outcome (Dialysis, doubling serum creatinine, changes in albuminuria and GFR)	NS over placebo	30

ARB: Angiotensin Receptor Blocker; GFR: Glomerular Filtration Rate; NS: not significant

Table 3. Clinical Trials in Patients with Diabetes Mellitus without Hypertension and Proteinuria (Primary Prevention)

DRI aliskiren is the newest addition to RAAS blocking agents[36]. Preclinical studies offered very attractive effect of aliskiren in renal protection in diabetic and non-diabetic models of CKD. Aliskiren has been shown to have antihypertensive and a renoprotective effect in diabetic experimental nephropathy[37]. The profound effect of aliskiren on renal RAAS was due to selective renal accumulation (aliskiren renal/plasma concentration ratio of 60)[37]. The promising preclinical renoprotective effect of aliskiren was then tested in clinical trials in patients with diabetic nephropathy. In the largest to date Aliskiren in the Evaluation of Proteinuria in Diabetes (AVOID) study, 599 patients with T2DM, hypertension and nephropathy were enrolled[38]. The addition of aliskiren to the maximum renoprotective dose of ARB losartan further reduced albuminuria by 20%[38]. The reduction of albuminuria was achieved despite a non-significant decrease in blood pressure, suggesting that the renoprotective effect of aliskiren was independent of the blood pressure control[38,39]. In the subsequent AVOID subanalysis, aliskiren was found to decrease urinary aldosterone level, which may be partially responsible for the additional renoprotective effect of aliskiren seen in the AVOID study[40]. The ongoing Aliskiren Trial in Type 2 Diabetic Nephropathy (ALTITUDE) study will give further insights into whether a dual RAAS blockade with either ACEIs or ARBs in combination with DRI aliskiren is beneficial in preventing progression of nephropathy in T2DM[41].

5. Controversies of dual RAAS blockade

5.1 Rationale for dual ACEI and ARB therapy

Despite proven efficacy of ACEIs and ARBs in decreasing the progression of renal decline and cardiovascular complications in patients with DM and nephropathy, residual cardiovascular and renal complications are still high[42]. Dual RAAS inhibition has a theoretical advantage over single therapy, since all classes of drugs that target RAAS have been proven to possess renal and cardiovascular protective effects. The rationale of dual blockade lies in the fact that inhibition of AngII production by ACEIs cause an increase in AngI levels, and increased levels of AngI lead to additional production of AngII via ACE-independent pathways (ACE escape). Blockade of AT1 receptors by ARBs leads to a compensatory increase of AngII[43], which may partly offset AT1 blockade by ARB (AngII escape). Dual blockade with ACEIs and ARBs has a theoretical advantage over monotherapy, since it may offer a more effective overall inhibition of RAAS. However, results from large clinical trials have been inconsistent. The results from the Combination treatment of angiotensin-II receptor blocker and angiotensin-converting-enzyme inhibitor in non-diabetic renal disease (COOPERATE) trial, which was the only large clinical trial so far showing improved renal outcomes with combination ACEI/ARB therapy, were recently retracted due to inconsistencies in the data[44,45]. In the OTNTARGET study, dual blockade with ACEI ramipril and ARB telmisartan was associated with worse renal outcomes and an increased risk of acute renal failure[27]. Subgroup analysis of the ONTARGET data showed that a dual blockade was harmful primarily in patients with a low renal risk, which does not exclude the potential benefit of a dual ACEI/ARB blockade in patients with high renal risk (i.e. patients with DM and nephropathy).

Ongoing studies on dual ACEI/ARB blockade in patients with DM and nephropathy: Combination Angiotensin Receptor Blocker and Angiotensin Converting Enzyme Inhibitor for Treatment of Diabetic Nephropathy (VA NEPHRON-D)[46] and the Long-term Impact of RAS Inhibition on Cardiorenal Outcomes (LIRICO)[47] are designed specifically to assess ACEI/ARB combination therapy in high risk patients. The VA-NEPHRON-D will assess combination of ACEI lisinopril and ARB losartan on the progression of kidney disease in patients with DM and nephropathy[46]. The LIRICO trial will evaluate the cardiovascular and renal effects of ACEI/ARB combination therapy in patients with preexisting albuminuria and at least one more cardiovascular risk factor (cigarette smoking, DM, HTN, visceral obesity, dyslipidemia, or family history of cardiovascular diseases)[47]. Results of these studies should provide more information on the usefulness of dual ACEI/ARB therapy in high risk patients.

5.2 Rationale for ACEI/ARB and DRI combination therapy

Both ACEI and ARB therapy cause a compensatory increase of plasma rennin activity (PRA) up to 15-fold[48,49]. High PRA has been shown to increase the risk of myocardial infarction in patients with HTN[50], and is associated with increased mortality in patients with heart failure[51]. DRI aliskiren inhibits ~75% of PRA, and selectively accumulates in the kidney[52]. Thus, combination therapy of aliskiren and either ACEIs or ARBs may provide an additional benefit especially in patients with preexisting renal impairment and high PRA. As previously mentioned, the AVOID study offered promising results of ARB and DRI combination therapy in T2DM patients with nephropathy[39,40]. The ongoing ALTITUDE study will assess combination therapy with either ACEI or ARB and DRI aliskiren in 8,600 T2DM patients with nephropathy and/or cardiovascular disease. The primary endpoint is the time to first event for the composite endpoint of cardiovascular death, resuscitated death, myocardial infarction, stroke, unplanned hospitalization for heart failure, onset of ESRD or doubling of baseline serum creatinine concentration[41].

A summary of the clinical trials evaluating combination RAAS therapy is presented in Table 4.

Study	Combination Therapy	Number of Patients	Renal Outcome	Risk Reduction (%)	Reference
COOPERATE	ACEI/ARB		RETRACTED (Inconsistency of data)		44,45
ONTARGET	Ramipril (ACEI), Telmisartan (ARB) or both	25,620	Composite of dialysis, doubling of serum creatinine, and death (primary endpoint) Dialysis, doubling serum creatinine (secondary endpoints)	HR 1.09 for primary outcome HR 1.24 for secondary outcome Worse renal outcome and increased risk of ARF in combination group	27
VA NEPHRON-D	Combination Lisinopril (ACEI) and Losartan (ARB)		Time to reduction in eGFR >50%, ESRD and death	Ongoing	46
LIRICO	Combination of ACEI and ARB	2,100	ESRD and Renal function (secondary outcome)	Ongoing	47
AVOID	Combination of losartan (ARB) and aliskiren (DRI)	599	Changes in UACR and eGFR (*post hoc* analysis)	Significant difference in number of patients with a >50% reduction in UACR from Baseline Reduction in eGFR decline only in group with HTN >140/90 mmHg at baseline	39, 40
ALTITUDE	Combination of aliskiren (DRI) with either ACEI or ARB	8,600	Time to first event for the composite endpoint of cardiovascular death, resuscitated death, myocardial infarction, stroke, unplanned hospitalization for heart failure, onset of ESRD or doubling of baseline serum creatinine concentration	Ongoing	41

ACEI: Angiotensin Converting Enzyme Inhibitor; ARB: Angiotensin Receptor Blocker; DRI: Direct Renin Inhibitor; AER: Albumin Excretion Rate; HR: hazard ratio; ARF: Acute Renal Failure; ESRD: End Stage Renal Disease; eGFR: estimated Glomerular Filtration Rate; UACR: Urinary Albumin Creatinine Ratio; NS: not significant

Table 4. Clinical Trials with Dual Renin Angiotensin System Blockade

Ongoing and future studies should answer questions regarding safety and efficacy of RAAS combination therapy, as well as to to assess specific patient populations that may benefit from a more intense RAAS blockade.

6. References

[1] Coresh J, Selvin E, Stevens LA, Manzi J, Kusek JW, Eggers P, Van Lente F, Levey AS: Prevalence of chronic kidney disease in the United States. JAMA 2007; 298: 2038-47

[2] Stojiljkovic L, Behnia R: Role of renin angiotensin system inhibitors in cardiovascular and renal protection: a lesson from clinical trials. Curr Pharm Des 2007; 13: 1335-45

[3] Ganne S, Arora S, Dotsenko O, McFarlane S, Whaley-Connell A: Hypertension in people with diabetes and the metabolic syndrome: Pathophysiologic insights and therapeutic update. Current Diabetes Reports 2007; 7: 208-217

[4] Velez JC: The importance of the intrarenal renin-angiotensin system. Nat Clin Pract Nephrol 2009; 5: 89-100

[5] Siamopoulos KC, Kalaitzidis RG: Inhibition of the renin-angiotensin system and chronic kidney disease. Int Urol Nephrol 2008; 40: 1015-25

[6] Effects of ramipril on cardiovascular and microvascular outcomes in people with diabetes mellitus: results of the HOPE study and MICRO-HOPE substudy. Heart Outcomes Prevention Evaluation Study Investigators. Lancet 2000; 355: 253-9

[7] Kannel WB, McGee DL: Diabetes and cardiovascular disease. The Framingham study. JAMA 1979; 241: 2035-8

[8] Creager MA, Luscher TF, Cosentino F, Beckman JA: Diabetes and vascular disease: pathophysiology, clinical consequences, and medical therapy: Part I. Circulation 2003; 108: 1527-32

[9] Messent JW, Elliott TG, Hill RD, Jarrett RJ, Keen H, Viberti GC: Prognostic significance of microalbuminuria in insulin-dependent diabetes mellitus: a twenty-three year follow-up study. Kidney Int 1992; 41: 836-9

[10] Lewis EJ, Hunsicker LG, Clarke WR, Berl T, Pohl MA, Lewis JB, Ritz E, Atkins RC, Rohde R, Raz I: Renoprotective effect of the angiotensin-receptor antagonist irbesartan in patients with nephropathy due to type 2 diabetes. N Engl J Med 2001; 345: 851-60

[11] Laffel LM, McGill JB, Gans DJ: The beneficial effect of angiotensin-converting enzyme inhibition with captopril on diabetic nephropathy in normotensive IDDM patients with microalbuminuria. North American Microalbuminuria Study Group. Am J Med 1995; 99: 497-504

[12] Randomised placebo-controlled trial of lisinopril in normotensive patients with insulin-dependent diabetes and normoalbuminuria or microalbuminuria. The EUCLID Study Group. Lancet 1997; 349: 1787-92

[13] Lewis EJ, Hunsicker LG, Bain RP, Rohde RD: The effect of angiotensin-converting-enzyme inhibition on diabetic nephropathy. The Collaborative Study Group. N Engl J Med 1993; 329: 1456-62

[14] Should all patients with type 1 diabetes mellitus and microalbuminuria receive angiotensin-converting enzyme inhibitors? A meta-analysis of individual patient data. Ann Intern Med 2001; 134: 370-9

[15] Mann JF, Gerstein HC, Yi QL, Franke J, Lonn EM, Hoogwerf BJ, Rashkow A, Yusuf S: Progression of renal insufficiency in type 2 diabetes with and without microalbuminuria: results of the Heart Outcomes and Prevention Evaluation (HOPE) randomized study. Am J Kidney Dis 2003; 42: 936-42

[16] Ruggenenti P, Fassi A, Ilieva AP, Bruno S, Iliev IP, Brusegan V, Rubis N, Gherardi G, Arnoldi F, Ganeva M, Ene-Iordache B, Gaspari F, Perna A, Bossi A, Trevisan R, Dodesini AR, Remuzzi G: Preventing microalbuminuria in type 2 diabetes. N Engl J Med 2004; 351: 1941-51

[17] Ruggenenti P, Fassi A, Ilieva AP, Iliev IP, Chiurchiu C, Rubis N, Gherardi G, Ene-Iordache B, Gaspari F, Perna A, Cravedi P, Bossi A, Trevisan R, Motterlini N, Remuzzi G: Effects of verapamil added-on trandolapril therapy in hypertensive type 2 diabetes patients with microalbuminuria: the BENEDICT-B randomized trial. J Hypertens 2011; 29: 207-16

[18] Marre M, Lievre M, Chatellier G, Mann JF, Passa P, Menard J: Effects of low dose ramipril on cardiovascular and renal outcomes in patients with type 2 diabetes and raised excretion of urinary albumin: randomised, double blind, placebo controlled trial (the DIABHYCAR study). BMJ 2004; 328: 495

[19] Parving HH, Lehnert H, Brochner-Mortensen J, Gomis R, Andersen S, Arner P: The effect of irbesartan on the development of diabetic nephropathy in patients with type 2 diabetes. N Engl J Med 2001; 345: 870-8

[20] Barnett AH, Bain SC, Bouter P, Karlberg B, Madsbad S, Jervell J, Mustonen J: Angiotensin-receptor blockade versus converting-enzyme inhibition in type 2 diabetes and nephropathy. N Engl J Med 2004; 351: 1952-61

[21] Brenner BM, Cooper ME, de Zeeuw D, Keane WF, Mitch WE, Parving HH, Remuzzi G, Snapinn SM, Zhang Z, Shahinfar S: Effects of losartan on renal and cardiovascular outcomes in patients with type 2 diabetes and nephropathy. N Engl J Med 2001; 345: 861-9

[22] Makino H, Haneda M, Babazono T, Moriya T, Ito S, Iwamoto Y, Kawamori R, Takeuchi M, Katayama S: The telmisartan renoprotective study from incipient nephropathy to overt nephropathy--rationale, study design, treatment plan and baseline characteristics of the incipient to overt: angiotensin II receptor blocker, telmisartan, Investigation on Type 2 Diabetic Nephropathy (INNOVATION) Study. J Int Med Res 2005; 33: 677-86

[23] Makino H, Haneda M, Babazono T, Moriya T, Ito S, Iwamoto Y, Kawamori R, Takeuchi M, Katayama S: Prevention of transition from incipient to overt nephropathy with telmisartan in patients with type 2 diabetes. Diabetes Care 2007; 30: 1577-8

[24] Makino H, Haneda M, Babazono T, Moriya T, Ito S, Iwamoto Y, Kawamori R, Takeuchi M, Katayama S: Microalbuminuria reduction with telmisartan in normotensive and hypertensive Japanese patients with type 2 diabetes: a post-hoc analysis of The Incipient to Overt: Angiotensin II Blocker, Telmisartan, Investigation on Type 2 Diabetic Nephropathy (INNOVATION) study. Hypertens Res 2008; 31: 657-64

[25] Bakris G, Burgess E, Weir M, Davidai G, Koval S: Telmisartan is more effective than losartan in reducing proteinuria in patients with diabetic nephropathy. Kidney Int 2008; 74: 364-9

[26] Sleight P: The ONTARGET/TRANSCEND Trial Programme: baseline data. Acta Diabetol 2005; 42 Suppl 1: S50-6

[27] Mann JF, Schmieder RE, McQueen M, Dyal L, Schumacher H, Pogue J, Wang X, Maggioni A, Budaj A, Chaithiraphan S, Dickstein K, Keltai M, Metsarinne K, Oto A, Parkhomenko A, Piegas LS, Svendsen TL, Teo KK, Yusuf S: Renal outcomes with telmisartan, ramipril, or both, in people at high vascular risk (the ONTARGET study): a multicentre, randomised, double-blind, controlled trial. Lancet 2008; 372: 547-53

[28] Molitch ME, DeFronzo RA, Franz MJ, Keane WF, Mogensen CE, Parving HH, Steffes MW: Nephropathy in diabetes. Diabetes Care 2004; 27 Suppl 1: S79-83

[29] Bilous R, Chaturvedi N, Sjolie AK, Fuller J, Klein R, Orchard T, Porta M, Parving HH: Effect of candesartan on microalbuminuria and albumin excretion rate in diabetes: three randomized trials. Ann Intern Med 2009; 151: 11-20, W3-4

[30] Mann JF, Schmieder RE, Dyal L, McQueen MJ, Schumacher H, Pogue J, Wang X, Probstfield JL, Avezum A, Cardona-Munoz E, Dagenais GR, Diaz R, Fodor G, Maillon JM, Ryden L, Yu CM, Teo KK, Yusuf S: Effect of telmisartan on renal outcomes: a randomized trial. Ann Intern Med 2009; 151: 1-10, W1-2

[31] Mauer M, Zinman B, Gardiner R, Suissa S, Sinaiko A, Strand T, Drummond K, Donnelly S, Goodyer P, Gubler MC, Klein R: Renal and retinal effects of enalapril and losartan in type 1 diabetes. N Engl J Med 2009; 361: 40-51

[32] Nguyen G, Delarue F, Burckle C, Bouzhir L, Giller T, Sraer JD: Pivotal role of the renin/prorenin receptor in angiotensin II production and cellular responses to renin. J Clin Invest 2002; 109: 1417-27

[33] Nguyen G, Burckle CA, Sraer JD: Renin/prorenin-receptor biochemistry and functional significance. Curr Hypertens Rep 2004; 6: 129-32

[34] Nguyen G: Renin/prorenin receptors. Kidney Int 2006; 69: 1503-6

[35] Huang Y, Wongamorntham S, Kasting J, McQuillan D, Owens RT, Yu L, Noble NA, Border W: Renin increases mesangial cell transforming growth factor-beta1 and matrix proteins through receptor-mediated, angiotensin II-independent mechanisms. Kidney Int 2006; 69: 105-13

[36] Pimenta E, Oparil S: Role of aliskiren in cardio-renal protection and use in hypertensives with multiple risk factors. Ther Clin Risk Manag 2009; 5: 459-64

[37] Feldman DL, Jin L, Xuan H, Contrepas A, Zhou Y, Webb RL, Mueller DN, Feldt S, Cumin F, Maniara W, Persohn E, Schuetz H, Jan Danser AH, Nguyen G: Effects of aliskiren on blood pressure, albuminuria, and (pro)renin receptor expression in diabetic TG(mRen-2)27 rats. Hypertension 2008; 52: 130-6

[38] Parving HH, Persson F, Lewis JB, Lewis EJ, Hollenberg NK: Aliskiren combined with losartan in type 2 diabetes and nephropathy. N Engl J Med 2008; 358: 2433-46

[39] Persson F, Lewis JB, Lewis EJ, Rossing P, Hollenberg NK, Parving HH: Aliskiren in combination with losartan reduces albuminuria independent of baseline blood pressure in patients with type 2 diabetes and nephropathy. Clin J Am Soc Nephrol 2011; 6: 1025-31

[40] Persson F, Lewis JB, Lewis EJ, Rossing P, Hollenberg NK, Parving HH: Impact of aliskiren treatment on urinary aldosterone levels in patients with type 2 diabetes and nephropathy: an AVOID substudy. J Renin Angiotensin Aldosterone Syst 2011; Aug 8 Epub ahead of print

[41] Parving HH, Brenner BM, McMurray JJ, de Zeeuw D, Haffner SM, Solomon SD, Chaturvedi N, Ghadanfar M, Weissbach N, Xiang Z, Armbrecht J, Pfeffer MA: Aliskiren Trial in Type 2 Diabetes Using Cardio-Renal Endpoints (ALTITUDE): rationale and study design. Nephrol Dial Transplant 2009; 24: 1663-71

[42] Slagman MC, Navis G, Laverman GD: Dual blockade of the renin-angiotensin-aldosterone system in cardiac and renal disease. Curr Opin Nephrol Hypertens 2010; 19: 140-52

[43] Mazzolai L, Maillard M, Rossat J, Nussberger J, Brunner HR, Burnier M: Angiotensin II receptor blockade in normotensive subjects: A direct comparison of three AT1 receptor antagonists. Hypertension 1999; 33: 850-5

[44] Nakao N, Yoshimura A, Morita H, Takada M, Kayano T, Ideura T: Combination treatment of angiotensin-II receptor blocker and angiotensin-converting-enzyme inhibitor in non-diabetic renal disease (COOPERATE): a randomised controlled trial. Lancet 2003; 361: 117-24

[45] Retraction--Combination treatment of angiotensin-II receptor blocker and angiotensin-converting-enzyme inhibitor in non-diabetic renal disease (COOPERATE): a randomised controlled trial. Lancet 2009; 374: 1226

[46] Fried LF, Duckworth W, Zhang JH, O'Connor T, Brophy M, Emanuele N, Huang GD, McCullough PA, Palevsky PM, Seliger S, Warren SR, Peduzzi P: Design of combination angiotensin receptor blocker and angiotensin-converting enzyme inhibitor for treatment of diabetic nephropathy (VA NEPHRON-D). Clin J Am Soc Nephrol 2009; 4: 361-8

[47] Maione A, Nicolucci A, Craig JC, Tognoni G, Moschetta A, Palasciano G, Pugliese G, Procaccini DA, Gesualdo L, Pellegrini F, Strippoli GF: Protocol of the Long-term Impact of RAS Inhibition on Cardiorenal Outcomes (LIRICO) randomized trial. J Nephrol 2007; 20: 646-55

[48] Koffer H, Vlasses PH, Ferguson RK, Weis M, Adler AG: Captopril in diuretic-treated hypertensive patients. JAMA 1980; 244: 2532-5

[49] Jones MR, Sealey JE, Laragh JH: Effects of angiotensin receptor blockers on ambulatory plasma Renin activity in healthy, normal subjects during unrestricted sodium intake. Am J Hypertens 2007; 20: 907-16

[50] Alderman MH, Ooi WL, Cohen H, Madhavan S, Sealey JE, Laragh JH: Plasma renin activity: a risk factor for myocardial infarction in hypertensive patients. Am J Hypertens 1997; 10: 1-8

[51] Latini R, Masson S, Anand I, Salio M, Hester A, Judd D, Barlera S, Maggioni AP, Tognoni G, Cohn JN: The comparative prognostic value of plasma neurohormones at baseline in patients with heart failure enrolled in Val-HeFT. Eur Heart J 2004; 25: 292-9

[52] Siragy HM: Rationale for combining a direct renin inhibitor with other renin-angiotensin system blockers. Focus on aliskiren and combinations. Cardiovasc Drugs Ther 2010; 25: 87-97

3

Parathyroid Hormone-Related Protein as a Mediator of Renal Damage: New Evidence from Experimental as well as Human Nephropathies

Ricardo J. Bosch et al.*
Laboratory of Renal Physiology and Experimental Nephrology, Department of Physiology
Spain

1. Introduction

End-stage renal disease (ESRD) is a public health problem worldwide, with an increasing incidence and prevalence, poor prognosis and high cost (Ministerio de Salud, 2005). In 2005 the prevalence of ESRD in the USA was 1,131 patients per million inhabitants, with an incidence of 296 new patients per year per million inhabitants. In 2008, the adjusted incident rate for patients age 45–64 fell to the same level seen in 1998 -605 per million population. The rate for those aged 75 and older declined 0.9 percent between 2007 and 2008. However, racial and ethnic discrepancies persist with 2008 incident rates in the African American and Native American populations 3.6 and 1.8 times greater, respectively, than the rate among whites, and the rate in the Hispanic population 1.5 times higher than that of non-Hispanics (U. S. Renal Data System, 2010).

Diabetic nephropathy (DN) is one of the major causes of ESRD in the Western world. The incidence of nephropathy owing to type 1 diabetes is declining; however, diabetes mellitus type 2 is now the most common single cause of renal insufficiency in the USA, Japan and Europe (Tisher & Hostetter, 1994). It has been estimated that 4% of the world's current population is diabetic, and that in Europe there will be more than 32 million patients with diabetes in 2010, causing an increase in related complications, such as DN. This pathology has been recognized as a worldwide medical catastrophe (Ziyadeh & Sharma, 2003).

DN appears clinically in 10-50% of diabetic patients after 10-20 years of evolution of the disease. These patients show a progressive increase in urinary excretion of protein, starting from an initial microalbuminuria to clear nephrotic syndrome with progressive decline of renal function (Cooper et al., 1999; Katoh et al., 2000; Tisher & Hostetter, 1994; Yotsumoto et al., 1997).

---

* María Isabel Arenas[1,2], Montserrat Romero[1], Nuria Olea[1], Adriana Izquierdo[1], Arantxa Ortega[1], Esperanza Vélez[1], Jordi Bover[3], Juan C. Ardura[4] and Pedro Esbrit[4]
[1]*Laboratory of Renal Physiology and Experimental Nephrology, Department of Physiology,*
[2]*Department of Cell Biology and Genetics, University of Alcalá, Alcalá de Henares,*
[3]*Nephrology Department, Fundació Puigvert, Barcelona*
[4]*Bone and Mineral Metabolism Laboratory, Instituto de Investigación Sanitaria-Fundación Jiménez Díaz, Madrid, Spain*

DN is characterized by hypertrophy of the glomerular and tubular structures of the kidneys, thickening of the basement membrane, glomerular hyperfiltration and accumulation of extracellular matrix components in the glomerular mesangium (glomeruloesclerosis) and tubular interstitium (tubulointerstitial fibrosis).

The thickening of the basement membrane as well as the expansion of mesangial matrix is associated with the deterioration of glomerular function (proteinuria) (Osterby et al., 2001, 2002; White & Bilous, 2000). Besides glomerulosclerosis, typically associated to DN, tubulointerstitial changes, including fibrosis, appear to be critical during the final progression of DN. In fact, tubulointerstitial fibrosis is the factor that best correlates with the progressive loss of renal function (White & Bilous, 2000). Although several aspects of DN are well known, its pathogenesis at molecular level is poorly understood.

Something similar occurs with acute renal injury (ARI). This pathology has a significant prevalence (5%) in hospitalized patients. The maintenance therapy in these patients, in which dialysis treatment is required, has important socio-economic implications (Nolan & Anderson, 1998). Thus, the survival range in the ARI has not improved in recent years. ARI is a potentially reversible multi-causal entity that is characterized by a tubuloepithelial renal necrosis, followed by an augmented proliferation and tubuloepithelial regeneration (Brady et al., 1996).

Depending on the intensity of and exposure time to the agent inducing the initial damage, ARI can progress to chronic renal disease - the evolution of which is an irreversible process characterized by the loss of nephrons and the development of fibrosis - and thus to ESRD (Chevalier, 2006; Remuzzi & Bertani, 1998).

The study of the mechanisms implicated in renal fibrosis, the final pathway to different nephropathies which can progress to ESRD, is very interesting as it involves the search for, and evaluation of, agents with therapeutic applications.

In the last decade several investigations have demonstrated the implication of the parathyroid hormone related protein (PTHrP) in renal injury. This protein was discovered at the end of the 1980s as the factor responsible for humoral hypercalcemia of malignancy, and today is the object of study as a possible new therapeutic target in some pathophysiological conditions (Clemens et al., 2001).

At present, it is well known that PTHrP is a widespread factor in normal tissues, including kidney, where it has autocrine/paracrine/intracrine actions through PTH/PTHrP type 1 receptor (PTH1R) (Clemens et al., 2001). Renal PTHrP overexpression is a common event in several acute as well as chronic nephropathies (Fiaschi-Taesch et al., 2004; Izquierdo et al., 2006; Largo et al., 1999; Lorenzo et al., 2002; Rámila et al., 2008; Santos et al., 2001). During the last years, studies to define the physiopathological role of PTHrP in the renal context have been carried out, using experimental models of tubulointerstitial or glomerular damage. In both entities the direct implication of PTHrP has been demonstrated, showing the important role of this protein in the mechanisms that regulate the cell cycle, inflammation and fibrosis, which indicates the possibility of new pathways of therapeutic intervention (Ortega et al., 2006; Rámila et al., 2008; Romero et al., 2010).

The following paragraphs describe the emerging role of the PTHrP system in acute and chronic renal injury, product of intense investigation for over a decade.

2. PTHrP in acute renal injury

Pioneer studies by Soifer et al. (1993) at the beginning of the 90´s suggested the implication of PTHrP in the mechanisms of injury and/or repair of the tubular epithelium after ischemic ARI. From then on, the majority of investigations have studied experimental nephropathies

characterized by tubular affectation (Fiaschi-Taesch et al., 2004; Largo et al., 1999; Lorenzo et al., 2002; Ortega et al., 2005; Santos et al., 2001).
Ischemic and toxic injury to renal tubular epithelial cells can cause both acute and chronic renal failure depending on the intensity of and exposure time to the damage (Humes et al., 1995; Lieberthal & Levine, 1996). Proliferation of injured tubule cells appears to be important for timely tubular recovery after renal injury, and for subsequent functional recovery of the damaged kidney. Several growth factors and cytokines, acting in an autocrine and paracrine manner, appear to participate in the repair process of the tubular epithelium in this setting (Fiaschi-Taesch et al., 2004; Gobe et al., 2000; Humes et al., 1995; Matsumoto & Nakamura, 2001; Vukicevic et al., 1998).
The mitogenic features of PTHrP and its early overexpression after renal injury in experimental models of acute renal failure (ARF), induced by either ischemia or nephrotoxins, initially suggested that PTHrP could participate in the regenerative process after ARI (Santos et al., 2001; Soifer et al., 1993). However, this putative role of PTHrP in the acutely damaged kidney was intriguing, since the PTH1R gene was found to be rapidly downregulated following ARI (Santos et al., 2001; Soifer et al., 1993). This is in sharp contrast to other well characterized renal mitogens, such as epidermal growth factor (EGF) and hepatocyte growth factor (HGF), whose receptors are upregulated after ARI (Humes et al., 1995; Matsumoto & Nakamura, 2001). Moreover, the PTH1R was also found to decrease in the kidney of protein-overloaded rats with tubulointerstitial damage (Largo et al., 1999). Current evidence suggests that factors other than PTHrP or Ang II are likely to account for the PTH1R downregulation associated with kidney damage (Fiaschi-Taesch et al., 2004; Lorenzo et al., 2002). It is interesting to mention in this context that spliced variants of this receptor showing low expression in the cell surface have shown to be present in the kidney (Jobert et al., 1996). In addition, the PTH1R can be internalized into the nucleus of renal tubular cells (Watson et al., 2000). The pathophysiological relevance of these mechanisms for the PTHrP action in the damaged kidney is presently unknown. The hypothetical beneficial effects of PTHrP as a mitogen in ARI was further questioned when considering that targeted delivery of PTHrP to the proximal tubule in mice failed to provide protection against renal ischemia or folic acid injury (Fiaschi-Taesch et al., 2004). Moreover, experimental data using the latter model in rats showed that pretreatment with Ang II blockers abolished the PTHrP upregulation but not tubular hyperplasia (Ortega et al., 2005). Thus, current evidence makes it unlikely that PTHrP plays a significant role in the regenerative process after ARI.
Renal PTHrP upregulation was also observed in other experimental nephropathies. Thus, chronic cyclosporin administration, which induces tubular atrophy and interstitial fibrosis, was shown to be associated with an increased PTHrP expression, at both mRNA and protein levels, in the rat renal cortex (Garcia-Ocaña et al., 1998). Moreover, PTHrP mRNA was found to increase sequentially in the renal cortex during the development of proteinuria in a rat model of tubulointerstitial damage after protein overload (Largo et al., 1999). Interestingly, in the latter model, dramatic PTHrP immunostaining was revealed in glomerular mesangial cells, associated with an increased mesangial growth and matrix expansion in those rats with intense proteinuria (Largo et al., 1999). These findings suggest that PTHrP could play a role in the mechanisms associated with progression of kidney damage.

3. Interaction between PTHrP and angiotensin II in the damaged kidney

The renin-angiotensin system is known to play an important pathogenic role in the mechanisms of renal injury (Egido, 1999; Harris & Martinez-Maldonado, 1995). In fact, the main agonist of this system, Ang II, can be envisioned as a growth factor which can promote the progression of kidney damage (Mezzano et al., 2001; Ruiz-Ortega & Egido, 1997). Activation of components of the renin-angiotensin system, including Ang II, locally in the kidney, has been shown to occur early in various experimental models of ARI, e.g., folic acid-induced nephrotoxicity or ischemia/reperfusion (Allred et al., 2000; Kontogiannis & Burns, 1998; Ortega et al., 2005; Santos et al., 2001). Moreover, Ang II antagonists exert beneficial effects on renal function in these models (Abdulkader et al., 1998; Long et al., 1993; Ortega et al., 2005).

Recent data strongly suggest that PTHrP might be involved in the mechanisms related to Ang II-induced renal injury. Exogenously administered Ang II, via its type 1 (AT1) receptor, increases PTHrP expression in glomerular and tubular cells as well as in vascular smooth muscle cells both *in vivo* and *in vitro* (Lorenzo et al., 2002; Noda et al., 1994; Pirola et al., 1993). Interestingly, a significant correlation between PTHrP overexpression and tubular damage and fibrosis was observed in the rat kidney after systemic Ang II infusion (Lorenzo et al., 2002). Furthermore, in nephrotoxic ARI, the improvement of renal function by Ang II antagonists was associated with inhibition of PTHrP overexpression (Ortega et al., 2005). Collectively, current data suggest that: 1) Ang II is a likely candidate responsible for PTHrP overexpression; and 2) PTHrP might contribute to the deleterious effects of Ang II, in the damaged kidney. These findings have established a new rationale for further studies focused on the putative contribution of PTHrP to the mechanisms of renal damage.

4. PTHrP in renal inflammation

Inflammation involves complex molecular and cellular mechanisms which are activated against physical, chemical or biological aggressions. This process normally serves a positive biological goal (e.g., to overcome invasion of potentially deleterious agents), but it may have detrimental effects in chronic pathological settings, such as progressive renal disease (Chevalier, 2006; Rees, 2006; Remuzzi & Bertani, 1998). Tubulointerstitial inflammation is a key event in a variety of nephropathies. Early after renal injury, damaged tubuloepithelial cells begin to overexpress proinflammatory cytokines and chemokines, which promote migration of monocytes/macrophages and T-lymphocytes to the renal interstitium (Muller et al., 1992; Rees, 2006). Both infiltrating leukocytes and damaged tubuloepithelial cells activate and induce proliferation of resident fibroblasts in the tubulointerstitial compartment. A severe and prolonged injury will determine a sustained activation of proinflammatory pathways, associated with overexpression of profibrogenic cytokines by tubulointerstitial cells leading to fibrogenesis and renal function loss (Strutz & Neilson, 2003).

Early studies suggested that PTHrP might act as an important mediator of proinflammatory cytokines, namely tumour necrosis factor and interleukin-6, in multi-organ inflammation and rheumatoid arthritis (Funk, 2001). More recent studies have shown that PTHrP activates nuclear factor NF-kB and the expression of NF-kB-dependent cytokines and chemokines [e.g., IL-6 and monocyte chemoattractant protein-1 (MCP-1)] in different cell types (Guillén et al., 2002; Martín-Ventura et al., 2003). PTHrP and MCP-1 were found to colocalize in smooth muscle cells in human atherosclerotic plaques (Ishikawa et al., 2000; Martín-Ventura et al., 2003; Nakayama et al., 1994).

Moreover, our results in mice with unilateral ureteral obstruction -a well characterized model of renal inflammation- have shown the critical role of PTHrP in this condition

(Rámila et al., 2008). In this study, PTHrP was found to be upregulated, even in PTHrP-overexpressing mice. In contrast to previous observations in ischemic or nephrotoxic renal injury (Rámila et al., 2008), PTH1R was not downregulated after ureteral obstruction in mice. Interestingly, an upregulation of both PTHrP and PTH1R was recently observed in the kidney of diabetic mice (Izquierdo et al., 2006). Furthermore, our recent in vitro findings indicate that PTHrP upregulates several proinflammatory factors in tubuloepithelial cells and promotes monocyte/macrophage migration. Moreover, ERK mediated NF-kB activation appears to be an important mechanism whereby PTHrP triggers renal inflammation. These data suggest that PTHrP might be envisioned as a new inflammation marker and a potential therapeutic target in the obstructed kidney (Rámila et al., 2008). Finally, since sustained renal inflammation is closely related to fibrogenesis, these data point to PTHrP as a likely pro-inflammatory and pro-fibrogenic cytokine in the damaged kidney.

5. PTHrP in renal cell apoptosis

Apoptosis is considered to be an important component of the acute response of the tubular epithelium to injury (Basnakian et al., 2002; Kaushal et al., 2004). Previous studies showed that PTHrP can inhibit apoptosis in several cell types like pancreatic β-cells and chondrocytes (Cebrián et al., 2002; Henderson et al., 1995). At least in the latter cells, this antiapoptotic effect appears to involve PTHrP interaction with the PTH1R, and also its internalization into the nucleus (Henderson et al., 1995). We recently found that PTHrP, interacting with the PTH1R, directly acts as a survival factor for renal tubulointerstitial cells by a dual mechanism involving Bcl-X_L upregulation and activation of the phosphatidylinositol-3 kinase/Akt/Bad pathway (Ortega et al., 2006). Our data, using PTHrP-overexpressing mice with folic acid-induced ARF, suggest that this PTHrP action might have detrimental consequences in the injured kidney. These mice showed a significant delay in renal function recovery and higher focal areas of tubulointerstitial fibrosis than normal mice, associated with a decrease in apoptotic tubulointerstitial cells (Ortega et al., 2006). The rationale for this association might come from the fact that apoptosis of interstitial fibroblasts appears to be a mechanism to prevent fibrogenesis (Lieberthal & Levine, 1996; Ortiz et al., 2000).

6. PTHrP in chronic renal injury: Diabetic Nephropathy (DN)

DN is characterized by the development of proteinuria and subsequent glomerulosclerosis, conditions which are always preceded by the development of an early hypertrophic process in the glomerular compartment (Wolf & Ziyadeh, 1999). Hypertrophy of podocytes, associated with a decrease in their number per glomerulus is known to occur in diabetes (Kriz et al., 1998; Mifsud et al., 2001; Pagtalunan et al., 1997). Over time, podocyte hypertrophy might become a maladaptive response leading to glomerulosclerosis.

Although the mechanisms by which high glucose (HG) leads to renal cell hypertrophy are still incompletely understood, it appears to involve cell entry into the cell cycle -associated to cyclin D_1 kinase activation early in G_1- and subsequent arrest at the G_1/S interphase implicating inhibition or insufficient activation of cyclin E kinase, to permit progression into S phase, and therefore, arrest of cell cycle progression followed by an increase in cell protein synthesis (Huang & Preisig, 2000).

Recent studies have shown that HG-induced hypertrophy involves an early activation of the renin-angiotensin system, followed by an induction of TGF-β_1, which in turn activates a cell cycle regulatory protein, the cyclin dependent kinase inhibitor (CDKI) $p27^{Kip1}$ (Pantsulaia, 2006; Wolf et al., 1998; Xu et al., 2005).The interaction of $p27^{Kip1}$ with the cyclin E kinase has been implicated in the inhibition of this late complex and thus the G_1 progression (Ekholm & Reed, 2000).

Previously we evaluated the expression of PTHrP in the kidney of mice with streptozotocin (STZ)-induced diabetes (Izquierdo et al., 2006). This animal model is characterized by development of renal hypertrophy and increased proteinuria early in the course of the disease (Gross et al., 2004). We found that diabetic mice showed a significant increase of both PTHrP and the PTH1R proteins expression associated with the development of both renal hypertrophy and proteinuria (Izquierdo et al., 2006). Interestingly, the regression analyses of these data also indicate that changes in the renal PTHrP/PTH1R system have predictive value on the early development of proteinuria in mice. Although the STZ model has limitations for assessing long-term histomorphological changes in the diabetic kidney (Gross et al., 2004); our findings might have pathophysiological implications since the amount of proteinuria is a reliable predictor of diabetic nephropathy (D'Amico & Bazzi, 2003; Hirschberg, 1996).

In a more recent study, Romero et al (2010) observed that PTHrP plays a key role in the mechanisms of HG-induced podocyte hypertrophy. In these studies, HG-induced podocyte hypertrophy was inhibited by the presence of a specific PTHrP neutralizing antibody. Interestingly, in this condition HG also failed to upregulate the expression of the hypertrophy factor TGF-β_1.

Although PTHrP does not seem to affect podocyte apoptosis, it was shown to be able to modulate the expression of several positive as well as negative cell cycle regulatory proteins. In this way, while PTHrP (1-36) was shown to stimulate cyclin $D_{1,}$ thus promoting podocytes to enter into G_1, it also downregulates cyclin E, hence blocking the cell cycle later in G_1. Moreover, PTHrP is able to upregulate the negative cell cycle regulatory protein $p27^{Kip1}$ which plays a key role in diabetic cell hypertrophy by preventing activation of cyclin E activity and arresting the cell cycle later in G_1 (Huang & Preisig, 2000; Romero et al., 2010). Interestingly, Romero et al (2010) found that the pharmacological blockade of the PTH1R inhibited the $p27^{Kip1}$ upregulation induced by both HG and AngII. Taken together, these data suggest that PTHrP might mediate the hypertrophic signalling acting in an autocrine/intracrine fashion through the PTH1R receptor.

To discern the mechanism involved in the stimulation of $p27^{kip1}$ induced by both PTHrP and TGF-$\beta_{1,}$ Romero et al (2010) performed two experimental approaches. First, they found that using a PTHrP siRNA inhibited the ability of HG and AngII to stimulate the upregulation of $p27^{Kip1}$, albeit it could not prevent the TGF-β_1 upregulation of this protein. Secondly, on TGF-β_1 siRNA transfected podocytes, PTHrP (1-36) failed to induce both $p27^{Kip1}$ overexpression and hypertrophy. Thus, suggesting that TGF-β_1 mediates both $p27^{Kip1}$ upregulation and the hypertrophy response induced by PTHrP on HG conditions.

Interestingly, Romero et al (2010) observed that the glomerular expression of both TGF-β_1 and $p27^{Kip1}$ are constitutively upregulated in PTHrP-overexpressing mice albeit, the latter was not accompanied by renal hypertrophy (Fiaschi-Taesch et al., 2004). This result seems plausible since the hypertrophic mechanism requires the entry into the cell cycle and subsequent arrest at the G_1/S interphase. Several studies have demonstrated that in glomerular cells grown in HG ambient, initially, self-limited proliferation occurs due to generation of HG-induced growth factors, followed by cell cycle arrest in the G_1 due to the expression of factors that block the checkpoint G1/S interphase and undergo cellular hypertrophy (Cosio, 1995; Huang & Preisig, 2000; Isono et al., 2000; Wolf et al., 1992). Of considerable interest is the fact that previous studies on PTHrP-overexpressing mice have revealed the constitutive upregulation of various proinflammatory mediators (Rámila et al., 2008), including the vascular endothelial growth factor-1 (Ardura et al., 2008) without evidence of kidney damage in the absence of renal insult. In any case, these data strongly suggest that PTHrP might participate in the upregulation of glomerular TGF-β_1 and p27^{Kip1}. Collectively, these results indicate that the renal PTHrP/PTH1R system is upregulated in streptozotozin-induced diabetes in mice, and appears to be involved with renal hypertrophy and adversely affects the outcome of DN. PTHrP also participates in the hypertrophic signalling triggered by HG on podocytes. In this condition, AngII induces the upregulation of PTHrP, which might induce the expression of TGF-β_1 and p27^{Kip1}. These findings provide new insights into the protective effects of AngII antagonists in DN, paving the way for new forms of intervention.

7. PTHrP in renal fibrosis

Renal fibrosis is recognized as the final common stage of main renal diseases, capable of progressing to chronic renal failure. Interstitial fibroblasts are the main cell type responsible for fibrogenesis, a process whereby these cells proliferate and become activated myofibroblasts (Ardura et al., 2008). Fibrosis of the kidney is known to be induced by both tubuloepithelial and infiltrating cells, as well as secretion of matrix compounds by both activated fibroblasts and tubular cells (Fan et al., 1999). In fact, an increased matrix synthesis and deposition, and loss of tubular structural integrity, are paramount events at later stages of fibrogenesis (Fan et al., 1999). Our previous studies indicate that the higher number of infiltrating macrophages was associated with increased fibroblast proliferation in the renal interstitium of folic acid-injured kidneys from PTHrP-overexpressing mice (Ortega et al., 2006). In these mice, an increased immunostaining for α-smooth muscle actin (α-SMA), a marker of activated fibroblasts or myofibroblasts (Strutz et al., 2002), was also observed in the renal interstitium after folic acid nephrotoxicity (Ortega et al., 2006). Consistent with the latter *in vivo* finding, PTHrP (1-36) was found to stimulate α-SMA expression in renal fibroblasts *in vitro* (Ortega et al., 2006). In addition, a higher immunostaining for both types I and IV collagens was observed in the renal interstitium of the obstructed kidneys from PTHrP-overexpressing mice than in their normal littermates (Ardura et al., 2008). In agreement with this finding, PTHrP (1-36) was found to stimulate the expression of both types of collagens, type-1 procollagen and fibronectin in tubuloepithelial cells and renal fibroblasts *in vitro*. At least part of these effects was abolished by a PTH1R antagonist (Ortega et al., 2006).

Tubuloepithelial cells might also contribute to development of renal fibrosis by directly generating myofibroblasts through a process known as epithelial-mesenchymal transition (EMT) (Ardura et al., 2008; Liu, 2004). EMT is a multiple step process that requires the integration of several extrinsic and intrinsic pathways including loss of epithelia polarity, rearrangement of the F-actin cytoskeleton, associated with upregulation of many genes used as EMT markers (Kalluri & Neilson, 2003). The latter includes, in addition to α-SMA, which increases cell contractility and motility, extracellular matrix proteins such as fibronectin and several types of collagens, metalloproteases (MMPs) and integrin linked kinase (ILK). In addition, a decrease in the expression of proteins that keep basolateral polarity, namely, cytokeratin, and intracellular junctions, including the adherent junction protein E-cadherin and β-catenin, takes place in the renal tubuloepithelium during EMT (Bonventre, 2003; Cheng & Lovett, 2003; Hinz et al., 2001; Kalluri & Neilson, 2003; Strutz et al., 2002; Strutz & Müller, 2006).

Activation of different signalling pathways acts as EMT intrinsic regulators: mitogen activated kinases (MAPKs), N-terminal c-Jun kinase (JNK), the RAS protein family, Wnt and Smad proteins and the transcription factors snail and slug (Kalluri & Neilson, 2003; Liu, 2004; Martínez-Estrada et al., 2006). Several studies support the important role of various pro-fibrogenic factors en the EMT process in the kidney. TGF-β is the best known factor studied in this regard, and seems to involve activation of MAPKs and Smad proteins. In addition, activation of EGF receptor (EGFR) tyrosine kinase can trigger EMT in renal tubuloepitelial cells (Gore-Hyer et al., 2002; Grände et al., 2002; Liu, 2004; Zhuang et al., 2004; Zhuang et al., 2005).

PTHrP has been reported to promote EMT through interaction with vascular endothelial growth factor (VEGF) (Ardura et al., 2008). Interestingly in this scenario, it has been suggested that TGF-β might act as a modulator of at least some PTHrP action through the PTH1R in renal cells. As previously mentioned, TGF-β is able to mediate PTHrP-induced hypertrophy in renal glomerular visceral epithelial cells -podocytes- where PTHrP can induce TGF-β upregulation (Romero et al., 2010). Furthermore, stimulation of the PTH1R may lead to EGFR transactivation, thus suggesting that PTHrP might play an important role in renal EMT (Ardura et al., 2010).

Recently, Ardura et al. (2010) expanded these studies and show that PTHrP is capable of inducing a variety of phenotypic changes related to EMT in tubuloephithelial cells. Hence, this peptide induced snail overexpression and its nuclear translocation, associated with the loss of ZO-1 and E-cadherin, key proteins in the maintenance of basolateral polarity and intercellular junction in renal tubuloepithelial cells. PTHrP also induced the phenotypic conversion to a fibroblast-like morphology, related to α-SMA and ILK upregulation.

Moreover, these authors observed that PTHrP can increase TGF-expression at both gene and protein expression in cultured tubuloepithelial cells. Moreover, TGF-β blockade by different manoeuvres was found to diminish renal fibrosis in both experimental models of renal damage and cultured renal cells, thus suggesting that TGF-β acts as a downstream mediator of PTHrP. Interestingly, the same interaction between these two factors was observed in PTHrP-induced podocyte hypertrophy. This study suggests that PTHrP, TGF-β, EGF and VEGF might cooperate through activation of ERK1/2 to induce EMT in renal tubuloepithelial cells.

Interestingly, some EMT-related changes occur associated with PTHrP overexpression in the mouse obstructed kidney as recently reported by the laboratory of Dr Esbrit. This group also found that two important EMT mediators such as TGF-β and p-EGFR proteins were elevated in this animal model associated with a targeted overexpression of PTHrP to the renal proximal tubule, thus suggesting that PTHrP might interact with TGF-β or EGFR to modulate EMT (Ardura et al., 2010).

Collectively, all the available data demonstrate a major role for PTHrP in renal fibrogenesis due to its capacity to induce the expression of extracellular matrix proteins as well as by modulating EMT in renal tubuloepithelial cells.

8. Conclusion

The upregulation of the renal PTHrP/PTH1R system represents a common event in several experimental nephropathies. Current data support the notion that AngII is a major factor responsible for PTHrP overexpression in both ARI and diabetic nephropathy. In the former condition, PTHrP appears to contribute to the progression of renal damage by increasing tubulointerstitial cell survival, promoting inflammation and fibrogenesis, including epithelia to mesenchyme transition. In diabetic nephropathy, PTHrP can favor renal hypertrophy and proteinuria (Fig. 1). Collectively, available data strongly support the implication of PTHrP as a pathogenic factor in kidney disease, and provide novel insights into the protective effects of Ang II antagonists in various nephropathies, paving the way for new therapeutic approaches.

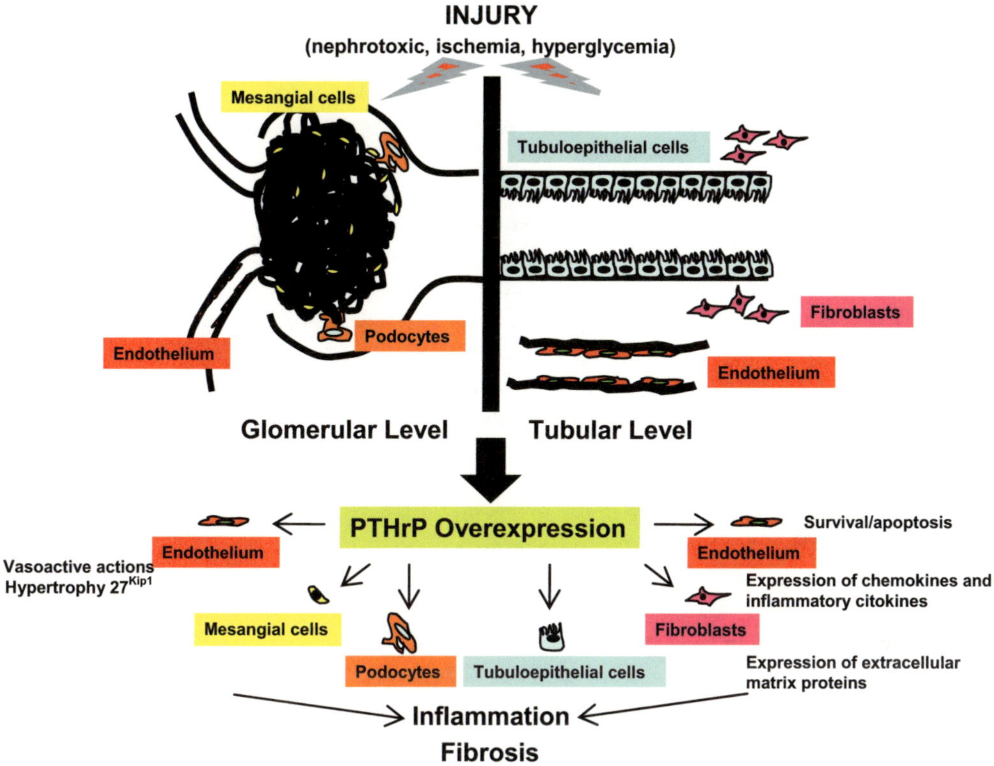

Fig. 1. Pathophysiology of PTHrP in acute and chronic renal injury.

9. Acknowledgment

A. Ortega was recipient of a research contract from Comunidad Autónoma de Madrid (S-BIO-2083-2006). A. Izquierdo is currently Assistant Professor at the Rey Juan Carlos University (Alcorcón, Madrid). E. Vélez is currently Professor at the Jiménez Diaz Foundation School of Nursing; J. A. Ardura was supported by Conchita Rábago Foundation and RETICEF, and is currently a post-doctoral researcher at the Department of Pharmacology and Chemical Biology (University of Pittsburgh, Pittsburgh, PA). This work was supported in part by grants from Ministerio de Educación y Cultura of Spain (SAF2002-04356-C03-01, -02, -03 and SAF2006-08747) and Ministerio de Ciencia e Innovación

(SAF2009-12009-C02-01), The Spanish Society of Nephrology, The Eugenio Rodríguez Pascual Foundation, and Instituto de Salud Carlos III (RETICEF RD06/0013/1002).

10. References

Abdulkader, R.C., Yuki, M.M., Paiva, A.C., & Marcondes, M. (1988). Prolonged inhibition of angiotensin II attenuates glycerol-induced acute renal failure. *Brazilian Journal of Medical and Biological Research*, Vol. 21, No. 2, (February 1981), pp. 233-239, ISSN 0100-879X.

Allred, A.J., Chappell, M.C., Ferrario, C.M., & Diz,D.I. (2000). Differential actions of renal ischemic injury on the intrarenal angiotensin system. *American Journal of Physiology. Renal Physiology*, Vol. 279, No. 4, (October 2000), pp. F636-F645, ISSN: 0363-6127.

Ardura J.A., Rayego-Mateos, S., Rámila D., Ortega-Ruiz, M., & Esbrit P. (2010). Parathyroid hormone-related protein promotes epithelial-mesenchymal transition. *Journal of the American Society of Nephrology*, Vol. 21, No. 2, (February 2010), pp. 237-248, ISSN 1046-6673.

Ardura, J.A., Berruguete, R., Rámila, D., Álvarez-Arroyo, V., & Esbrit, P. (2008). Parathyroid hormone-related protein interacts with vascular endothelial growth factor to promote fibrogenesis in the obstructed mouse kidney. *American Journal of Physiology. Renal Physiology*, Vol. 295, No. 2, (June 2008), pp. F415-F425, ISSN 0363-6127.

Basnakian, A.G., Kaushal, G.P., & Shah, S.V. (2002). Apoptotic pathways of oxidative damage to renal tubular epithelial cells. *Antioxidant & Redox Signaling*, Vol. 4, No. 6, (December 2002), pp. 915-924, ISSN 1523-0864.

Bonventre, J.V. (2003). Dedifferentiation and proliferation of surviving epithelial cells in acute renal failure. *Journal of the American Society of Nephrology*, Vol. 14, No. Suppl 1, (June 2003), pp. S55-S61, ISSN 1046-6673.

Brady, H.R., Brenner, B.M., & Lieberthal, W. (1996). Acute Renal Failure, In: *The Kidney*, 5th B.M. Brenner, F.C. Rector (Eds.), pp. 1200-1252, W.B. Saunders ISBN-10: 9781416031055 ISBN-13: 978-1416031055, Philadelphia.

Cebrián, A., García-Ocaña, A., Takane, K.K., Sipula, D., Stewart, A.F., & Vasavada, R.C. (2002). Overexpression of parathyroid hormone-related protein inhibits pancreatic beta-cell death in vivo and in vitro. *Diabetes*, Vol. 51, No. 10, (October 2002), pp. 3003-3013, ISSN 0012-1797.

Cheng, S., & Lovett, D.H. (2003). Gelatinase A (MMP-2) is necessary and sufficient for renal tubular cell epithelial-mesenchymal transformation. *The American Journal of Pathology*, Vol. 162, No. 6, (June 2003), pp. 1937-1949, ISSN 1479-398.

Chevalier, R.L. (2006). Obstructive nephropathy: towards biomarker discovery and gene therapy. *Nature Clinical Practice. Nephrology*, Vol. 3, No. 2, (March 2006), pp. 157-168, ISSN 1745-8323, 1745-8331.

Clemens, T.L., Cormier, S., Eichinger, A., Endlich, K., Fiaschi-Taesch, N., Fischer, E., Friedman, P.A., Karaplis, A.C., Massfelder, T., Rossert, J., Schlüter, K.D., Silve, C., Stewart, A.F., Takane, K., & Helwig, J.J. (2001). Parathyroid hormone-related protein and its receptors: nuclear functions and roles in the renal and cardiovascular systems, the placental trophoblasts and the pancreatic islets. *British Journal of Phamacology*, Vol. 134, No. 6, (November 2001), pp. 1113-1136, ISSN 1476-5381.

Cooper, M.E., Vranes, D., Youssef, S., Stacker, S.A., Cox, A.J., Rizkalla, B., Casley, D.J., Bach, L.A., Kelly, D.J., & Gilbert, R.E. (1999). Increased renal expression of vascular endothelial growth factor (VEGF) and its receptor VEGFR-2 in experimental diabetes. *Diabetes*, Vol. 48, No. 11 (November 1999), pp. 2229-2239, ISSN: 0012-1797.

Cosio, F.G. (1995). Effects of high glucose concentrations on human mesangial cell proliferation. *Journal of the American Society of Nephrology*, Vol. 5, No. 8, (February 1995), pp. 1600-1609, ISSN 1046-6673.

D'Amico, G., & Bazzi, C. (2003). Pathophysiology of proteinuria. *Kidney International*, Vol. 63, No. 3, (March 2003), pp. 809-25, ISSN 0085-2538.

Egido, J. (1996). Vasoactive hormones and renal sclerosis. *Kidney International*, Vol. 49, No. 2, (February 1996), pp. 578-597, ISSN 0085-2538.

Ekholm, S.V., & Reed, S.I. (2000). Regulation of G(1) cyclin-dependent kinases in the mammalian cell cycle. *Current Opinion in Cell Biology*, Vol. 12, No. 6, (December 2000), pp. 676-684, ISSN 0955-0674.

Fan, J.M., Ng, Y.Y., Hill, P.A., Nikolic-Paterson, D.J., Mu, W., Atkins, R.C., & Lan, H.Y. (1999). Transforming growth factor-beta regulates tubular epithelial-myofibroblast transdifferentiation in vitro. *Kidney International*, Vol. 56, No. 4, (October 1999), pp. 1455-1467, ISSN 0085-2538.

Fiaschi-Taesch, N.M., Santos, S., Reddy, V., Van Why, S.K., Philbrick, W.F., Ortega, A., Esbrit, P., Orloff, J.J., & Garcia-Ocaña, A. (2004). Prevention of acute ischemic renal failure by targeted delivery of growth factors to the proximal tubule in transgenic mice: the efficacy of parathyroid hormone-related protein and hepatocyte growth factor. *Journal of the American Society of Nephrology*, Vol. 15, No. 1, (January 2004), pp. 112-125, ISSN 1046-6673.

Funk, J.L. (2001). A role for parathyroid hormone-related protein in the pathogenesis of inflammatory/autoimmune diseases. *International Immunopharmacology*, Vol. 1, No. 6, (June 2001), pp. 1101-1121, ISSN 1567- 5769.

García-Ocaña, A., Gómez-Casero, E., Peñaranda, C., Sarasa, J.L., & Esbrit, P. (1998). Cyclosporine increases renal parathyroid hormone-related protein expression in vivo in the rat. *Transplantation*, Vol. 65, No. 6, (March 1998), pp. 860-863, ISSN 0041-1337.

Gobe, G., Zhang, X.J., Willgoss, D.A., Schoch, E., Hogg, N.A., & Endre, Z.H. (2000). Relationship between expression of Bcl-2 genes and growth factors in ischemic acute renal failure in the rat. *Journal of the American Society of Nephrology*, Vol. 11, No. 3, (March 2000), pp. 454-467, ISSN 1046-6673.

Gore-Hyer, E., Shegogue, D., Markiewicz, M., Lo, S., Hazen-Martin, D., Greene, E.L., Grotendorst, G., & Trojanowska, M. (2002). TGF-beta and CTGF have overlapping and distinct fibrogenic effects on human renal cells. *American Journal of Physiology. Renal Physiology*, Vol. 283, No. 4, (October 2002), pp. F707-F716, ISSN 0363-6127.

Grände, M., Frazen, A., Karlsson, J.O., Ericson, L.E., Heldin N.E., & Nilsson, M. (2002). Transforming growth factor-beta and epidermal growth factor synergistically stimulate epithelial to mesenchymal transition (EMT) through a MEK-dependent mechanism in primary cultured pig thyrocytes. *Journal of Cell Science*, Vol. 115, No. Pt 22, (November 2002), pp. 4227-4236, ISSN 0021-9533.

Gross, M.L., Ritz, E., Schoof, A., Adamczak, M., Koch, A., Tulp, O., Parkman, A., El Shakmak, A., Szabo, A., & Amann, K. (2004). Comparison of renal morphology in the Streptozotocin and the SHR/N-cp models of diabetes. *Laboratory Investigation*, Vol. 84, No. 4, (April 2004), pp. 452-464, ISSN 0023-6837.

Guillén, C., Martínez, P., de Gortázar, A.R., Martínez, M.E., & Esbrit, P. (2002). Both N- and C-terminal domains of parathyroid hormone-related protein increase interleukin-6 by nuclear factor-kappa B activation in osteoblastic cells. *Journal of Biological Chemistry*, Vol. 277, No. 31, (August 2002), pp. 28109-28117, ISSN 0021-9258.

Harris, R.C., & Martínez-Maldonado, M. (1995). Angiotensin II-mediated renal injury. *Mineral and Electrolyte Metabolism*, Vol. 21, No. 4-5, (August 1995), pp. 328-335, ISSN 0378-0392.

Henderson, J.E., Amizuka, N., Warshawsky, H., Biasotto, D., Lanske, B.M., Goltzman, D., & Karaplis, A.C. (1995). Nucleolar localization of parathyroid hormone-related peptide enhances survival of chondrocytes under conditions that promote apoptotic cell death. *Molecular and Cell Biology*, Vol. 15, No. 8, (August 1995), pp. 4064-4075, ISSN 0270- 7306.

Hinz, B., Celetta, G., Tomasek, J.J., Gabbiani, G., & Chaponnier, C. (2001). Alpha-smooth muscle actin expression upregulates fibroblast contractile activity. *Molecular Biology of the Cell*, Vol. 12, No. 9, (September 2001), pp. 2730-2741, ISSN 1059-1524.

Hirschberg, R. (1996). Bioactivity of glomerular ultrafiltrate during heavy proteinuria may contribute to renal tubulo-interstitial lesions: evidence for a role for insulin-like growth factor I. *Journal of Clinical Investigation*, Vol. 98, No. 1, (July 1996), pp. 116-124, ISSN 0021-9738.

Huang, H.C., & Preisig P.A. (2000). G1 kinases and transforming growth factor-beta signaling are associated with a growth pattern switch in diabetes-induced renal growth. *Kidney International*, Vol. 58, No. 1, (July 2000), pp. 162-172, ISSN 0085-2538.

Humes, H.D., Lake, E.W., & Liu, S. (1995). Renal tubule cell repair following acute renal injury. *Mineral and Electrolyte Metabolism*, Vol. 21, No. 4-5, (August 1995), pp. 353-365, ISSN 0378-0392.

Ishikawa, M., Akishita, M., Kozaki, K., Toba, K., Namiki, A., Yamaguchi, T., Orimo, H., & Ouchi, Y. (2000). Expression of parathyroid hormone-related protein in human and experimental atherosclerotic lesions: functional role in arterial intimal thickening. *Atherosclerosis*, Vol. 152, No. 1, (September 2000), pp. 97-105, ISSN 0021-9150.

Isono, M., Mogyorósi, A., Han, D.C., Hoffman, B.B., & Ziyadeh, F.N. (2000). Stimulation of TGF-beta type II receptor by high glucose in mouse mesangial cells and in diabetic kidney. *American Journal of Physiology. Renal Physiology*, Vol. 278, No. 5, (May 2000), pp. F830-F838, ISSN 0363-6127.

Izquierdo, A., López-Luna, P., Ortega, A., Romero, M., Gutiérrez-Tarrés, M.A., Arribas, I., Esbrit P., & Bosch, R.J. (2006). The parathyroid hormone-related protein system and diabetic nephropathy outcome in streptozotocin-induced diabetes. *Kidney International*, Vol. 69, No. 12, (June 2006), pp. 2171-2178. ISSN 0085-2538.

Jobert, A.S., Fernandes, I., Turner, G., Coureau, C., Prie, D., Nissenson, R.A., Friedlander, G., & Silve, C. (1996). Expression of alternatively spliced isoforms of the parathyroid hormone (PTH)/PTH-related peptide receptor messenger RNA in human kidney and bone cells. *Molecular Endocrinology*, Vol. 10, No. 9, (September 1996), pp. 1066-1076, ISSN 0888-8809.

Kalluri, R., & Neilson E.G. (2003). Epithelial-mesenchymal transition and its implications for fibrosis. *Journal of Clinical Investigation*, Vol. 112, No. 12, (December 2003), pp. 1776-1784. ISSN 0021-9738.

Katoh, M., Ohmachi, Y., Kurosawa, Y., Yoneda, H., Tanaka, N., & Narita, H. (2000). Effects of imidapril and captopril on streptozotocin-induced diabetic nephropathy in mice. *European Journal of Pharmacology*, Vol. 398, No. 3, (June 2000), pp. 381-387, ISSN 0014- 2999.

Kaushal, G.P., Basnakian, A.G., & Shah, S.V. (2004). Apoptotic pathways in ischemic acute renal failure. *Kidney International*, Vol. 66, No. 2, (August 2004), pp. 500-506, ISSN 0085-2538.

Kontogiannis, J., & Burns, K.D. (1998). Role of AT1 angiotensin II receptors in renal ischemic injury. *American Journal of Physiology. Renal Physiology*, Vol. 274, No. 1-Pt2, (January 1998), pp. F79-F90, ISSN 0363-6127.

Kriz, W., Grezt, N., & Lemley, K.V. (1998). Progression of glomerular diseases: is the podocyte the culprit?. *Kidney International*, Vol. 54, No. 3, (Septiembre 1998), pp. 687-697, ISSN 0085-2538.

Largo, R., Gómez-Garré, D., Santos, S., Peñaranda, C., Blanco, J., Esbrit, P., & Egido, J. (1999). Renal expression of parathyroid hormone-related protein (PTHrP) and PTH/PTHrP receptor in a rat model of tubulointerstitial damage. *Kidney International*, Vol. 55, No. 1, (January 1999), pp. 82-90, ISSN 0085-2538.

Lieberthal, W., & Levine, J.S. (1996). Mechanisms of apoptosis and its potential role in renal tubular epithelial cell injury. *American Journal of Physiology. Renal Physiology* Vol. 271, No. 3 Pt2 (September 1996), pp. F477-F488, ISSN 0363-6127.

Liu, Y. (2004). Epithelial to mesenchymal transition in renal fibrogenesis: pathologic significance, molecular mechanism, and therapeutic intervention. *Journal of the American Society of Nephrology*, Vol. 15, No. 1, (January 2004), pp. 1-12, ISSN 1046-6673.

Long, G.W., Misra, D.C., Juleff, R., Blossom, G., Czako, P.F., & Glover, J.L. (1993). Protective effects of enalaprilat against postischemic renal failure. *Journal of Surgical Research*, Vol. 54, No. 3, (March 1993), pp. 254-257, ISSN 0022-4804.

Lorenzo, O., Ruiz-Ortega, M., Esbrit, P., Rupérez, M., Ortega, A., Santos, S., Blanco, J., Ortega, L., & Egido, J. (2002). Angiotensin II increases parathyroid hormone-related protein (PTHrP) and the type 1 PTH/PTHrP receptor in the kidney. *Journal of the American Society of Nephrology*, Vol. 13, No. 6, (June 2002), pp. 1595-1607, ISSN 1046-6673.

Martínez-Estrada, O.M., Cullerés, A., Soriano, F.X., Peinado, H., Bolós, V., Martínez, F.O., Reina, M., Cano, A., Fabre, M., & Vilaró, S. (2006). The transcription factors Slug and Snail act as repressors of Claudin-1 expression in epithelial cells. *Biochemical Journal*, Vol. 394, No. Pt2 (March 2006), pp. 449-457, ISSN 0264-6021.

Martín-Ventura, J.L., Ortego, M., Esbrit, P., Hernández-Presa, M.A., Ortega, L., & Egido, J. (2003). Possible role of parathyroid hormone-related protein as a proinflammatory cytokine in atherosclerosis. *Stroke*, Vol. 34, No. 7, (July 2003), pp. 1783-1789, ISSN 0039-2499.

Matsumoto, K., & Nakamura, T. (2001). Hepatocyte growth factor: renotropic role and potential therapeutics for renal diseases. *Kidney Internacional*, Vol. 59, No. 6, (June 2001), pp. 2023-2038, ISSN 0085-2538.

Mezzano, S.A., Ruiz-Ortega, M., & Egido, J. (2001). Angiotensin II and renal fibrosis. *Hypertension*, Vol. 38, No. 3 Pt 2, (Sep 2001), pp. 635-638, ISSN 0194911X.

Mifsud, S.A., Allen, T.J., Bertram, J.F., Hulthen, U.L., Kelly, D.J., Cooper, M.E., Wilkinson-Berka, J.L., & Gilbert, R.E. (2001). Podocyte foot process broadening in experimental diabetic nephropathy: amelioration with renin-angiotensin blockade. Diabetologia, Vol. 44, No. 4, (July 2001), pp. 878-882, ISSN 0012-186X.

Ministerio de Salud. (2005). *Guía Clínica Insuficiencia Renal Crónica Terminal,* (1st Ed.), Minsal, Santiago, Chile.

Muller, G.A., Markovic-Lipkovski, J., Frank, J., & Rodemann, H.P. (1992). The role of interstitial cells in the progression of renal diseases. *Journal of the American Society of Nephrology*, Vol. 2, No. 10 Suppl, (April 1992), pp. S198-S205, ISSN 1046-6673.

Nakayama, T., Ohtsuru, A., Enomoto, H., Namba, H., Ozeki, S., Shibata,Y., Yokota, T., Nobuyoshi,M., Ito, M., & Sekine, I. (1994). Coronary atherosclerotic smooth muscle cells overexpress human parathyroid hormone-related peptides. *Biochemical and Biophysical Research Communications*, Vo. 200, No. 2, (April 1994), pp. 1028-1035, ISSN 0006-291X.

Noda, M., Katoh, T., Takuwa, N., Kumada, M., Kurokawa, K., & Takuwa, Y. (1994). Synergistic stimulation of parathyroid hormone-related peptide gene expression by mechanical stretch and angiotensin II in rat aortic smooth muscle cells. *Journal of Biological Chemistry*, Vol. 269, No. 27, (July 1994), pp. 17911-17917, ISSN 0021-9258.

Nolan, C.R., & Anderson, R.J. (1998). Hospital-acquired acute renal failure. *Journal of the American Society of Nephrology*, Vol. 9, No. 4, (April 1998), pp. 710-718, ISSN 1046-6673.

Ortega, A., Rámila, D., Izquierdo, A., González, L., Barat, A., Gazapo, R., Bosch, R.J., & Esbrit, P. (2005). Role of the renin-angiotensin system on the parathyroid hormone-related protein overexpression induced by nephrotoxic acute renal failure in the rat. *Journal of the American Society of Nephrology*, Vol. 16, No. 4, (April 2005), pp. 939-949, ISSN 1046-6673.

Ortega, A., Rámila, D., Ardura, J.A., Esteban, V., Ruiz-Ortega, M., Barat, A., Gazapo, R., Bosch, R.J., & Esbrit, P. (2006). Role of parathyroid hormone-related protein in tubulointerstitial apoptosis and fibrosis after folic acid-induced nephrotoxicity. *Journal of the American Society of Nephrology*, Vol. 17, No. 6, (June 2006), pp. 1594-15603, ISSN 1046-6673.

Ortiz, A., Lorz, C., Catalán, M.P., Danoff, T.M., Yamasaki, Y., Egido, J., & Neilson, E.G. (2000). Expression of apoptosis regulatory proteins in tubular epithelium stressed in culture or following acute renal failure. *Kidney International*, Vol. 57, No. 3, (March 2000), pp. 969-981, ISSN 0085-2538.

Osterby, R., Hartmann, A., Nyengaard, J.R., & Bangstad, H.J. (2002). Development of renal structural lesions in type-1 diabetic patients with microalbuminuria. Observations by light microscopy in 8-year follow-up biopsies. *Virchows Archiv*, Vol. 440, No. 1, (January 2002), pp. 94-101, ISSN 0945-6317.

Osterby, R., Tapia, J., Nyberg, G., Tencer, J., Willner, J., Rippe, B., & Torffvit, O. (2001). Renal structures in type 2 diabetic patients with elevated albumin excretion rate. *Acta Pathologica Microbiologica et Immunologica Scandinavica*, Vol. 109, No. 11, (November 2001), pp. 751-761, ISSN 1600-0463.

Pagtalunan, M.E., Miller, P.L., Jumping-Eagle, S., Nelson, R.G., Myers, B.D., Renke, H.G., Coplon, N.S., Sun, L., & Meyer, T.W. (1997). Podocyte loss and progressive glomerular injury in type II diabetes. *Journal of Clinical Investigation*, Vol. 99, No. 2, (January 1997), pp. 342-348, ISSN 00219738.

Pantsulaia, T. (2006). Role of TGF-beta in pathogenesis of diabetic nephropathy. *Georgian Medical News*, Vol. 131, No. N2, (February 2006), pp. 13-18, ISSN 0016-5751.

Pirola, C.J., Wang, H.M., Kamyar, A., Wu, S., Enomoto, H., Sharifi, B., Forrester, J.S., Clemens, T.L., & Fagin, J.A. (1993). Angiotensin II regulates parathyroid hormone-related protein expression in cultured rat aortic smooth muscle cells through transcriptional and post-transcriptional mechanisms. *Journal of Biological Chemistry*, Vol. 268, No. 3, (January 1993), pp. 1987-1994, ISSN 0021-9258.

Rámila, D., Ardura, J.A., Esteban, V., Ortega, A., Ortega-Ruiz, M., Bosch, R.J, & Esbrit, P. (2008). Parathyroid hormone-related protein promotes inflammation in the kidney with an obstructed ureter. *Kidney International*, Vol. 73, No. 7, (April 2008), pp. 835-847. ISSN 0085-2538.

Rees, A.J. (2006). The role of infiltrating leukocytes in progressive renal disease: implications for therapy. *Nature Clinical Practice. Nephrology*, Vol. 2, 7, (July 2006), pp. 348-349, ISSN 1745-8331.

Remuzzi, G., & Bertani, T. (1998). Pathophysiology of progressive nephropathies. *The New England Journal of Medicine*, Vol. 339, No. 20, (November 1998), pp. 1448-1456, ISSN 0028-4793.

Romero, M., Ortega, A., Izquierdo, A., López-Luna, P., & Bosch, R.J. (2010). Parathyroid hormone-related protein induces hypertrophy in podocytes via TGF-beta(1) and p27(Kip1): implications for diabetic nephropathy. *Nephrology, Dialysis, Transplantation*, Vol. 25, No. 8, (August 2010), pp. 2447-2457, ISSN 0931- 0509.

Ruiz-Ortega, M., & Egido, J. (1997). Angiotensin II modulates cell growth-related events and synthesis of matrix proteins in renal interstitial fibroblasts. *Kidney International*, Vol. 52, No. 6, (December 1997), pp. 1497-1510, ISSN 0085-2538.

Santos, S., Bosch, R.J., Ortega, A., Largo, R., Fernández-Agulló, T., Gazapo, R., Egido, J., & Esbrit, P. (2001). *Kidney International*, Vol. 60, No. 3, (September 2001), pp. 982-995, ISSN 0085-2538.

Soifer, N.E., Van Why, S.K., Ganz, M.B., Kashgarian, M., Siegel, N.J., & Stewart, A.F. (1993). Expression of parathyroid hormone-related protein in the rat glomerulus and tubule during recovery from renal ischemia. *Journal of Clinical Investigation*, Vol. 2, No. 6, (December 1993), pp. 2850-2857, ISSN 00219738.

Strutz, F., & Müller, G.A. (2006). Renal fibrosis and the origin of the renal fibroblast. *Nephrology, Dialysis, Transplantation*, Vol. 21, No. 12, (December 2006), pp. 368-3370, ISSN 0931- 0509.

Strutz, F., & Neilson, E.G. (2003). New insights into mechanisms of fibrosis in immune renal injury. *Springer Seminars in Immunopathology*, Vol. 24, No. 4, (May 2003), pp. 459-476, ISSN 0172-6641.

Strutz, F., Zeisberg, M., Ziyadeh, F.N., Yang, C.Q., Kalluri, R., Muller, G.A., & Neilson, E.G. (2002). Role of basic fibroblast growth factor-2 in epithelial-mesenchymal transformation. *Kidney International*, Vol. 61, No. 5, (May 2002), pp. 1714-1728, ISSN 0085-2538.

Tisher, C.C., & Hostetter, T.H. (1994). Diabetic nephropathy, In: *Renal Pathology*, C.C. Tisher, B.M. Brenner (Eds.), pp. 1387-1412, J.B. Lippincott Company, ISBN 0-397-51240-6, Philadelphia, USA.

U. S. Renal Data System, USRDS (2010), *Annual Data Report Atlas of Chronic Kidney Disease and End Stage Renal Disease in the United States*. National Institutes of Health, National Institute of Diabetes and Digestive and Kidney Diseases, Bethesda, MD, USA.

Vukicevic, S., Basic, V., Rogic, D., Basic, N., Shih, M.S., Shepard, A., Jin, D., Dattatreyamurty, B., Jones, W., Dorai, H., Ryan, S., Griffiths, D., Maliakal, J., Jelic, M., Pastorcic, M., Stavljenic, A., & Sampath,T.K. (1998). Osteogenic protein-1 (bone morphogenetic protein-7) reduces severity of injury after ischemic acute renal failure in rat. *Journal of Clinical Investigation*, Vol. 102, No. 1, (July 1998), pp. 202-214, ISSN 00219738.

Watson, P.H., Fraher, L.J., Hendy, G.N., Chung, U.I., Kisiel, M., Natale, B.V., & Hodsman, A.B. (2000). Nuclear localization of the type 1 PTH/PTHrP receptor in rat tissues. *Journal of Bone and Mineral Research*, Vol. 15, No. 6, (June 2000), pp. 1033-1044, 0884-0431.

White, K.E., & Bilous, R.W. (2000). Type 2 diabetic patients with nephropathy show structural-functional relationships that are similar to type 1 disease. *Journal of the American Society of Nephrology*, Vol. 11, No. 9, (September 2000), pp. 1667-1673, ISSN 1046-6673.

Wolf, G., Schroeder, R., Thaiss, F., Ziyadeh, F.N., Helmchen, U., & Stahl, R.A. (1998). Glomerular expression of $p27^{Kip1}$ in diabetic db/db mouse: role of hyperglycemia. *Kidney International*, Vol. 53, No. 4, (April 1998), pp. 869-879, ISSN 0085-2538.

Wolf, G., Sharma, K., Chen, Y., Ericksen, M., & Ziyadeh, F.N. (1992). High glucose-induced proliferation in mesangial cells is reversed by autocrine TGF-beta. *Kidney International*, Vol. 42, No. 3, (September 1992), pp. 647-656, ISSN 0085-2538.

Wolf, G., & Ziyadeh, F.N. (1999). Molecular mechanisms of diabetic renal hypertrophy. *Kidney International*, Vol. 56, No. 2, (August 1999), pp. 393-405. ISSN 0085-2538.

Xu, Z.G., Yoo, T.H., Ryu, D.R., Cheon Park, H., Ha, S.K., Han, D.S., Adler, S.G., Natarajan, R., & Kang, S.W. (2005). Angiotensin II receptor blocker inhibits $p27^{Kip1}$ expression in glucose-stimulated podocytes and in diabetic glomeruli. *Kidney International*, Vol. 67, No. 3, (March 2005), pp. 944-952, ISSN 0085-2538.

Yotsumoto, T., Naitoh, T., Shikada, K., & Tanaka, S. (1997). Effects of specific antagonists of angiotensin II receptors and captopril on diabetic nephropathy in mice. *Japanese Journal of Pharmacology*, Vol. 75, No. 1, (September 1997), pp. 59-64, ISSN 0021-5198.

Zhuang, S., Yan, Y.,Han, J., & Schnellmann, R.G. (2005). p38 kinase-mediated transactivation of the epidermal growth factor receptor is required for dedifferentiation of renal epithelial cells after oxidant injury. *Journal of Biological Chemistry*, Vol. 280, No. 22, (June 2005), pp. 21036-21042, ISSN 0021-9258.

Zhuang, S., Dang, Y., & Schnellmann, R.G. (2004). Requirement of the epidermal growth factor receptor in renal epithelial cell proliferation and migration. *American Journal of Physiology*. Renal Physiology, Vol. 287, No. 3, (September 2004), F365-F372, ISSN 0363-6127.

Ziyadeh, F.N., & Sharma, K. (2003). Overview: combating diabetic nephropathy. *Journal of the American Society of Nephrology*, Vol. 14, No. 5, (May 2003), pp. 1355-1357, ISSN 1046-6673.

4

Psychological and Social Aspects of Living with Chronic Kidney Disease

Daphne L. Jansen[1], Mieke Rijken[1], Monique J.W.M. Heijmans[1], Ad A. Kaptein[2] and Peter P. Groenewegen[1]
[1]*NIVEL (Netherlands Institute for Health Services Research)*
[2]*Leiden University Medical Centre (LUMC)*
The Netherlands

1. Introduction

Chronic Kidney Disease (CKD) draws heavily on patients' daily functioning. The disease, treatment and associated demands have a great impact on physical and emotional well-being and interfere with patients' social roles. Patients with CKD who are being prepared for, or receive renal replacement therapy often experience difficulties in participating in various domains of life, such as paid work, sports and other social and leisure activities (Heijmans & Rijken, 2004). A study among Dutch renal transplant patients revealed that these patients participate less in employment and sports compared with the general Dutch population (Van der Mei et al., 2007). For CKD patients on dialysis it seems in particular difficult to perform paid work, and it is notable that people who are being prepared for renal replacement therapy (pre-dialysis patients) already experience work related problems. Restrictions with respect to performing daily activities, including work, might impede people's feelings of autonomy and self-esteem. Recognising the importance of these aspects for people's well-being, we conducted a series of studies during the last six years with the aim of providing more insight into the psychological and social aspects of living with CKD. More specifically, we investigated the extent to which pre-dialysis patients and patients on dialysis feel autonomous, experience self-esteem and perform paid work, and the extent to which variation in these aspects is related to differences in patients' perceptions of illness and treatment (personal factors) and social support (external factors). Furthermore, we developed an intervention programme aimed at supporting patients' participation in daily activities, including paid work, and feelings of autonomy and self-esteem, by means of influencing illness perceptions, treatment perceptions and social support.

In this chapter we provide an overview of the results of our studies and reflect upon the findings. In the next section the key findings of our empirical research on this topic will be discussed in the context of previous research and existing theories. In the third section the development of the psychological intervention programme will be described. Furthermore, findings of the evaluation of the intervention on feasibility and initial experiences will be discussed, and areas of attention for the development and implementation of interventions in general will be addressed.

2. Review key findings empirical research

In this section we provide an overview of the main findings of our empirical studies carried out during the period 2006-2011 among pre-dialysis patients (CKD stage 4) and patients on dialysis (end-stage renal disease (ESRD), CKD stage 5) in the Netherlands. Data were gathered within a national cohort of pre-dialysis patients (PREPARE-2 study) and a national cohort of patients on dialysis (NECOSAD-2 study) by means of survey research. The findings will be placed in the context of previous research and existing theories.

2.1 Autonomy and self-esteem in patients with CKD

According to Deci and Ryan's Self-Determination Theory (SDT; 1985), autonomy is one of the basic psychological needs for optimal functioning. Autonomy refers to regulation by the self (Ryan et al., 2009). When autonomous, a person experiences his or her behaviour as self-organised and endorsed (Ryan et al., 2009). SDT postulates that the need for autonomy can energise human activity, and must be satisfied for long-term psychological health (Deci & Ryan, 2000). Reis et al. (2000) found that daily variations in the fulfilment of the need for autonomy, independently predicted daily variations in well-being. When the fulfilment of the need for autonomy is hindered, one's experience of self-worth is also damaged, leading to either insecure or low self-esteem (Ryan & Brown, 2003). Research demonstrated that both high self-esteem and stable self-esteem are associated with greater psychological well-being (Paradise & Kernis, 2002). Our study findings demonstrated that both patients in the pre-dialysis phase and patients on dialysis have, on average, moderate feelings of autonomy (Jansen et al., 2010). This indicates that they do not often feel that they can do the things they like to do in everyday life, because of their health condition or otherwise. Despite this, both groups of patients have high mean levels of self-esteem. In our research we have not examined the stability of patients' self-esteem. A Dutch study by Abma et al. (2007) revealed that people with renal disease also consider the maintenance and increase of their self-governance with respect to living their lives, as one of the most important themes that need more attention in renal care.

2.2 Labour participation in patients with CKD

People often regard participation in paid work as an important life activity. It generates income which in turn makes it possible to participate in other life domains as well. Moreover, a literature review by Waddell and Burton (2006) provided evidence that work is generally good for physical and mental health and well-being, and that unemployment is associated with negative health effects. Within our sample of 109 pre-dialysis patients, 42% (N = 45) were younger than 65 years and therefore were part of the potential labour force. Fifty-one percent of these patients had a paid job for at least 12 hours per week (definition of labour participation as applied by Statistics Netherlands (CBS)) in 2006 (Jansen et al., 2010). Furthermore, the results showed that, despite of their health condition, patients of working age placed relatively high importance on carrying out a paid job. It should be noted here that employers in the Netherlands must pay at least 70% of the salaries of sick employees for the first two years. Consequently people who are on long-term sick leave are in fact still employed. This means that our employed sample may also include patients on long-term sick leave. Fritschka et al. (2000) found a higher employment rate in their study among pre-dialysis patients in Germany, and demonstrated that 63% of the patients aged 18-64 years were employed on a full-time basis. A more recent Danish study by Sondergaard and Juul

(2010) revealed a labour participation rate of 57%, irrespective of the number of working hours, in pre-dialysis patients aged below 65. Of our sample of 166 patients on dialysis, 37% (N = 62) were younger than 65 years. Within this group 24% had a paid job for at least 12 hours per week (in 2006; Jansen et al., 2010). Previous studies among working-age patients on dialysis carried out in Europe as well as in the United States found comparable labour participation rates, however, some studies found higher rates (Table 1). It should be noted that the studies vary with respect to the labour participation definitions and age ranges used.

Sample	Labour participation rate	Country	
Dialysis patients < 65 yrs	20%	Sweden	Theorell et al., 1991
Haemodialysis patients < 60 yrs	22%	Denmark	Molsted et al., 2004
Dialysis patients < 63 yrs	24%	United States	Braun Curtin et al., 1996
Dialysis patients < 55 yrs	19%	United States	Kutner et al., 2008
Dialysis patients < 65 yrs	38%	Netherlands	De Wit et al., 2001
Haemodialysis patients	34% (full-time)	Germany	Fritschka et al., 2000

Table 1. Labour participation rates of working-age patients on dialysis

Previous research among renal patients has detected specific predictors of employment of patients on dialysis, and showed that occupational status before dialysis, a higher educational level and a good physical condition are important determinants (see Heijmans & Rijken et al., 2004; see Kutner et al., 2008). Kutner et al. (2008) investigated the association between dialysis facility characteristics and employment rates. They found that offering a late dialysis shift, as well as peritoneal dialysis or home haemodialysis training and more frequent haemodialysis were associated with higher facility employment rates, after adjusting for patient/social worker ratio, rurality of unit location, and unit size. However, patient-level characteristics were not taken into account, and due to the design of the study the associations observed between facility characteristics and patient employment could not be interpreted as cause-and-effect relationships. Another study by Kutner et al. (2010) revealed that higher levels of energy expenditure reflected in usual activity levels were associated with increased likelihood of continued employment after dialysis start.

The labour participation rate of 24% found in our study among Dutch dialysis patients of working age is considerably lower than that of the general Dutch population in the ages of 15-64 years, of which 65% were employed for at least 12 hours per week in 2006. Compared to a representative sample of people with a chronic illness in the Netherlands, the dialysis patients' employment rate found in our study is also low. Among this sample of chronically ill people (aged 15-64 years) 35% had a paid job for at least 12 hours per week in 2006 (Van den Brink-Muinen et al., 2009). The labour participation rate of pre-dialysis patients deviates to a lesser extent from the Dutch labour participation rate. This is plausible, since the restrictions of the illness and treatment are less profound in this phase of the illness, compared to the dialysis phase. We wish to mention here that the working-age groups in our studies among (pre-)dialysis patients comprised a high percentage of older patients. Notwithstanding that, our results suggest that labour participation in (pre-)dialysis patients is indeed lower than in the general Dutch population. We also compared the (pre-)dialysis patients' employment rates of the group aged below 55 years and the group aged 55-64 years with rates of the general population by age (Table 2). The employment rates of the patients on dialysis still lag behind. The employment rate of the pre-dialysis patients aged

55-64 years appears to be comparable with the employment rate of the general population aged 55-64 years. The employment rate of the patients aged below 55 years is however considerably lower compared to the employment rates in the general population aged between 25 and 54 years.

	Dutch general population (15-64 years)*	Sample pre-dialysis patients (19-64 years)	Sample dialysis patients (32-64 years)
15-24 yrs	39%		
25-34 yrs	82%		
35-44 yrs	80%	57%	32%
45-54 yrs	75%		
55-64 yrs	40%	41%	19%
Total group	65%	51%	24%

Table 2. Labour participation (paid job ≥ 12 hrs pw) in the Dutch general population, the sample of pre-dialysis patients (N=45) and patients on dialysis (N=62) of working age in 2006; * source: CBS, Statistics Netherlands

Looking at the labour participation rates found in our studies among dialysis and pre-dialysis patients, the findings indicate that people already resign from their jobs in the pre-dialysis phase. These findings are in line with the findings of the study by Van Manen et al. (2001) among 659 dialysis patients aged 18-64 years. This study revealed that drop out of the labour market already occurs before patients start with dialysis treatment: at the start of the dialysis treatment, 35% of the patients had a paid job compared to 61% in the general Dutch population in 1997, the year the study was carried out. This is alarming, since research identified prior occupational status as an important predictor of employment in dialysis patients. In addition, Van Manen et al. found that labour participation in dialysis patients decreased as patients were on dialysis for a longer time: the percentage of employed patients on dialysis decreased from 31% to 25% in patients on haemodialysis, and from 48% to 40% in patients on peritoneal dialysis after one year on dialysis. Our results also suggest that resignation from paid work further continues in the dialysis phase. Findings from a study conducted by Kutner et al. (2010) also point to job resignation during the pre-dialysis phase and the initiation phase of dialysis treatment. Their study showed that, among 585 incident patients who were working for pay during the year before dialysis, only 191 (32.6%) continued working approximately 4 months after dialysis start.

These results point to the importance and necessity of work-related support and guidance at an early stage of the illness process. Research indicates that renal patients themselves also report to have problems with respect to work. The study by Abma et al. (2007) revealed that patients struggle with whether they can work and what kind of work they can do. A Swedish study among pre-dialysis patients and patients on dialysis demonstrated that around 30% of the pre-dialysis patients, and more than 50% of the patients on dialysis reported problems with respect to work and regarding leisure time (Ekelund & Anderson, 2007).

What have we learned from scientific research?

- patients in the pre-dialysis and dialysis phase, on average, have moderate feelings of autonomy and high levels of self-esteem
- patients in the pre-dialysis phase already resign from paid work, and resignation from paid work further continues in the dialysis phase

- patients themselves consider self-governance with respect to living their lives as an important topic and report difficulties with respect to work and leisure time

What is important for clinical practice?

- it is important that patients are being supported in their efforts to carry out paid work, and - more generally - in their sense of autonomy, in an early phase of the illness process in order to prevent drop out of paid work and other daily activities

What needs to be investigated further?

- it is recommended that research investigates why patients, who have a comparable clinical status, differ in the extent to which they feel autonomous, experience self-esteem and participate in paid work; it is then important to focus on potentially modifiable factors; by gaining insight into this matter, starting points can be generated for the development of interventions

2.3 The role of perceptions of illness and treatment

One of the objectives of our studies was to investigate (pre-)dialysis patients' illness perceptions and treatment perceptions in relation to employment, and more generally perceived autonomy and self-esteem. The findings of two previous studies inspired us to investigate these relationships. First, the study by Braun Curtin et al. (1996) which demonstrated that dialysis patients with and without a paid job differed regarding their attitudes towards work. Employed patients did not feel limited by their health in the hours they worked or the kind of work in which they could engage. Patients without work on the other hand, perceived their health as a barrier to find work. These findings are interesting since both patient groups did not differ with respect to objective health indicators. Second, a study by Petrie et al. (1996) among myocardial infarction (MI) patients, which showed that illness perceptions are related to return to work. In particular, perceptions of the duration and the consequences of the illness predicted the speed of return to work.

Patients' perceptions of their illness are the central concepts of the Common Sense Model (CSM; Leventhal et al., 1984), which is a self-regulation model of health threat. According to this model people make sense of a health threat by developing their own cognitive and emotional representations of that threat. These representations or perceptions develop from exposure to a variety of social and cultural sources of information – news stories, education in schools, personal experiences of illness, witnessing illness experiences of others, portrayals of illness in books and movies, and other experiences (Cameron & Moss-Morris, 2004). CSM postulates that both cognitive and emotional representations determine how patients cope with their illness and adapt to their illness. The representations generally consist of the following components:

- *identity* - patients' beliefs about the label of the illness and associated symptoms;
- *cause* - patients' beliefs about factors or conditions that have caused the illness;
- *timeline* - patients' beliefs about the expected duration of the illness;
- *personal control* - patients' beliefs about how much their own actions will help to control the illness;
- *treatment control* - patients' beliefs about how much their prescribed treatment will be effective in controlling or curing the condition;
- *consequences* - patients' beliefs about the impact of the illness on their physical, social and psychological well-being;
- *coherence* - patients' beliefs about how well they understand the illness;

- *representation of emotional reaction* - patients' beliefs about how much they are emotionally affected by the illness, e.g. whether they experience fear or worry.

These cognitive and emotional representations can be activated and developed at the same time (Broadbent et al., 2009a; Cameron & Moss-Morris, 2004). Two important aspects of illness perceptions are, that patients' beliefs about their condition are often at variance from those who are treating them, and secondly, patients' perceptions vary widely, even in patients with the same medical condition (Petrie et al., 2007). Many studies have investigated the relationships between illness perceptions and outcomes in different patient populations. A meta-analysis of 45 empirical studies among patients with various medical conditions, demonstrated that perceptions that the illness was curable/controllable were significantly and positively related to the adaptive outcomes of psychological well-being, social functioning and vitality, and negatively related to psychological distress and disease state. Conversely, perceptions of illness consequences, timeline and identity exhibited significant, negative relationships with psychological well-being, role and social functioning and vitality (Hagger & Orbell, 2003). In addition, studies provided evidence that illness perceptions are associated with eating and exercise self-efficacy in patients with coronary heart disease, attending rehabilitation in MI patients, and self-management in patients with diabetes (see Petrie et al., 2007). Besides representations of illness, patients' beliefs about their prescribed medical treatment (i.e. beliefs about necessity and concerns) also play a role in how patients cope with and adapt to their illness. Studies have demonstrated that beliefs about treatment are related with adherence and treatment decisions (Horne et al., 2007; Horne & Weinman, 2002).

2.3.1 Content of CKD patients' illness and treatment perceptions

From the findings of our studies, among pre-dialysis patients and patients on dialysis, it is notable that both patient groups on average reported relatively low levels of perceived personal control over the illness (Jansen et al., 2010). Personal control over the illness refers to the feeling that one can influence the course of the illness, and one can fit the illness and its treatment into daily life. In a study by Broadbent et al. (2006), using the same measurement instrument, people with diabetes and people with asthma both reported higher mean levels of personal control (M=6.7, on a scale from 0 to 10) compared with the mean personal control levels found in our studies among pre-dialysis patients (M=4.7) and patients on dialysis (M=4.9). Previous studies have shown that dialysis patients' beliefs of personal control are important for patients' health related quality of life (Covic et al., 2004; Timmers et al., 2008). In order to manage their illness, pre-dialysis patients and dialysis patients obviously depend on medical treatment, i.e. pharmacotherapy and dialysis. Our findings also show that, on average, patients believe that their treatment positively influences their illness, this is particularly true for patients on dialysis. However, the fact that patients are dependent on medical treatment does not mean that there are no opportunities for personal control. For dialysis patients it is very important to engage in self-care behaviours. Virtually all patients with ESRD are likely to be required to monitor food and fluid intake and to take multiple medications, in addition to following a generally healthy lifestyle overall with regard to smoking, alcohol, weight maintenance, regular exercise, etc. (Braun Curtin et al., 2005). However, the extreme dependence on the dialysis treatment might predominate and overshadow the extent to which one self can influence the course of the illness. For pre-dialysis patients it is of great importance as well to practice self-care behaviours, such as following a healthy diet and performing daily exercise in order to optimise their health condition (Sijpkens et al., 2008). Patients in this stage of the illness, however, got the news that they have to start with renal replacement therapy in the near future, which indicates that despite of their self-care activities they apparently were not able to maintain sufficient renal function. This knowledge might have a negative effect on patients' personal control beliefs. Sijpkens et al. (2008) state that in the pre-dialysis phase the long foreseen implications of kidney disease become immediate and many patients experience feelings of helplessness and hopelessness. Moreover, our study results showed that pre-dialysis patients are quite worried about their illness, which also could be related to the prospect that one has to start with the dialysis treatment soon.

In addition, the results of our studies revealed that dialysis patients, on average, believe that their illness has rather serious consequences for their daily life. Pre-dialysis patients also believe that their illness affects their daily life, but to a somewhat lesser extent. Furthermore, the mean scores indicated that patients on dialysis perceive moderate disruption from their treatment in daily life, and pre-dialysis patients perceive mild disruption from their current treatment. Previous studies among patients with ESRD have emphasised the importance of beliefs related to the experienced impact of ESRD and its treatment for patients' quality of life (Fowler & Baas, 2006; Griva et al., 2009; Timmers et al., 2008). Moreover, the type of treatment might also play a role in patients' perceptions of personal control. The study by Timmers et al. (2008) among haemodialysis (HD) patients and peritoneal dialysis (PD) patients showed that patients on PD experienced more personal control, compared to HD patients.

2.3.2 Patterns of CKD patients' illness and treatment perceptions

Leventhal et al. have emphasised the potential value of examining interrelations between combinations of illness perceptions in relation to outcomes in patients with chronic physical illness (Kaptein et al., 2010). In our studies we therefore also looked at interrelations between illness and treatment perceptions. We found similar patterns of significant interrelations in both patient groups. As (pre-) dialysis patients perceive more consequences from their illness, they experience less personal control, more physical symptoms, greater concern, higher levels of emotional response, and greater disruption from the treatment. However, different patterns were observed as well. It is notable that pre-dialysis patients' feelings of greater personal control are associated with both cognitive and emotional representations (i.e. lower illness consequences, higher treatment control, lower concern and emotional response scores). Whereas dialysis patients' feelings of personal control are solely associated with cognitive representations (i.e. lower illness consequences, higher treatment control, lower identity, higher understanding, and lower treatment disruption scores). It is furthermore notable that pre-dialysis patients' beliefs of greater treatment disruption are associated with beliefs that the treatment cannot control the illness. Whereas dialysis patients, beliefs of greater treatment disruption are associated with beliefs that they themselves cannot control the illness. Like Griva et al. (2009) we found relationships between the illness perception dimensions and treatment (disruption) beliefs hereby, in addition to Griva and colleagues, providing support for extending the Common Sense Model with treatment related beliefs (Horne & Weinman, 2002). It seems important to take the patterns of interrelations into account when focusing on influencing perceptions shown to be related to better outcomes.

2.3.3 CKD patients' illness and treatment perceptions and outcomes

As already discussed in the previous sections, several studies have investigated the relationship between illness perceptions and treatment perceptions of patients with ESRD on the one hand, and quality of life on the other hand (e.g. Covic et al., 2004; Fowler & Baas, 2006; Griva et al., 2009; Timmers et al., 2008). From all these studies, it can be concluded that more perceived personal control, less perceived (negative) consequences (from both the illness and treatment), and a lower emotional response are generally associated with better outcomes in patients on dialysis. Covic et al. (2006) investigated whether illness perceptions of patients on haemodialysis, reported at a certain point in time, could actually explain subsequent changes in quality of life outcomes over time. Their results showed that baseline emotional response, personal control and coherence explained changes in the physical component of quality of life over a two year period. Baseline illness consequences appeared to explain changes in the mental component of quality of life during the two year follow-up period. Horne et al. (2001) investigated the treatment beliefs of patients on haemodialysis with respect to medication and fluid-diet restrictions, and found associations between these specific treatment beliefs and adherence to these treatments.

In our studies we have investigated whether differences in patients' illness and treatment perceptions are associated with variation in autonomy and self-esteem. We did this by means of multivariate analyses in which we controlled for differences in socio-demographic and clinical characteristics (Jansen et al., 2010). The results demonstrated that the illness and treatment beliefs explained a substantial amount of variance in autonomy and self-esteem, after controlling for background characteristics. With respect to pre-dialysis patients, the results illustrated that less perceived disruption from the treatment upon life is a significant contributor to self-esteem, and makes a close to significant contribution to autonomy (global measure). Treatment in the pre-dialysis phase in most cases includes taking pharmacotherapy and following a diet. Although these treatments may be less disruptive than dialysis treatment, the findings show that the way patients perceive their treatment is already a significant theme in this stage of the illness. According to Leventhal et al. (1984) illness representations are constantly updated as new experiences and knowledge are acquired. In this transition phase of treatments, in which patients receive information on all available renal replacement therapies, it therefore can be expected that patients are occupied with treatment in general, both their current treatment as well as their future treatment.

With respect to the patients on dialysis, the results showed that the perception of personal control over the illness is an important contributor to patients' feelings of autonomy (global measure). Thus, the belief that one's own actions will help to control the illness is related with global autonomy feelings. In light of these findings it is important to point out the difference between *personal control* and *autonomy*, since autonomy is often incorrectly equated with ideas of internal locus of control (Deci & Ryan, 2000). Beliefs of personal control reflect beliefs regarding the extent to which one feels that one can control or influence an outcome. However, people are autonomous when they act in accordance with their authentic interests or values. Furthermore, the results showed that beliefs that the illness and treatment have little impact on daily life are positively associated with autonomy (health related measure). Thus, patients who do not feel that the illness and treatment impede their lives, do not feel that their health stops them from doing the things they would like to do. Lastly, less concern about the illness, and less perceived treatment disruption were significant contributors to a higher self-esteem in patients on dialysis. It should be noted that a large amount of variation in people's autonomy and self-esteem levels remained unexplained. Braun Curtin et al. (1996) provided evidence for the role of another psychological factor. They found that patients who themselves believed that dialysis patients should work, and had this notion reinforced by significant others were more likely to be employed. This suggests that the extent to which people in patients' social environment (e.g. patients' partners or doctors) support patients in their efforts to carry out activities, including work, also plays an important role.

We also examined the relationships between (pre-)dialysis patients' illness perceptions and treatment perceptions on the one hand, and labour participation (defined as the performance of paid work for at least 12h per week) on the other hand within the working-age group (18-64 years). We were not able to demonstrate clear relationships between illness and treatment perceptions and labour participation. However, the results of the bivariate analyses showed some trends. Employed dialysis patients perceived less severe physical symptoms from the illness, less impact from the illness, greater personal control, and less disruption from the treatment compared with unemployed patients. It is noteworthy that employed dialysis patients also reported less treatment control and less understanding compared with unemployed patients. This might indicate that employed patients are less focused on, or occupied with factors that lie outside of their control or reach. Pre-dialysis patients who were employed perceived their illness as better controllable by self-care and medical care, and their treatment as less disruptive than unemployed patients. However, employed patients had a stronger emotional response compared with unemployed patients. A possible explanation for this latter finding might be that these patients are more upset or scared for the future consequences in view of their work, for example whether they can continue working. Previous studies also have provided evidence for the role of illness perceptions in employment. As described earlier, Petrie et al. (1996) found a relationship between illness perceptions regarding duration and the consequences of the illness and return to work in MI patients. Recently, Hoving et al. (2010) conducted a literature review on illness perceptions and work participation in patients with somatic diseases and complaints. The findings showed that, overall, non-working patients perceived more serious consequences, expected their illness to last a longer time, and reported more symptoms and emotional responses. Working patients on the other hand had a stronger belief in the controllability of their condition and a better understanding of their disease. The authors concluded that the findings suggest that illness perceptions play a role in the work participation of patients with somatic diseases or complaints, although it is not clear how strong this relationship is and which illness perception dimensions are most useful.

The absence of clear relationships in our sample of pre-dialysis and dialysis patients might be caused by the small group sizes. The number of (pre-)dialysis patients of working age was low. A possible additional explanation might be that patients of older age or patients in this stage of the illness do not value a paid job as that important anymore, i.e. performing paid work does not contribute to their feelings of autonomy, and in turn their self-esteem. According to Self-Determination Theory, one of the requirements for need satisfaction, including the need for autonomy, is that people engage in an activity because they find the activity interesting and enjoyable or accept the value of the activity as personally important (autonomous motivation) (see Deci & Ryan, 2000). Renal patients in advanced illness stages may be aware of the fact that they are seriously ill, and therefore other life domains or life goals might have become more important, and work moves to the background. Consequently, a possible negative impact of for example a low degree of perceived personal control over the illness is not reflected in one's employment status. In this line of reasoning, we are assuming that people who place less value on doing work, might be less affected by the work limitations caused by their illness. Patients who on the other hand regard work as an important activity might be more affected by limitations, and therefore, perhaps more inclined to resign from work. Therefore, pre-dialyses patients were asked about the importance of performing paid work, and the results indicated that these patients regard paid work still as of considerable importance. When trying to increase feelings of autonomy and self-esteem, it seems important to take into account the life domains people find really important, explore their corresponding goals and focus on these goals.

On the whole, our results show that beliefs of more personal control, less impact of the illness and its treatment and less concern were the most important contributors to perceived autonomy and self-esteem. With respect to labour participation similar trends were observed, i.e. beliefs of greater personal control and less impact of the illness and treatment were associated with employment. These findings point to the likely importance of positively influencing these perceptions in order to improve patients' autonomy, self-esteem and labour participation. The results are in line with the findings from previous studies, which showed that beliefs of more personal control, less perceived (negative) consequences from the illness and treatment, and a lower emotional response were generally associated with better quality of life outcomes in patients on dialysis.

2.3.4 The course of CKD patients' illness and treatment perceptions

Identifying perceptions related to adaptive outcomes is a first step. In view of developing interventions aimed at altering (unhelpful) perceptions, it is additionally important to know whether these perceptions can be influenced in order to improve adaptive functioning. We investigated the illness perceptions and treatment disruption beliefs across the trajectory of CKD, in pre-dialysis patients and patients on dialysis (Jansen et al., in preparation). In so doing we aimed to elucidate the dynamics of patients' illness and treatment perceptions across the illness trajectory. This knowledge is important for determining whether perceptions vary and, consequently, whether interventions could potentially target perceptions of patients with CKD stage 4 and 5.

As mentioned previously, it is assumed that illness representations are constantly being updated as new illness knowledge and illness experience are acquired (Leventhal et al., 1984). Some years ago, a pilot study was conducted to change treatment beliefs of patients on haemodialysis who used phosphate-binding medication, by means of a psycho-educational intervention (Karamanidou et al., 2008). This brief intervention seemed to be able to change treatment beliefs immediately after the intervention. Randomised controlled trial studies by Petrie et al. (2002) and Broadbent et al. (2009b) among myocardial infarction (MI) patients suggest that perceptions of illness can be changed by means of a psychological intervention, and showed that the intervention resulted in improved outcomes, including an earlier return to work.

Two interesting longitudinal studies in patients with ESRD have provided knowledge about how perceptions of illness and treatment change over time. Covic et al. (2006) investigated the illness representations of patients on established haemodialysis with low co-morbidity over a 2-year period. Following this 2-year period, patients had fewer negative emotional reactions to the disease, a better understanding, and the perception that dialysis is more efficient in controlling their illness. Chilcot et al. (2010) revealed a similar trajectory for illness understanding in dialysis patients over their first year on dialysis: over a one year follow-up, patients' understanding significantly increased. In addition, illness identity decreased suggesting that individuals tended to identify their illness with fewer somatic symptoms over time. Previous research in other patient populations also demonstrated longitudinal changes in illness perceptions, as well as associated changes in health outcomes (see Kaptein et al., 2010). Another indication of the dynamic nature of illness and treatment perceptions of patients with CKD comes from a study by Griva et al. (2008). This longitudinal study suggests that changes in clinical state and treatment bring about changes in illness and treatment perceptions. In this study the researchers compared the illness perceptions and treatment perceptions of 41 patients with ESRD pre to post kidney transplantation (i.e., still on dialysis compared to six months after transplantation). After the transplantation, patients expressed different perceptions, including lower illness and treatment disruptiveness, and stronger control beliefs. Cross-sectional studies have also demonstrated differences in illness and treatment perceptions between patients who receive different treatments for their ESRD (Griva et al., 2009; Griva et al., 2010; Timmers et al., 2008). Treatment is of particular importance in CKD, since treatments differ significantly across the different phases of the illness (pre-dialysis, dialysis, transplantation), and are associated with different intense demands.

We examined whether patients who received different treatments (pre-dialysis treatment, haemodialysis treatment and peritoneal dialysis treatment) and who were on dialysis treatment for different lengths of time differed in their beliefs about the illness and treatment (for pre-dialysis patients the value regarding time on dialysis was set to zero years). In these analyses we adjusted for socio-demographic characteristics. We investigated these relationships using data provided by the sample of pre-dialysis patients at one measurement point and data provided by the sample of dialysis patients at two measurement points (either at only measurement point one, only measurement point two or at both measurement point one and two with an interval of eight months). We analysed the data by means of an analysis in which we could combine the multiple measurements (pooled cross-sectional analysis). Because of the multiple observations over time for a part of the dialysis patient group, we also took the dependency of these observations into account when analysing the data. We did this by controlling for the correlation between the measurements within individuals.

The results of the analyses demonstrated an association between time on dialysis treatment on the one hand and beliefs about *understanding* and beliefs about *treatment disruption* on the other hand. The association between time on dialysis and perceived understanding of the illness indicated that patients who just started dialysis reported lower levels of understanding than pre-dialysis patients; patients who are on dialysis for a moderate amount of time reported higher levels of understanding compared with patients who just started dialysis, and patients who are on dialysis for long lengths of time (quadratic association).

The association between time on dialysis and perceived treatment disruption indicated that patients who are on dialysis for a longer period of time perceive their treatment as more disruptive for daily life compared to patients who are not yet on dialysis or who are on dialysis for a shorter time. These findings indicate that perceptions of treatment disruption and understanding vary between patients as a function of time on dialysis.

The results of the analyses also provided insight into the extent to which perceptions vary within patients on dialysis over an interval of eight months, based upon the correlation between the perceptions measured at time point one and time point two. The results showed that the correlation of perceptions of *personal control* and perceptions of *treatment control* was r= 0.37 and r= 0.31, respectively. These findings suggest that these perceptions vary within patients over an interval of eight months. The correlations regarding the other perception dimensions were higher and ranged from r= 0.50 to r=0.79.

The findings that perceptions of understanding and perceptions of treatment control vary are in line with the (longitudinal) research findings of Covic et al. (2006) and Chilcot et al. (2010). These studies however also revealed changes in illness perceptions which we did not observe in our study and vice versa. The different findings might have been caused by the fact that different research designs were used, or by the fact that patients in these studies were exposed to other conditions which may have influenced their perceptions.

Our results furthermore demonstrated that perceptions of *illness consequences, treatment disruption* and *treatment control* vary between patients as a function of treatment type. Patients on HD and PD perceived more illness consequences compared with patients in the pre-dialysis phase. These differences are plausible, since the dialysis phase is characterised by specific disease aspects and intensive and time-consuming treatment demands. Moreover, various studies have demonstrated impaired functioning with respect to physical, mental, and social domains in patients on dialysis treatment (e.g. Khan et al., 1995; Molsted et al., 2007). Furthermore, patients on HD perceived more treatment disruption compared with patients in the pre-dialysis phase and patients on PD. It should be noted that, since we were not able to control for clinical characteristics and due to the cross-sectional design, this disruption cannot be simply attributed to HD.

Lastly, patients on HD and PD believed more strongly that their treatment controls the illness than patients who receive a pre-dialysis treatment. For patients on dialysis, dialysis is not an option but a vital need. Treatment control for these patients has a different meaning than for many other patients with a chronic disease. This may also explain the stronger beliefs in treatment control in patients on dialysis compared to pre-dialysis patients who use medication or follow a diet, and are much less dependent on their treatment compared to patients on dialysis.

Our study findings suggest that certain beliefs (pre-)dialysis patients hold about their illness and treatment vary across the illness trajectory, and therefore offer starting points for the development of interventions to target illness and treatment perceptions of patients with CKD. One of the perceptions that varies across the illness trajectory is the perception of treatment disruption. It seems important that interventions focus particularly on reducing the perceived negative impact of treatment on daily life, since our findings suggest that greater treatment disruption is negatively associated with perceived autonomy and self-esteem in both pre-dialysis patients and patients on dialysis. In addition, patients' illness perceptions regarding personal control, illness consequences and concern also seem to play an important role in patients' perceived autonomy and self-esteem. Moreover, patients in the pre-dialysis phase and/or dialysis phase, on average, reported unfavourable scores with respect to these illness perceptions. From our investigation of the relationships between the illness and treatment perceptions, it was also noticed that pre-dialysis patients' beliefs about greater treatment disruption were associated with beliefs of less treatment control, but not with personal control. Whereas a reverse pattern was found for patients on dialysis. Based on these findings it seems important to promote awareness among pre-dialysis patients regarding the opportunities to integrate treatment in daily life by means of their own efforts. In addition, it was notable that pre-dialysis patients' beliefs of little personal control were associated with higher levels of concern and emotional impact. It is therefore advised to, besides enhance personal control beliefs, reduce feelings of concern regarding the illness and treatment to more 'realistic standards'. However, because some perceptions of illness seem to be more stable than others, it is recommended to intervene on these perceptions as early as possible, preferably when people are likely to form their perceptions. The illness perception intervention study by Petrie et al. (2002) in MI patients also suggests that it is important to intervene in an early stage of the illness process.

What have we learned from scientific research?

- patients in the pre-dialysis phase and dialysis phase, on average, have relatively low levels of personal control over the illness; pre-dialysis patients are, generally, quite worried about their illness; patients on dialysis, on average, experience rather serious consequences of their illness in daily life
- on the whole, beliefs of more personal control, less (negative) impact of the illness and its treatment, and less concern were the most important contributors to perceived autonomy and self-esteem (taking into account socio-demographic and clinical characteristics); with respect to labour participation similar trends were observed
- perceptions of treatment disruption and understanding vary between (pre-) dialysis patients as a function of time on (dialysis) treatment
- perceptions of personal control and treatment control vary within dialysis patients over an interval of eight months
- perceptions of illness consequences, treatment disruption and treatment control vary between (pre-)dialyis patients as a function of treatment type (pre-dialysis, haemodialysis, peritoneal dialysis)

What is important for clinical practice?

- the findings point to the importance of self-management support on combining CKD and its (dialysis) treatment with daily activities, including paid work; by giving realistic information and providing tools and support on fitting the illness and (future) treatment into daily life, positive (realistic) beliefs might be stimulated and unhelpful illness and treatment related beliefs may be prevented or challenged; this might contribute to a greater sense of autonomy and self-esteem as well as to participation in general
- it seems important that such interventions focus particularly on reducing the perceived (negative) impact of dialysis treatment on daily life, in addition to reducing perceived (negative) consequences of the illness and concerns about the illness, as well as increasing perceptions of personal control over the illness
- the best moment to offer interventions to alter unhelpful or maladaptive beliefs in patients with CKD seems to be when people are likely to form their perceptions of illness and treatment, e.g. in the pre-dialysis phase (preferably even before CKD stage 4) or at the start of dialysis treatment

What needs to be investigated further?

- the formation process of CKD patients' illness and treatment perceptions, and the further development of these perceptions over time and phases of the illness, by means of longitudinal research; by comparing patients' perceptions at different points in time, this research can furthermore provide information about *when* patients' perceptions are most variable, and, consequently, most likely susceptible to change
- the course of illness and treatment perceptions in relation to autonomy, self-esteem and employment outcomes, by means of longitudinal research among CKD patients; this research can gain insight into causal relationships

- with respect to research in patients on dialysis, it would be interesting to take into account a broader range of dialysis modality characteristics, such as whether patients dialyze at night; this research can shed light on whether these characteristics have a positive effect on patients' outcomes, for example patients' sense of autonomy

2.4 The joint role of social support and illness perceptions

As stated before, previous research among patients on dialysis has shown that, besides patients' own attitudes towards employment, the attitudes towards work of people in patients' social environment (such as spouses or doctors) play an important role in patients' labour participation: patients who themselves believed that dialysis patients should work, and had this notion reinforced by significant others were more likely to be employed (Braun Curtin et al., 1996). These findings suggest that patients' social environment can support patients in their efforts to carry on with daily activities, which in turn might support patients' sense of autonomy and self-esteem. A prerequisite for providing this support is that the social environment also has positive (realistic) beliefs regarding the illness in relation to being active. A recent study by Grunfeld et al. (2010) among patients with cancer and (unlinked) employers demonstrated that employers in general held more negative illness perceptions of cancer in relation to work than patients. The authors foresaw that such a discrepancy could impact on an employees' management of their work and on employers' responsiveness to the needs of employees.

Self-determination theory, by Deci and Ryan (1985), postulates that social contexts can indeed support a person's basic psychological need for autonomy. According to Williams et al. (2006) autonomy support, in a health related context, refers to practitioners eliciting and acknowledging patients' perspectives, supporting their initiatives, offering choice about treatment options, and providing relevant information, while minimizing pressure and control. Studies have shown that autonomy support has resulted in improved health-related behaviours (see Ryan et al., 2008) and psychological well-being (Deci et al., 2006; Kasser & Ryan, 1999). Studies also provided evidence for relationships between well-being and other types of social support (see Cohen, 2004) and overprotection (Buunk et al., 1996; Thompsom & Sobolew-Shubin, 1993). In patients with ESRD, social support has also been linked to depressive affect and quality of life (see Patel et al., 2005). However, there are studies that did not demonstrate relationships between support and well-being in patient populations (e.g. Buunk et al., 1996; De Ridder et al., 2005).

A possible explanation for the inconsistent findings is that social support is only beneficial for those experiencing adversity, but does not play a role for those without highly stressful demands (stress-buffering hypothesis, see Cohen, 2004). Another explanation is that not all types of support are equally beneficial in face of the demands (Cohen, 2004). Research has shown that emotional support worked in the face of a variety of stressful events, whereas other types of support (e.g. instrumental, informational) responded to specific needs elicited by an event (Cohen, 2004). The main-effect hypothesis of social support, on the other hand, argues that support is beneficial irrespective of whether one is under stress (see Cohen, 2004). In line with this, Ryan and Solky (1996) conclude that autonomy-support not just buffers one from negative outcomes during distress, but actually facilitates development, expression and integration of the self, such as increased self-esteem, self-confidence, achievement, volition, and vitality. Taking this into account, we aimed to investigate the role of emotional support and overprotection in perceived autonomy and self-esteem of patients with ESRD on dialysis. We chose to investigate the relationships in this patient group, since patients on dialysis and their significant others are highly required to actively deal with the illness demands on a daily basis. More specifically, we investigated whether support is more beneficial for patients with specific illness perceptions. Thereby assuming that illness perceptions can function as indicators for whether patients experience adversity from their illness, and for whether they could (additionally) benefit from coping resources provided by their social environment. We looked at two specific illness perceptions, namely perceptions of *personal control* and *concern*. Assuming that for those who believe that they cannot personally control their illness and those who are highly concerned about their illness, the ESRD is likely to be stressful. It is particularly important to gain insight into these relationships in view of interventions focusing on enhancing social support interactions. In addition, this insight is valuable for the purpose of simultaneously intervening on both patients' illness perceptions and experienced support.

2.4.1 Emotional support combined with perceptions of concern and personal control

First of all, we found that, generally taken, dialysis patients now and then experience emotional support from significant others (including general emotional support, e.g. 'being affectionate', and problem-oriented emotional support, e.g. 'giving a nudge in the right direction') (Jansen et al., submitted). The results furthermore showed that the patient group as a whole does not experience significant lack of emotional support. Moreover, the findings of the regression analyses indicated that the extent to which general emotional support is beneficial for patients' sense of autonomy, depends on the way patients perceive their illness. Looking at concern, we found that general emotional support was positively related to autonomy solely in highly concerned patients. However, looking at personal control we did not find such a relationship between general emotional support and autonomy in patients low in control. General emotional support, however, might not be the most relevant type of support in case people feel that they cannot control or influence their illness. Perhaps other types of support, such as informational support, are more relevant under these circumstances. This is in line with the idea that support functions have to match with the stressors or needs faced with (Cohen, 2004). According to Cohen and Wills (1985) informational support that helps one reappraise a stressor as benign or suggests appropriate coping responses would counter a perceived lack of control. In light of our results that patients in the pre-dialysis phase report considerable worry about their disease, the finding that general emotional support is positively associated with autonomy in high concerned patients is particularly interesting. It was notable, that in patients reporting lower levels of concern, the experience of general emotional support was associated with lower levels of perceived autonomy (though this association was not significant). Due to the cross-sectional design of our study this could be explained in two ways, namely that for people with low levels of concern, the experience of more support results in feeling less autonomous, or that people who feel less autonomous generate more support from their social environment. In contrast to autonomy, one's self-esteem always seems to benefit from general emotional support and furthermore suffers from a lack of it, irrespective of illness perceptions. This might reflect satisfaction or dissatisfaction of the general need for belongingness or relatedness which is important for people's self-esteem (Deci & Ryan, 2000; Leary & Baumeister, 2000). It is further notable that emotional support in case of problems showed no associations at all (no main or buffer effects) with autonomy and self-esteem. This type of support is offered in the face of problems and it could be that this support type cannot boost feelings of autonomy and self-esteem, in light of the problems one is faced with.

2.4.2 Overprotection combined with perceptions of concern and personal control

The patient group as a whole experienced little overprotection by significant others. Experienced overprotection appeared to be associated with lower levels of autonomy and self-esteem. This is a plausible finding, since overprotection refers to unwanted and unnecessary help, and therefore likely detracts from one's feelings of autonomy and self-esteem. Moreover, the negative association between overprotection and autonomy appeared to be stronger in patients experiencing more personal control. This finding indicates that experienced overprotection is most harmful for patients' feelings of autonomy, as they experience high levels of personal control over the illness. However, we did not find such a relationship in patients with low levels of concern. People high in personal control over the illness in particular believe that they can manage the illness themselves. The experience of overprotection therefore might have an extra negative impact, because it gives the impression that others believe that one is not capable in managing the illness.

What have we learned from scientific research?

- the role of support (emotional support and overprotection) in patients' perceived autonomy seems to depend on patients' illness perceptions
- the role of support in patients' self-esteem does not seem to depend on the way patients perceive their illness
- the findings suggest that patients' perceptions of their illness provide insight into whether patients actually experience adversity from their illness, and whether they could (additionally) benefit from support provided by their social environment
- the findings point to the relevance of specifying illness related needs, since the results suggest that patients who are worried or experience little personal control regarding their illness do not benefit from the same support interactions, when it comes to their feelings of autonomy

What is important for clinical practice?

- the findings with respect to autonomy, indicate that the provision of support should be tailored to dialysis patients' individual needs, and that patients' needs should be monitored; the findings should be taken into account when developing interventions focused on supporting patients in their efforts to maintain a sense of autonomy and self-esteem

What needs to be investigated further?

- more research is needed to unravel the interaction effects of illness perceptions and (other) types of social support on outcomes related to patients' well-being (including patients' perceived autonomy and self-esteem)
- the relationships between illness perceptions and social support in relation to outcomes should be investigated longitudinally; this research can provide insight into causal relationships
- research should take into account a broader range of social interactions, such as attitudes and provided support of health care providers, employers, and colleagues

3. Development and evaluation of a psychological intervention

We developed a psychological intervention programme for patients who are being prepared for renal replacement therapy (i.e. pre-dialysis patients) and patients on dialysis for a maximum period of twelve months (for details see Jansen et al., 2011). The intervention assists patients and their partners in integrating the renal disease and treatment into their daily lives, and aims at maintaining or widening patients' daily activities, including paid work, and thereby increasing patients' feelings of autonomy and self-esteem. The intervention also focused on patients' partners, since family members play an important role in patients' recovery from and adjustment to chronic illness, and are also affected by patients' symptomatology, activity restriction, and need for emotional support or physical assistance (Martire, 2005). It can be expected that this is particularly true for patients' spouses. The intervention focused on patients in the mentioned stages for three reasons: 1) patients in the pre-dialysis phase already seem to experience problems from their illness and treatment in their daily lives, and resignation from paid work seems to occur particularly in this stage of the illness as well as the initiation phase of the dialysis treatment; 2) patients' perceptions regarding their illness and treatment are already maladaptive in the pre-dialysis phase; 3) it seems essential to intervene on perceptions in an early stage of the illness process.

Three theoretical models served as a framework for our intervention: the Common Sense Model of self-regulation of health and illness by Leventhal et al. (CSM; 1984); Social Learning Theory by Bandura (1977a); and Self-Determination Theory by Deci and Ryan (SDT; 1985). The content of the intervention is based on the results of our empirical studies among (pre-)dialysis patients, and targets the psychological factors which showed to be associated with perceived autonomy, self-esteem and labour participation. Additionally, knowledge and experiences of experts in the field of research and practice were used. More specifically, the programme focuses on three aspects:

- The first is stimulating positive but realistic beliefs about the illness, treatment, and the opportunities to stay active in both patients and partners - and in so doing, to change unhelpful, maladaptive beliefs. Partners' beliefs are also addressed, because in order to provide support it seems important that the perceptions of the support providers are constructive and not in conflict with patients´ perceptions. A study by Broadbent et al. (2009a) among spouses of MI patients indicates that a brief intervention can change spouses' illness perceptions. Spouses in the intervention group had, amongst other aspects, a higher illness understanding compared to the control group, and they had lower anxiety about their spouses' doing physical activity;
- The second aspect is enhancing patients' beliefs in self-efficacy;
- The final aspect concerns stimulating behaviour that supports autonomy in both patients and partners.

The intervention was pilot tested on feasibility and evaluated on initial experiences of participants, course leaders and health care providers involved (for details see Jansen et al., 2011). The intervention as implemented in the pilot phase, consisted of a group course for a minimum of five patients aged 18-64 years and their partners. Patients from three different dialysis centres were invited to participate via the social workers working in the centres. The course comprised six 2.5-hour sessions every two weeks, and one return session after three months, led by a health psychologist in cooperation with a nephrologist and an employment expert familiar with patients with CKD. Social workers of the participating dialysis centres were also present at one or more sessions. Course material for participants included a handbook which contains assignments and practical and theoretical information. Material for the course leaders included a detailed manual for delivering the course.

3.1 Components of the intervention programme

For the first three sessions the method developed by Petrie et al. (2002) was followed. In these sessions, information is provided about the illness and treatment in relation to the performance of daily activities, paid work in particular. This specific information is given by a nephrologist and an employment expert. Beliefs patients hold about their illness, treatment, and about the importance and attainability of activities related to work and private life are explored and discussed within the group. Special attention is given to perceptions which seem important for patients' feelings of autonomy, self-esteem, and labour participation. These include perceptions of consequences (particularly beliefs that activities including working cannot be combined with dialysis treatment), and beliefs about personal control (particularly beliefs that one cannot influence the course of the illness and one cannot fit the illness and dialysis treatment into daily life). Negative beliefs and misperceptions are challenged, and positive (realistic) beliefs are stimulated. Hereby, broadening participants' views on the opportunities available. Furthermore, the sessions focus on reducing existing concerns about the illness by means of addressing questions and providing information. Techniques that are used to influence beliefs are observational learning techniques, such as didactic teaching, written material, examples of personal stories from peers, and group discussion about personal experiences, wishes and perceived opportunities. The choice for the applied techniques stems from the Common Sense Model (CSM) of illness representations and Social Learning Theory. Illness perceptions are formed on the basis of personal and observed encounters with illness, as well as information from for example medical sources, friends, the Internet, and fellow patients (Kaptein et al., 2008). Social Learning Theory postulates that human beings learn by observing attitudes, behaviours and behavioural outcomes of others (Bandura, 1977a). Furthermore, participants are asked to set a main goal and related sub goals, with respect to employment and private life by the end of the third session. Patients have to evaluate these goals on personal importance and attainability, hereby taking into account the importance of autonomous motivation for the initiation and maintenance of behaviours (see Deci & Ryan, 2000), and the importance of perceived self-efficacy (see Bandura, 1977a, 1977b) or perceived competence (see Deci & Ryan, 2000) for behaviour change. Subsequently, the chosen goals are discussed within the group and adjusted if necessary, and participants learn how to develop action plans in order to reach the sub goals, and ultimately their main goals. From the third session onwards, the participants develop and carry out an action plan every two weeks, helped by their partners.

Changing maladaptive perceptions and stimulating constructive perceptions regarding illness and treatment are first steps towards behaviour change. Support for self-efficacy (Bandura, 1977a, 1977b) and support for autonomy (Deci & Ryan, 1985) are necessary to actually perform the intended behaviour. In sessions four to six, the focus is on these aspects. Beliefs in self-efficacy in relation to activities, including employment, are explored and enhanced using techniques such as self-monitoring, guided mastery of skills through the two-weekly action plans and feedback on progress, modelling of self-management behaviours and problem-solving strategies. These techniques are based on Social Learning Theory, which argues that personal experiences, modelling, social persuasions and physiological states are sources for affecting self-efficacy beliefs (Bandura, 1977b). In the context of self-efficacy, attention is furthermore given to fatigue. Fatigue is a common complaint in patients with chronic kidney disease, and might interfere with the performance of daily activities (Bonner et al., 2010). Patients are asked to keep a fatigue diary in order to gain insight into existing fatigue complaints and its patterns. The experiences are discussed and advice is given, so that a framework is provided for structuring and prioritising activities and for making the activities more accessible. In so doing, the threshold for carrying out activities is lowered and beliefs of self-efficacy are supported. Resulting in a greater chance of successful implementation of the action plans.

Our study findings showed that the experience of overprotection was associated with lower levels of autonomy and self-esteem, and highlight the importance of promoting autonomy-supportive behaviours. Autonomy-support is enhanced by means of discussing supportive and unsupportive behaviours, by exchanging ways to provide support, to prevent overprotection and to ask for support in an adequate way. These elements were partly derived from the family partnership intervention of Clark and Dunbar (2003). Moreover, autonomy-supportive behaviours in patients and partners are encouraged by means of the implementation of the developed action plans, which enable patients to carry out activities that they personally value with support from their social environment (partners or family members, friends). Furthermore, our findings indicated that the extent to which general emotional support is beneficial and overprotection is harmful for patients' sense of autonomy depends on the way patients view their illness (i.e. perceptions regarding concern and personal control). This suggests that the provision of support has to be tailored to patients' individual illness-related needs and patients' needs have to be monitored. This knowledge should be taken into account when stimulating supportive interactions. In session six, the focus is on the development of an action plan for an employment goal for the next three months, which is personally important and attainable. Patients develop the action plan together with their partners, under guidance of the course leader and employment expert. The plans are discussed within the group, and advice is given on which steps to take and how to contact relevant parties, such as employers and company doctors. During the return session, the outcome of the action plans regarding the employment goal are discussed and evaluated within the group, under guidance of the course leader and employment expert. The participants discuss what the course has given to them, paying attention to how one can maintain or widen the goals that have been achieved.

3.2 Evaluation of the intervention programme

The developed psychological intervention was theory driven. The three theories, providing a framework for our intervention, all focus on different aspects important for self-regulatory processes, including cognitive, emotional, behavioural and contextual aspects. An important component within the intervention is the focus on goals or activities which patients themselves choose and value, i.e. autonomous motivation (instead of controlled motivation), which is associated with greater behavioural persistence and more effective performance (see Deci & Ryan, 2000). According to Michie et al. (2008) there are three main reasons for advocating the use of theory in designing interventions: 1) interventions are likely to be more effective if they target causal determinants of behaviour and behaviour change; 2) theory can be tested and developed by evaluations of interventions only if those interventions and evaluations are theoretically informed; 3) theory-based interventions facilitate an understanding of what works and thus a basis for developing better theory across different contexts, populations and behaviours. Within our intervention we have combined three theories. It could be argued that the number of theoretical frameworks and corresponding components used is relatively high. Behaviour change and its maintenance are however complex processes, and several aspects seem to underlie these processes. We believe that the components provided by the separate theories are all important for behaviour change, and complement each other well. Another important aspect of our intervention is the multidisciplinary aspect, pooling the knowledge of experts including nephrologists, employment experts, social workers, and peers. The contribution of the employment expert was particularly greatly appreciated by both participants and involved social workers, and should therefore be an integral part of the course.

The intervention mainly has a proactive character. It focuses on prevention of the development of negative beliefs with respect to the illness, treatment and opportunities to stay active in both patients and partners. It stresses anticipating possible future problems due to changing conditions with respect to treatment, physical condition, work situation, and ultimately prevention of unnecessary resignation from paid work and other daily activities.

The participating three dialysis centres endorsed the necessity of this type of assistance. Together the centres approached enough patients eligible for participation (N=28), however the rate of participation was lower than expected (7 participating patients and 5 participating partners). The reasons for not responding indicated that it is important for the course to be fitted into participants' daily schedules. It is therefore advised to be flexible with respect to scheduling future courses (in terms of days / times / locations). Preferences for course times seem to be very personal, since patients differ regarding dialysis and work schedules. One could think of giving the intervention to participants at the dialysis centre while they are on dialysis, or adapting dialysis or work schedules in cooperation with health care providers or employers. It was further notable that no participants younger than 30 years took part, although some were approached. More efforts are needed to reach these younger patients by emphasising that besides employment, attention is given to education and training.

Another issue is that patients may not always see the need for a proactive approach. In particular, those patients who have not experienced any problems in the past. The involved course leaders however stressed that it is important that patients are referred to the course as early as possible, preferably even before CKD stage 4, in order to work preventatively. These patients often have no insight into the consequences of the illness and treatment for their daily life. As a result they are not able to anticipate necessary adjustments in order to prevent problems with employment. Therefore this group of patients are likely to benefit the most from the assistance offered in the course. Thus, there is a perceived need for widening the target group to the earlier stages of CKD (e.g. CKD stage 3). Following this, it seems appropriate to stress the importance of participating in the course, in view of future changes regarding the physical condition, treatment, and employment situation. Patients on dialysis in the more advanced stages of CKD stage 5 were not included in the pilot study. These patients may, however, also benefit from the practical assistance provided during the course. Any existing problems with daily functioning could be addressed. Moreover, possible future changes in circumstances regarding patients' physical condition, treatment modality, or work may bring about new problems.

Furthermore, it seems important that, besides social workers, more different health care providers (e.g. nephrologists, dialysis nurses) are involved in highlighting the course among patients so that the course becomes more integrated into regular care. Naturally, the individual needs of the patients must remain the starting point and taken into consideration at all times. Patients can be too overwhelmed by all the demands imposed by the illness and treatment, and may feel that they are not able to participate in the course on top of all the other tasks they have to undertake. This may particularly be the case for people who have to start with the dialysis treatment at short notice, or for people who just started with the dialysis treatment. It is then advised that health care providers continue to follow these patients and offer the course again at a later point in time. Furthermore, it would be helpful for health care providers if they have an instrument at their disposal, by which they at a given time can get insight into the most vulnerable patients, i.e. the patients who could benefit the most from the assistance provided by the course and consequently should be included in the course. Connecting to this, it is also important to reflect on whether the course should be offered to all eligible patients, or only to those who may benefit the most from it. Implementation of these types of interventions requires efforts from health care providers and requires financial resources. The health care providers involved in the pilot study reported no unfavourable consequences from their cooperation with the course. Moreover, in the long run, health care providers, especially social workers, might experience favourable consequences, since an intervention of this kind may prevent problems, or anticipates problems, which social workers normally encounter in their regular care.

Regarding the process and content of the intervention, there are both strengths and points for improvement to mention. Important elements within the course included group discussion, giving examples of practice, and didactic teaching. These elements were strategies to broaden participants' views on the available opportunities and, in so doing, to promote positive realistic beliefs. This was also endorsed by one of the participants, who stated that the course gave insight into how "healthy" you still are, and what and how much you still can do. The focus on influencing patients' perceptions can be regarded as an important ingredient of the intervention, and we advise to maintain these elements. The focus on influencing beliefs was also the reason for choosing a group format instead of an individual format, since peer modelling and peer support are useful strategies to influence beliefs. All participants held positive attitudes towards the group element, indicating that they valued the opportunity to exchange knowledge and experiences and had learned from it. The mixture of experiences and information of both patients who were being prepared for dialysis and patients on dialysis was particularly highly valued. The course leaders also indicated that there was a lot of open discussion, cooperation and mutual interest, and thought that it was important to increase the opportunities for discussion and cooperation in order to improve the group process and, in turn, the learning process. This should be achieved by increasing the number of participating patients to at least eight. However, when working with larger groups it is essential to have two main course leaders so that the process with respect to both content and the group will be warranted. A prerequisite for a successful group process, however, is that a trustful, confidential atmosphere is created from the first moment by means of an extensive group introduction, and occasionally putting participants together in smaller groups. Participants are asked to share their feelings and thoughts and these should be reviewed in a non judgmental way.

The topics addressed (e.g. dialysis, employment legislation) within the course appeared to be relevant to all participants. However, an area for attention is how the information given, is tailored to individual preferences. The differences in these preferences may be partly caused by differences in participants' stages of illness and/or treatment. Therefore, the amount of orally presented, discussed general information should be reduced. This information can be offered in the form of written information or on a website instead. On the other hand more time should be spent on exploring and discussing individual needs for information. This can be done throughout the course or by organising separate question times.

The attitudes of the participants towards the exercises were good, particularly the fatigue diary and the action plans. These exercises were tools to enhance beliefs about self-efficacy. Participants indicated that these exercises meant they were more able to divide their time and energy during the day, and one participant stated that creating plans to reach goals gave peace of mind. Based on these experiences, it seems important to preserve these exercises as part of the course. However, some participants encountered difficulties with the exercises: it is recommended tackling this problem by working in small groups, paying more attention to discussion of the exercises and giving more examples regarding the interpretation of the exercises, so that participants are able to relate to them better. It is furthermore advised to reduce the number of action plans.

An advantage of the course was the involvement of partners and attention for the role of the social environment. These aspects were appreciated by both patients and partners. However, increased attention is needed for partners and how they cope with the illness. Participating partners themselves indicated that more opportunities should be created for partners to exchange experiences with respect to how they deal with their partners' illness. Partners for example could work in separate groups occasionally, so that they can talk about their experiences more freely. Clark and Dunbar (2003) stress the importance of taking into account family members' experiences and their own needs for support.

Lastly, patients' self-observed results were encouraging. One patient reported that he found a job and generally became more active. Patients reported that they were able to divide their time and energy better during the day, they learned to involve their social environment in their illness and treatment, and they were more aware of the possible consequences of their illness and were better prepared for possible complications.

What have we learned?

- findings from the pilot study are encouraging and suggest that a theory driven multiple approach - focusing on cognitive, emotional, behavioural, and contextual aspects - is promising
- on the whole it can be concluded that the ingredients of the intervention all have value, however, the total course programme appears very intensive and parts of the sessions should be shortened
- issues that deserve attention are the need for larger course groups, two main course leaders, tailoring information to individual needs, increasing opportunities for discussion, and increasing attention for the needs of the participating partners
- a successful implementation process in regular care is not easy to achieve, despite the efforts of motivated health care providers; many conditions must be met in order to implement interventions successfully

What is important for clinical practice?

- the study elucidated factors that need specific attention when implementing interventions of this kind: the need for insight into patient groups that could benefit from the intervention, awareness of the importance of a proactive approach, early referral, flexibility in scheduling interventions, the need for broad support and cooperation among health professionals for organising and embedding interventions into regular care, the importance of the direct involvement of a multidisciplinary team of experts (i.e. employment expert, social worker, nephrologist, dialysis nurse)

What needs to be investigated further?

- the study meets the emerging need for research regarding development and evaluation of self-regulatory based interventions aimed at improving patient outcomes and CKD patient outcomes in particular; future research needs to evaluate whether the developed and refined intervention leads to lower rates of job resignation, increased feelings of autonomy, and whether the benefits outweigh the efforts, both in the short-term and in the long run
- research needs to address the question at which point in time (i.e. which illness phases) interventions of this kind should be offered to patients
- instruments should be developed by which health care providers can identify patients who could benefit from this type of intervention
- implementation of interventions requires a specific and separate route, which identifies success factors and bottlenecks and takes into account all necessary conditions

4. Acknowledgements

The studies were supported by a grant from the Dutch Kidney Foundation and the Institute Gak Foundation, Netherlands. We would like to thank the members of the advisory board regarding the studies, the participating hospitals, and the health care providers and patients who participated in the studies. Furthermore, we would like to thank the trial nurses and data managers of the Hans Mak Institute for data monitoring and data management. Lastly, we wish to thank Dr. Elisabeth W. Boeschoten and the Dutch Kidney Patient Association for their cooperation in the organisation and delivery of the intervention.

5. References

Abma, T., Nierse, C., Van de Griendt, J., Schipper, K. & Van Zadelhoff, E. (2007). *Leren over lijf en leven. Een agenda voor sociaal-wetenschappelijk onderzoek door Nierpatiënten. [Learning about life and body. An agenda for social science research by patients with kidney disease.]*, Maastricht University, Maastricht, The Netherlands

Bandura, A. (1977a). *Social Learning Theory*, Prentice Hall, ISBN 9780138167448, Englewood Cliffs, NJ

Bandura, A. (1977b). Self-efficacy: toward a unifying theory of behavioral change. *Psychological Review*, Vol.84, No.2, pp. 191-215

Bonner, A., Wellard, S. & Caltabiano, M. (2010). The impact of fatigue on daily activity in people with chronic kidney disease. *Journal of Clinical Nursing*, Vol.19, No.21-22, pp. 3006-3015

Braun Curtin, R., Mapes, D., Schatell, D. & Burrows-Hudson, S. (2005). Self- management in patients with end stage renal disease: Exploring domains and dimensions. *Nephrology Nursing Journal*, Vol.32, No.4, pp. 389-395

Braun Curtin, R., Oberly, E.T., Sacksteder, P. & Friedman, A. (1996). Differences between employed and non-employed dialysis patients. *American Journal of Kidney Diseases*, Vol.27, No.4, pp. 533-540

Broadbent, E., Ellis, C.J., Thomas J., Gamble, G. & Petrie, K.J. (2009a). Can an illness perception intervention reduce anxiety in spouses of myocardial infarction patients? A randomised controlled trial. *Journal of Psychosomatic Research*, Vol.67, No.1, pp. 11-15

Broadbent, E., Ellis, C.J., Thomas, J., Gamble G. & Petrie, K.J. (2009b). Further development of an illness perception intervention for myocardial infarction patients: A randomised controlled trial. *Journal of Psychosomatic Research,* Vol.67, No.1, pp. 17-23

Broadbent, E., Petrie, K.J., Main, J. & Weinman, J. (2006). The brief illness perception questionnaire. *Journal of Psychosomatic Research,* Vol.60, No.6, pp. 631-637

Buunk, B.P., Berkhuysen, M.A., Sanderman, R., Nieuwland, W. & Ranchor, A.V. (1996). Active engagement, protective buffering, and overprotection. Measurements for assessing spousal support in heart revalidation. *Gedrag en Gezondheid: Tijdschrift voor Psychologie en Gezondheid,* Vol.24, No.6, pp. 304-313

Cameron, L.D. & Moss-Morris, R. (2004). Illness-related cognition and behaviour, In: *Health Psychology,* A.A. Kaptein & J. Weinman, (Eds.), pp. 84-110, Blackwell Publishers, ISBN 0631214410, Oxford, UK

CBS, Statistics Netherlands (2006). Labor and social security, In: *StatLine,* 23.05.2011, Available from http://statline.cbs.nl/statweb

Chilcot, J.J. (2010) *Studies of depression and illness representations in end-stage renal disease, PhD thesis,* University of Hertfordshire, Hertfordshire, United Kingdom

Clark, P.C. & Dunbar, S.B. (2003). Family partnership intervention: a guide for a family approach to care of patients with heart failure. *AACN Clinical Issues,* Vol.14, No.4, pp. 467-476

Cohen, S. (2004). Social relationships and health. *American Psychologist,* Vol.59, No.8, pp. 676-684

Cohen, S. & Wills, T.A. (1985). Stress, social support, and the buffering hypothesis. *Psychological Bulletin,* Vol.98, No.2, pp. 310-357

Covic, A., Seica, A., Gusbeth-Tatomir, P., Gavrilovici, O. & Goldsmith, D.J. (2004). Illness representations and quality of life scores in haemodialysis patients. *Nephrology Dialysis Transplantation,* Vol.19, No.8, pp. 2078-2083

Covic, A., Seica, A., Mardare, N. & Gusbeth-Tatomir, P. (2006). A longitudinal study on changes in quality of life and illness representations in long-term hemodialysis patients with low comorbidity. *Medica – A Journal of Clinical Medicine,* Vol.1, No.4, pp. 12-19

Deci, E.L., La Guardia, J.G., Moller, A., Scheiner, M.J. & Ryan, R.M. (2006). On the benefits of giving as well as receiving autonomy support: Mutuality in close friendships. *Personality and Social Psychology Bulletin,* Vol.32, No.3, pp. 313–327

Deci, E.L. & Ryan, R.M. (1985). *Intrinsic motivation and self-determination in human behaviour,* Plenum, ISBN 0306420228, New York

Deci, E.L. & Ryan, R.M. (2000). The "what" and "why" of goal pursuits: Human needs and the self-determination of behavior. *Psychological Inquiry,* Vol.11, No.4, pp. 227-268

De Ridder, D., Schreurs, K. & Kuijer, R. (2005). Is spousal support always helpful in asthma and diabetes? A longitudinal study. *Psychology and Health,* Vol.20, No.4, pp. 497-508

De Wit, G.A., Polder, J.J., Jager, K.J. & De Charro, FTh. (2001). Social costs of renal diseases in the Netherlands. *Tijdschrift voor Gezondheidswetenschappen,* Vol.79, No.1, pp. 49-54

Ekelund, M.L. & Andersson, S.I. (2007). Elucidating issues stressful for patients in predialysis and dialysis: From symptom to context. *Journal of Health Psychology,* Vol.12, No.1, pp. 115-126

Fowler, C. & Baas, L.S. (2006). Illness representations in patients with chronic kidney disease on maintenance hemodialysis. *Nephrology Nursing Journal*, Vol.33, No.2, pp. 173-186

Fritschka, E., Mahlmeister, J., Liebscher-Steinecke, R. et al. (2000). Rehabilitation bei patienten mit chronischer niereninsuffizienz, dialysepatienten und nach nierentransplantation. *Nieren- und Hochdruckkrankheiten*, Vol.29, No.11, pp. 555-565

Griva, K., Davenport, A., Harrison, M. & Newman, S. (2008). A longitudinal investigation of illness and treatment cognition pre to post kidney transplantation. *Psychology & Health abstracts book*, Vol.23, Suppl. 1, pp.134

Griva, K., Davenport, A., Harrison, M. & Newman, S. (2010). An evaluation of illness, treatment perceptions, and depression in hospital- vs. home-based dialysis modalities. *Journal of Psychosomatic Research*, Vol.69, No.4, pp. 363-370

Griva, K., Jayasena, D., Davenport, A., Harrison, M. & Newman, S.P. (2009). Illness and treatment cognitions and health related quality of life in end stage renal disease. *British Journal of Health Psychology*, Vol.14, No.1, pp. 17-34

Grunfeld, E.A., Low, E., & Cooper, A.F. (2010). Cancer survivors' and employers' perceptions of working following cancer treatment. *Occupational Medicine*, Vol.60, No.8, pp. 611-617

Hagger, M.S. & Orbell, S. (2003). A meta-analytic review of the common-sense model of illness representations. *Psychology and Health*, Vol.18, No.2, pp. 141-184

Heijmans, M.J.W.M. & Rijken, P.M. (2004). *Social participation of people with chronic renal insufficiency. A literature study on experienced obstacles and opportunities*, NIVEL, ISBN 9069056763, Utrecht, The Netherlands

Horne, R., Cooper, V., Gellaitry, G., Leake Date, H. & Fisher, M. (2007). Patients' perceptions of highly active antiretroviral therapy in relation to treatment uptake and adherence. *Journal of Acquired Immune Deficiency Syndromes*, Vol.45, No.3, pp. 334-341

Horne, R., Sumner, S., Jubraj, B., Weinman, J. & Frost, S. (2001). Haemodialysis patients' beliefs about treatment: implications for adherence to medication and fluid-diet restrictions. *International Journal of Pharmacy Practice*, Vol.9, No.3, pp. 169–175

Horne, R. & Weinman, J. (2002). Self-regulation and self-management in asthma: exploring the role of illness perceptions and treatment beliefs in explaining non-adherence to preventer medication. *Psychology and Health*, Vol.17, No.1, pp. 17–32

Hoving, J.L., Van der Meer, M., Volkova, A.Y.& Frings-Dresen, M. H. W. (2010). Illness perceptions and work participation: a systematic review. *International Archives of Occupational and Environmental Health*, Vol. 83, No.6, pp. 595-605

Jansen, D.L., Grootendorst, D.C., Rijken, M., Heijmans, M., Kaptein, A.A., Boeschoten, E.W. & Dekker, F.W., the PREPARE-2 Study Group (2010). Pre-dialysis patients' perceived autonomy, self-esteem and labor participation: associations with illness perceptions and treatment perceptions. A cross-sectional study. *BMC Nephrology*, Vol.11, No.35

Jansen, D.L., Heijmans, M., Rijken, M. & Kaptein, A.A. (2011). The development of and first experiences with a behavioural self-regulation intervention for end-stage renal disease patients and their partners. *Journal of Health Psychology*, Vol.16, No.2, pp. 274-283

Jansen, D.L., Rijken, M., Heijmans, M. & Boeschoten, E.W., for the NECOSAD Study Group (2010). Perceived autonomy and self-esteem in Dutch dialysis patients: The importance of illness and treatment perceptions. *Psychology and Health,* Vol.25, No.6, pp. 733-749

Jansen, D.L., Rijken, P.M., Kaptein, A.A., Boeschoten, E.W., Dekker, F.W. & Groenewegen, P.P. The role of social support in dialysis patients' feelings of autonomy and self-esteem: is support more beneficial for patients with specific illness perceptions? (submitted)

Kaptein, A.A., Bijsterbosch, J., Scharloo, M., Hampson, S.E., Kroon, H.M. & Kloppenburg, M. (2010). Using the common sense model of illness perceptions to examine osteoarthritis change: a 6-year longitudinal study. *Health Psychology,* Vol.29, No.1, pp. 56-64

Kaptein, A.A., Scharloo, M., Fischer, M.J., Snoei, L., Cameron, L.D., Sont., J.K., et . (2008). Illness perceptions and COPD: an emerging field for COPD patient management. *Journal of Asthma,* Vol.45, No.8, pp. 625-629

Karamanidou, C., Weinman, J. & Horne, R. (2008). Improving haemodialysis patients' understanding of phosphate-binding medication: A pilot study of a psycho-educational intervention designed to change patients' perceptions of the problem and treatment. *British Journal of Health Psychology,* Vol.13, No.2, pp. 205-214

Kasser, V.G. & Ryan, R.M. (1999). The relation of psychological needs for autonomy and relatedness to health, vitality, well-being and mortality in a nursing home. *Journal of Applied Social Psychology,* Vol.29, No.5, pp. 935–954

Khan, I.H., Garratt, A.M., Kumar, A., Cody, D.J., Catto, G.R.D., Edward, N., et al. (1995). Patients' perception of health on renal replacement therapy: Evaluation using a new instrument. *Nephrology Dialysis Transplantation,* Vol.10, No.5, pp. 684-689

Kutner, N., Bowles, T., Zhang, R., Huang, Y. & Pastan, S. (2008). Dialysis facility characteristics and variation in employment rates: A National study. *Clinical Journal of the American Society of Nephrology,* Vol.3, No.1, pp. 111–116

Kutner, N.G., Zhang, R., Huang, Y. & Johansen, K.L. (2010). Depressed mood, usual activity level, and continued employment after starting dialysis. *Clinical Journal of the American Society of Nephrology,* Vol.5, No.11, pp. 2040-2045

Leary, M.R. & Baumeister, R.F. (2000). The nature and function of self-esteem: Sociometer Theory, In: *Advances in experimental social psychology,* M.P. Zanna, (Ed.), pp. 1-62, Academic Press, San Diego, CA

Leventhal, H., Nerenz, D.R. & Steele, D.J. (1984). Illness representations and coping with health threats, In: *Handbook of Psychology and Health,* A. Baum, S.E. Taylor & J.E. Singer, (Eds.), pp. 219-252, Lawrence Erlbaum Associates, Hillsdale, New Jersey

Martire, L.M. (2005). The "relative" efficacy of involving family in psychosocial interventions for chronic illness: are there added benefits to patients and family members? *Families, Systems & Health,* Vol.23, No.3, pp. 312-328

Michie, S., Johnston, M., Francis, J., Hardeman, W. & Eccles, M. (2008). From theory to intervention: mapping theoretically derived behavioural determinants to behaviour change techniques. *Applied Psychology: An International Review,* Vol.57, No.4, pp. 660-680

Molsted, S., Aadahl, M., Schou, L. & Eidemak, I. (2004). Self-rated health and employment status in chronic haemodialysis patients. *Scandinavian Journal of Urology and Nephrology,* Vol.38, No.2, pp. 174-178

Molsted, S., Prescott, L., Heaf, J. & Eidemak, I. (2007). Assessment and clinical aspects of health-related quality of life in dialysis patients and patients with chronic kidney disease. *Nephron Clinical Practice,* Vol.106, pp. c24-c33

Paradise, A.W. & Kernis, M.H. (2002). Self-esteem and psychological well-being: Implications of fragile self-esteem. *Journal of Social and Clinical Psychology,* Vol.21, No.4, pp. 345-361

Patel, S.S., Peterson, R.A. & Kimmel, P.L. (2005). The impact of social support on end-stage renal disease. *Seminars in Dialysis,* Vol.18, No.2, 98-102

Petrie, K.J., Cameron, L.D., Ellis, C.J., Buick, D. & Weinman, J. (2002). Changing illness perceptions after myocardial infarction: An early intervention randomized controlled trial. *Psychosomatic Medicine,* Vol.64, No.4, pp. 580-586

Petrie, K.J., Jago, L.A. & Devcich, D.A. (2007). The role of illness perceptions in patients with medical conditions. *Current Opinion in Psychiatry,* Vol.20, No.2, pp. 163-167

Petrie, K.J., Weinman, J., Sharpe, N. & Buckley, J. (1996). Role of patients' view of their illness in predicting return to work and functioning after myocardial infarction: longitudinal study. *British Medical Journal,* Vol.312, No.7040, pp. 1191-1194

Reis, H.T., Sheldon, K.M., Gable, S.L., Roscoe, J. & Ryan, R.M. (2000). Daily well-being: The role of autonomy, competence, and relatedness. *Personality and Social Psychology Bulletin,* Vol.26, No.4, pp. 419-435

Ryan, R.M. & Brown, K.W. (2003). Why we don't need self-esteem: On fundamental needs, contingent love, and mindfulness. *Psychological Inquiry,* Vol.14, No.1, pp. 71-76

Ryan, R.M., Patrick, H., Deci, E.L. & Williams, G. C. (2008). Facilitating health behaviour change and its maintenance: interventions based on self-determination theory. *The European Health Psychologist,* Vol.10, pp. 2-5

Ryan, R.M. & Solky, J.A. (1996). What is supportive about social support? On the psychological needs for autonomy and relatedness, In: *Handbook of social support and the family,* G. R. Pierce, B.R. Sarason & I.G. Sarason, (Eds.), pp. 249-267, Plenum Press, ISBN 0-306-45232-4, New York

Ryan, R.M., Williams, G.C., Patrick, H. & Deci, E.L. (2009). Self-determination theory and physical activity: the dynamics of motivation in development and wellness. *Hellenic Journal of Psychology,* Vol.6, No. 2, pp. 107-124

Sijpkens, Y.W. J., Berkhout-Byrne, N.C. & Rabelink, T.J. (2008). Optimal predialysis care. *Nephrology Dialysis Transplantation Plus,* Vol.1, Issue suppl. 4, pp. iv7–iv13

Sondergaard, H. & Juul, S. (2010). Self-rated health and functioning in patients with chronic renal disease. *Danish Medical Bulletin,* Vol.57, No.12, pp. A4220

Theorell, T., Konarski-Svensson, J.K., Ahlmen, J. & Perski, A. (1991). The role of paid work in Swedish chronic dialysis patients—a nation-wide survey: paid work and dialysis. *Journal of Internal Medicine,* Vol.230, No.6, pp. 501–509

Thompson, S.C. & Sobolew-Shubin, A. (1993). Perceptions of overprotection in ill adults. *Journal of Applied Social Psychology,* Vol.23, No.2, pp. 85-97Timmers, L., Thong, M., Dekker, F.W., Boeschoten, E.W., Heijmans, M., Rijken, M., et al. (2008). Illness perceptions in dialysis patients and their association with quality of life. *Psychology and Health,* Vol.23, No.6, pp. 679-690

Timmers, L., Thong, M., Dekker, F.W., Boeschoten, E.W., Heijmans, M., Rijken, M., et al. (2008). Illness perceptions in dialysis patients and their association with quality of life. *Psychology and Health,* Vol.23, No.6, pp. 679-690

Van den Brink-Muinen, A., Rijken, P.M., Spreeuwenberg, P. & Heijmans, M.J.W.M. (2008). *Key data social situation 2008 (Dutch National Panel of the Chronically Ill and Disabled)*, NIVEL, ISBN 9789069059631, Utrecht, The Netherlands

Van der Mei, S.F., Van Sonderen, E.L., Van Son, W.J., De Jong, P.E., Groothoff, J.W. & Van den Heuvel, W.J. (2007). Social participation after successful kidney transplantation. *Disability and Rehabilitation,* Vol.29, No.6, pp. 473-483

Van Manen, J.G., Korevaar, J.C., Dekker, F.W., Reuselaars, M.C., Boeschoten, E.W. & Krediet, R.T., NECOSAD Study Group. (2001). Changes in employment status in end-stage renal disease patients during their first year of dialysis. *Peritoneal Dialysis International,* Vol.21, No.6, pp. 595-601

Waddell, G. & Burton, A.K. (2006). *Is work good for your health and well-being?*, The Stationery Office, ISBN 0117036943, London, England

Williams, G.C., McGregor, H.A., Sharp, D., Levesque, C, Kouides, R.W., Ryan, R.M. & Deci, E.L. (2006). Testing a self-determination theory intervention for motivating tobacco cessation: supporting autonomy and competence in a clinical trial. *Health Psychology,* Vol.25, No.1, pp. 91-101

5

Role of Fermentable Carbohydrate Supplements in the Course of Uremia

Hassan Younes
Institut Polytechnique Lasalle Beauvais
France

1. Introduction

During the past few years, considerable attention has been given to the impact of nutrition on kidney disease. Interventions that restrict protein intake lower the plasma urea concentration, alleviate adverse clinical symptoms, and may slow the progression of chronic renal failure (CRF). Although these studies provide a logical explanation for a relationship between a low protein diet and altering the progression of functional renal deterioration, this beneficial effect is often accompanied by some muscle wasting and malnutrition. The question arises whether the effect of a moderate dietary protein restriction could be reinforced by enrichment of the diet with fermentable carbohydrates, since these carbohydrates may stimulate the extra-renal route of nitrogen (N) excretion, via the fecal route.

At a physiological level, there is two routes to eliminate N: urine and feces. Our results show that it is possible to increase the N fecal route excretion by reducing the protein supply and increasing fermentable carbohydrate availability. This additional dietary manipulation seems to be very interesting in case of renal deficiency in animal models and in humans. The modification of the urea N enterohepatic cycling by fermentable carbohydrates is likely to promote proliferation of the large intestine microflora, which could be an interesting approach to deviate a part of the N excretion to feces as a consequence of N utilization by the bacteria. Conversely, a large proportion of the N released by urea hydrolysis in the digestive tract may be recycled, via the reabsorption of ammonia, and could contribute thus to reduce the need of N.

In the domain of preventive nutrition, the first recognized effect of dietary fibers was to regularize the digestive transit, especially in the case of constipation. However, during the past decades, some other interesting effects have been reported, especially lipid-lowering effects, improvement of blood glucose control, reduction of colon cancer risk and increase of the availability of some cations. In contrast, the efficacy of the dietary fibers in the treatment of CRF has been less investigated although the availability of dietary fibers should profoundly alter the microflora metabolism and proliferation, and as a result N metabolism.

The aim of this chapter is to review, for the course of CRF, the capacity of an additional manipulation of diet in increasing fermentable carbohydrates which can stimulate the transfer of urea into the large intestine and shift N excretion from the urine to the feces.

2. Relationship between fermentable carbohydrate intake and symbiotic fermentations in the large intestine

Originally, fiber was defined to be the components of plants that resist human digestive enzymes, a definition that includes lignin and polysaccharides (cellulose, hemicellulose, pectin). The definition was later changed to also include resistant starches, along with inulin and other oligosaccharides. Pectin is 90 -100% degradable (by the bacteria in the colon), hemicellulose is 50-80%, and cellulose is 30-50%. Lignin is completely indigestible. Therefore, depending on the concentration of these components in the fiber, the digestibility and calorie value of fiber food varies (Anderson et al., 2009; Cummings et al., 2009).

There is now substantial evidence that fermentative processes similar to those occurring in non-ruminant herbivorous and omnivorous species also take place in the human large intestine (Cummings, 1984; Macfarlane & Macfarlane, 2009). In many animal species, the colon has an important digestive role to recover energy from non-available dietary carbohydrates that are not hydrolyzed and absorbed in the upper digestive tract. Traditionally, the human large intestine has been considered of as an organ that conserves minerals and water, and controls the disposal of indigested products. In recent years, research has also focused on the metabolic and digestive effects of various dietary fibers. In humans, it has been shown that the development of symbiotic fermentations had beneficial effects via the absorption and the utilization of short-chain fatty acids (SCFAs) (Macfarlane & Cummings, 1991; Elia & Cummings, 2007).

The breakdown of nutriments transfered from the ileum into the large intestine is carried out by diverse population of bacteria. In fact, bacteria are ubiquitous in the digestive tract, but the main part of them is confined in the large intestine. In humans, there are from 10^{11} to 10^{12} germs/g of content which are divided up into no less than 400 various species, this represents 35 to 55% of the digestive contents weight (Stephen & Cummings, 1980). This flora, mainly anaerobic, establishes relationships of symbiosis with the host. In addition, they probably fulfills a protective effect towards pathogenic species. The principal substrates for the bacteria are dietary fibers (non-starch polysaccharides, 10 to more 50 g/day), resistant starches (8 to 40 g/day) and oligosaccharides, and as well as proteins. Concerning the quantity of mucus (coming from the higher parts of the digestive tract or secreted in "situ") and the sloughed epithelial cells, there is still an uncertainty about their quantitative contribution.

In humans, the major end-products of carbohydrate breakdown are SCFA (essentially acetate, propionate and butyrate), and the gases H_2 and CO_2 (Fig. 1). The total concentration in SCFA is relatively stable in the large intestine: in the proximal part (cecum, proximal colon), they are generally found in the range of 80 to 150 mmol/L and, in the distal colon, they may be lower (from 50 to 100 mmol/L) (Macfarlane & Cummings, 1991). The SCFA are the main anions in the large intestine. For some osmotic reasons, it is expectable that they could hardly exceed 130-150 mmol/L. However, when the pH of fermentation is very acid (close to 5), the proportion of SCFA under protoned form becomes very important and then, it is possible to find concentrations higher than 150 mmol/L for SCFA alone or, more often, for SCFA + lactate (Macfarlane & Cummings, 1991).

The availability of fermentable carbohydrate influences the molar proportions of SCFA in the colon. Schematically, fermentations with a pH higher than 6.5 are relatively slow and favor the production of acetic acid. Fermentations close to a pH 6.0-6.5 are generally favorable to high propionic acid fermentations, while acidic fermentations (close to 5.5) give rise to the appearance of notable concentrations of lactate. Other products of the fermentation include branched-SCFA from the deamination of branched-chain amino acids, ammonia, various carboxylic and phenolic acids, and amines (Cummings & Macfarlane, 1991). The branched-SCFA (isobutyrate, isovalerate, 2-methylbutyrate) are very low in the proximal part of the large intestine (less than 10% of the total SCFA) where takes place a very active bacterial anabolism. In the distal part of the large intestine, the exhaustion of fermentable carbohydrates and the rise of the luminal pH favor proteolysis which chiefly affects bacterial protein, together with desaminations of AAs and production of the branched-SCFA. In humans, these last could be 35-40% of the total SCFA in the distal colon (Macfarlane & Cummings, 1991; Tarini & Wolever, 2010).

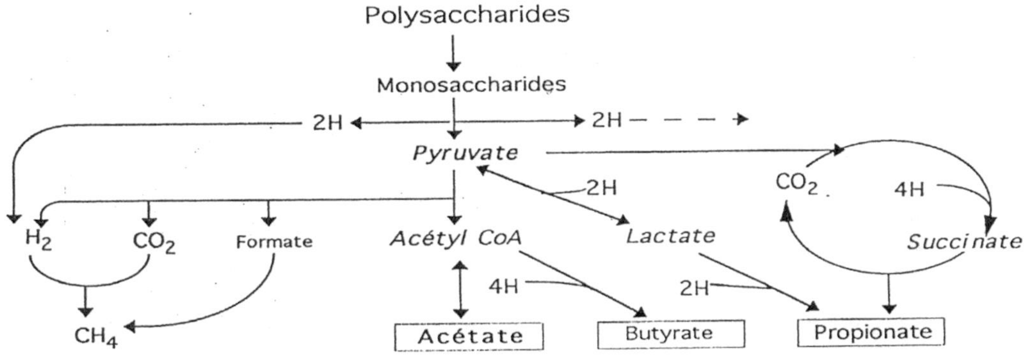

Fig. 1. Conversion stages of polysaccharides in SCFAs and other fermentation products by microflora in the large intestine

On the other hand, active fermentation stimulates the bacterial growth and leads to a considerable enlargement of the colonic contents and an hypertrophy of the cecal wall in rat (Levrat et al., 1991; Younes et al., 1995a). These changes results in an enlargement of the exchange surface area between blood and the luminal fluid, together with an increase of colonic blood flow. This in turn stimulates the exchanges of urea and ammonia N between blood and digestive lumen (Rémésy & Demigné, 1989; Levrat et al., 1991; Younes et al., 1995b; 1997). The relative hypertrophy of the cecal wall in rat fed fermentable carbohydrates can be ascribed to high concentrations of SCFA, especially butyrate, which is considered as a particularly potent trophic factor (Young & Gibson, 1995; Canani et al., 2011). In this view, it must be noticed that resistant starch exerts a marked trophic effect on colonic mucosa (Demigné & Rémésy, 1982; Bauer-Marinovic et al., 2006). Data on the action of fiber on colonic wall in humans are lacking, but it is possible that fermentable carbohydrates exert similar trophic effect (Jahns et al., 2011).

Dietary fibers contribute to reduce transit time in the large intestine by exerting a bulk effect directly or indirectly by the increase of bacterial mass (Luria, 1960). In fact, there is a direct relationship between an accelerated transit time, an enhanced fecal bacterial mass and fecal N excretion (Stephen et al., 1987). Furthermore, we have shown that the increase in fecal N excretion was compensated for by a decrease in urinary urea (Younes et al, 1995a,b, 1996a, 1997). The laxative effects of fermentable carbohydrate are particularly interesting to prevent and to treat the constipation (frequent in patients with CRF) (Burkitt et al., 1974; Eastwood, 1983; Turnbull et al., 1986).

3. Relationship between fermentable carbohydrate intake and enterohepatic cycling of urea and ammonia

How do these changes in bacterial mass and stool bulk affect N metabolism? Fermentation, by stimulating microbial growth, increases the N requirements of microorganisms. Nitrogen reaching the colon is mainly of endogenous origin, protein coming from the small intestine, or urea coming either directly from the blood or from the small intestine. Indeed, with diets which provide a small quantity of fermentable carbohydrates, only small amount of undigested dietary proteins and endogenous proteins (pancreatic enzymes and sloughed micosal cells) reach the large intestine. Here, they will be hydrolyzed and used for the microbial proliferation in the large bowel, but many of the end-products of protein fermentation are undesirable. However, when the intake of fermentable carbohydrates increases, N transfer may be not enough to promote an optimal bacterial growth. In such conditions, several investigations (Demigné & Rémésy, 1979; Langran, 1992; Younes et al. 1995a, 1995b, 1996a, 1997; Geboes et al., 2006) have shown that the blood urea constitutes the largest and the most available source of N for bacterial protein synthesis. As a result, fecal N excretion is significantly increased by comparison with fiber-free diets. (Younes et al., 1995a, 1995b, 1996a, 1997; Geboes et al., 2006; Wutzke, 2010)

In the 1980s, several hypothesis have been put forward for the manner in which fermentable carbohydrates brings about this effect : (i) the fecal N could originate from structural proteins of plant cell wall (Saunders & Betschart, 1980), and (ii) the fiber could decrease the digestibility of dietary protein in small intestine (Bender et al., 1979; Schneeman & Gallaher, 1986). Although these N sources may be significant, another source of fecal N is bacterial proliferation (Stephen, 1987). Bacteria make up ~ 55% of dry stool weight in humans on a western diet (Stephen & Cummings, 1980), and because bacteria are composed of 7-8% of N (dry weight) (Stephen, 1987), any increase in their colonic proliferation will increase fecal mass and N excretion.

Urea disposal in the large intestine has been shown in various species including humans (Demigné & Rémésy, 1979; Viallard, 1984; Forsythe & Parker, 1985; Moran & Jackson, 1990; Langran et al., 1992). In humans, it has been estimated that the urea hydrolyzed in the large intestine could represent approximately one-third of total urea produced by the liver (Richards, 1972). Various factors control the urea hydrolysis: the rate of urea transfer to the site(s) of hydrolysis, the activity of the bacterial urease, the demand of ammonia for the bacterial protein synthesis, and the availability of other N sources (Langran et al., 1992). However, some studies suggest that the human colon, unlike the colon of many animals, is relatively impermeable to urea and at most, a passive flux might allows diffusion of about 20% of the amount of urea destroyed (Bown et al., 1975; Moran & Jackson, 1990). But, these studies have entailed preliminary cleansing of the colon; yet removal of digestive constituents (bacterial urease, SCFA, carbon dioxide) is known to affect gastrointestinal permeability to urea (Dobbins & Binder, 1979; Kennedy & Milligan, 1980). Another study has shown, by direct measurements of the contribution of endogenous urea to fecal ammonia, that urea is a relatively minor source (8%) of fecal ammonia in healthy subjects with intact renal function (Wrong et al., 1985). The intensity of urea contribution to colonic ammonia is certainly dependent on the fermentable carbohydrate availability for maintaining highly active urease activity. Indeed, the transfer of urea is proportional to the concentration gradient of urea across the colonic wall; this explains the stimulatory effect of colonic bacteria via their ureolytic activity to promote urea uptake by the colon.

Consequently, in the presence of fermentable carbohydrates (particularly oligosaccharides which exerts osmotic effects and favors the ureolytic activity) and in case of hyperuremia, this transfer into the colon may become considerable (Fig.2A) (Younes et al., 2001). Some urea could be utilized in the distal ileum which presents a high permeability for this molecule (Gibson et al., 1976). However, the bacterial population in the terminal ileum is only one thousandth or so of that in the colon. Although the permeability of human ileum to urea is higher than that of the colon, the transfer of urea to the colon may be substantial because the transit time in the colon is longer.

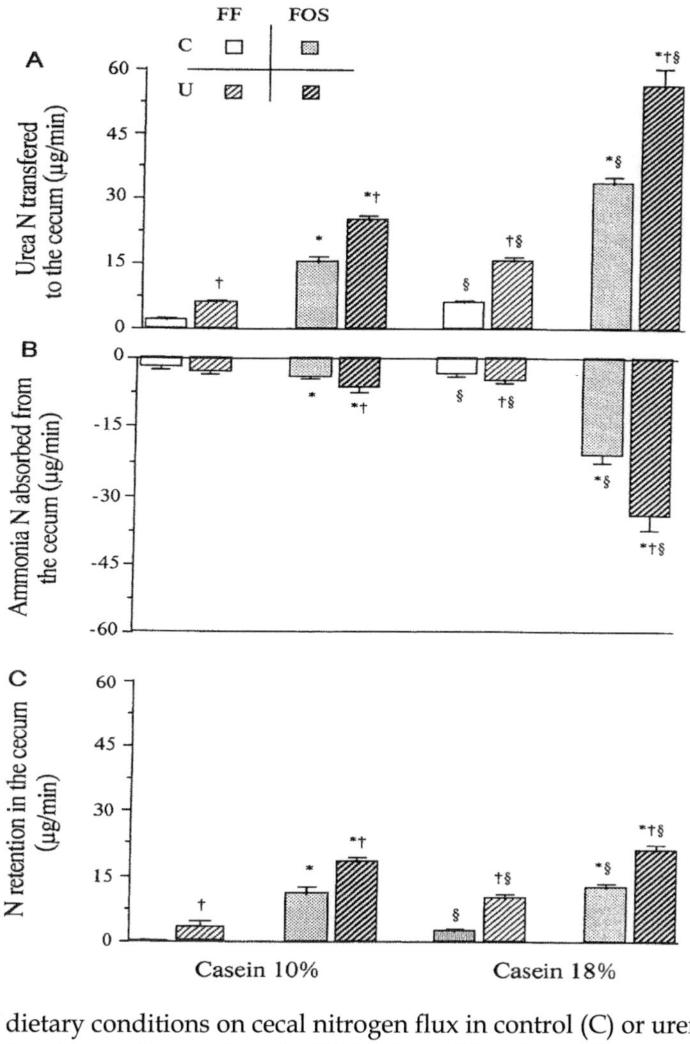

Fig. 2. Effects of dietary conditions on cecal nitrogen flux in control (C) or uremic (U) rats fed fiber-free (FF) or fructooligosaccharide (FOS) diets. * Significat difference (P<0.05) between groups of rats fed FF diets and groups of rats fed FOS diets. t Significat difference (P< 0.05) between groups of control rats and uremic rats. § Significat difference (P< 0.05) between groups of rats fed the moderately low protein level and those fed the moderately high protein level.

A part of ammonia produced from urea will be used for bacterial protein synthesis which will be eliminated in the stool, and therefore fecal N excretion is increased (Younes et al., 1995; Bliss et al., 1996; Younes et al., 1997). Another part of ammonia will be absorbed and converted in the liver to urea or recycled by different ways for non-essential AAs synthesis such as glutamate and glutamine (Rémésy et al., 1997). Moreover, some AAs coming from bacterial metabolism could be recovered by the host, but the importance of this way is still poorly documented (Jackson, 1995, Aufreiter et al., 2011). In fact, the incorporation of ammonia into bacterial protein mainly leads to an irreversible loss of N via the fecal route and it is more significant when the quantity of fermentable carbohydrates is high.
Our results support the view that there is a close relationship between the net flux of urea N towards large intestine and fecal N excretion, hence a lowering of plasma urea (Fig. 3) (Younes et al., 2001). A high rate of urea transfer into the cecum is favored by an enlarged surface area of exchange between blood and the luminal fluid and by an accelerated blood flow in the cecum (Rémésy & Demigné, 1989; Younes et al., 1997). All these parameters are enhanced by feeding various fermentable carbohydrates. In turn, a high supply of urea elevates the cecal pool of ammonia and elicits a substantial absorption of ammonia in spite of a marked acidification of cecal contents (Fig. 2B) (Younes et al., 2001). In fact, ammonia and SCFAs are generally considered to be transported across biological membranes as uncharged molecules (Bödeker et al., 1992). In colonocytes (intracellular pH 7.0-7.1) SCFAs and ammonia will be dissociated again, and it is conceivable that protons required for NH_4+ formation arise from SCFA dissociation.

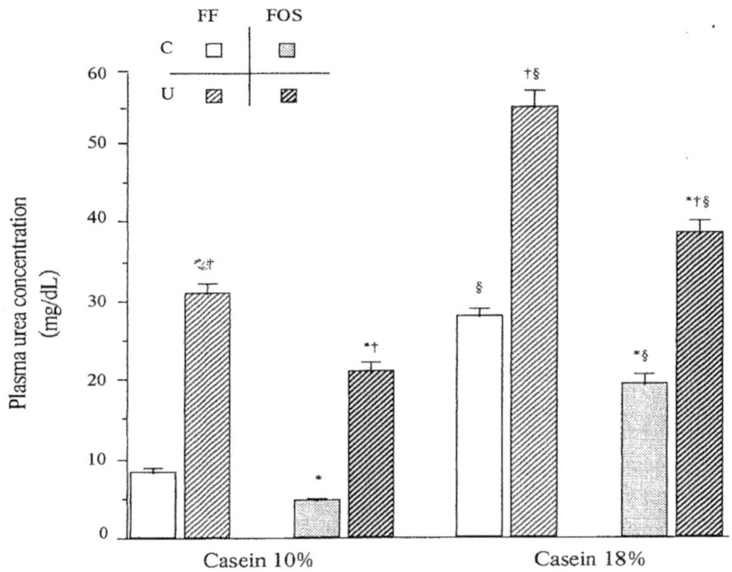

Fig. 3. Effects of dietary conditions on plasma urea concentration in control (C) or uremic (U) rats fed fiber-free (FF) or fructooligosaccharide (FOS) diets. * Significat difference (P<0.05) between groups of rats fed FF diets and groups of rats fed FOS diets. t Significat difference (P< 0.05) between groups of control rats and uremic rats. § Significat difference (P< 0.05) between groups of rats fed the moderately low protein level and those fed the moderately high protein level.

Thus, the enterohepatic cycle of urea and ammonia N observed in numerous works, (Stephen & Cummings, 1980; Forsythe & Parker,1985; Rémésy & Demigné, 1989; Moran & Jackson, 1990; Jackson, 1995) and as represented in Fig 4, suggests that this process is not necessarily a futile cycle. It participates in both the elimination of urea N by the fecal route and in the N salvage, particularly with a low protein diet enriched with fermentable carbohydrate.

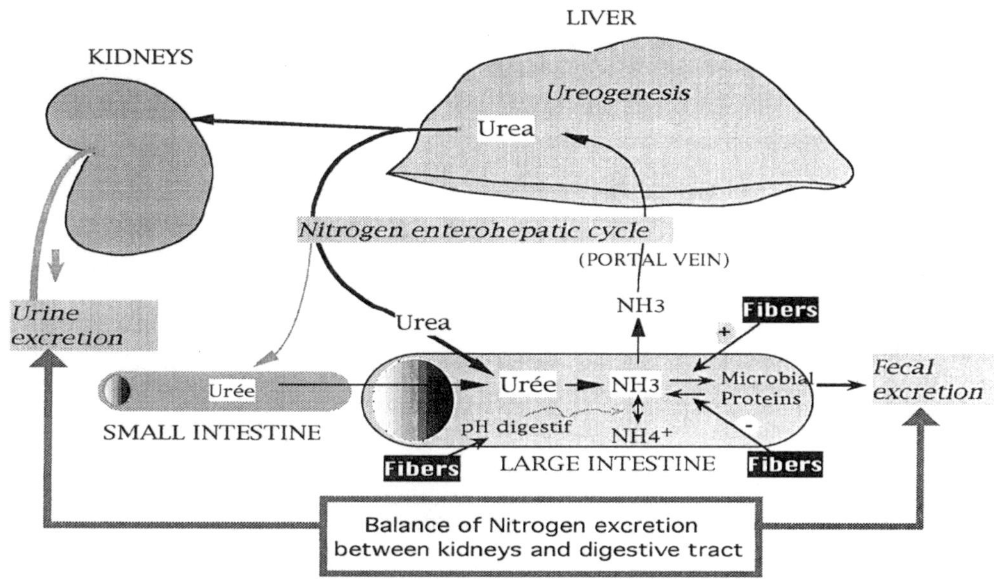

Fig. 4. Impact of fermentable carbohydrate intake on N enterohepatic cycle.

4. Present dietary approach to treat the patient with chronic renal failure

Until now, researches and dietetic propositions for CRF patients were based on the nephroprotection concept, making an attempt to maintain a satisfactory nutritional state. In other words, the aim of these researches and dietetic propositions were to delay the progression of renal deterioration, reduce urea toxicity and limit muscle wasting. Numerous studies have reported a reduction of the renal failure progression with a low protein diet. In fact, a linkage between glomerular hyperperfusion, hyperfiltration, and structural changes was suggested in studies involving dietary protein restriction (Brenner, 1985; Levey et al., 1996a, 1996b; Fouque et al., 2011, Garneata L & Mircescu G, 2011).

The relationship between the dietary protein restriction and renal failure progression is known for a long time. Approximately 60 years ago, Addis speculated that the severity of CRF could be improved by reducing the dietary protein level (Addis, 1948). Since then, a considerable body of evidence has been accumulated suggesting the slowing or temporary halting of the progression of CRF. In fact, a large number of diets have been proposed and more or less widely used during the last decades. The overall strategy was to reduce N intake by selecting foods of vegetable origin and by supplementing this "basal diet" with small amounts of protein of high biological value to satisfy the requirement for essentials amino-acids (AAs). Another approach was to use a supplementation of essentials AAs or

keto acids (KAs) (Giovannetti, 1989; Lin, 2009), however, the use of these KAs was not particularly convincing (Klahr, 1994; Aparicio et al ., 2009).
Studies in CRF patients (randomized trial or not) reported that starting a restriction of dietary protein and phosphate early in the course of CRF has a considerable influence on the rate of progression of this disease (Mitch, 1991 ; Levey et al., 1996a, 1996b ; William & Maroni, 1998 ; Mackenzie & Brenner, 1998, Garneata & Mircescu, 2010; Kalista-Richards, 2011; Fouque et al., 2011a). In experimental models, dietary protein restriction reduces the load of N metabolism end-products for excretion, limits the adaptive changes in remnant nephrons, and slows the tendency to renal disease progression (Hostetter, 1986). Despite the unambiguous support from experimental studies, the conclusive results are often regarded as unconvincing and as they do not meet strict statistical rules (Gretz & Strauch, 1986; Garneata & Mircescu, 2010).
Other works carried on within MDRD study (The Modification of Diet in Renal Disease: a randomized and controlled trials), it appeared that the protein restriction gives only a slight benefit for the patients with a moderate renal failure (Mackenzie & Brunner, 1998). Moreover, when the renal failure was at an advanced stage, the protein restriction, even severe and supplemented with KAs, did not really reduce the progression of the disease (Klahr, 1994). In fact, there is an initial diet-induced decline in GFR followed by a long-term beneficial effects of dietary protein restriction (appeared after 4 months), with an improvement of functioning nephrons conservation (Mackenzie & Brunner, 1998). This initial rapid reduction in GFR, accompanied by a reduction in protein excretion rates, is a functional effect and does not reflect a further loss of nephrons (levey et al, 1996c). In second MDRD study, the authors concluded that the addition of KAs did not exert a beneficial effects (Klahr et al., 1994), and that for patients with a low GFR (< 25 mL/min/1.73 m^2), a dietary protein intake of 0.6 g/kg/day should be prescribed (Levey et al., 1996a).
The question arises therefore on to the degree of the protein restriction. For health maintenance, a minimum daily supplies in protein was defined by the FAO in the range of 0.5 g/kg/day (FAO/WHO/UNU, 1985). In practice, in patients who are pre-dialysis and treated by a maintenance method, a protein supply lower than 0.6 g/kg/day has been proposed in association with KAs supplementation (El Nahas & Coles, 1986). However, the risk of protein malnutrition, and the constraints inherent to this supplementation led to recommend a moderate dietary protein supply of about 0.8 g/kg/day (Klahr et al., 1994 ; Tom et al., 1995 ; Levey et al., 1996a; Dumler, 2011; Fouque et al., 2011a).
In dialysis patients, the protein restriction question is more complex because there is a aggravated risk of protein-caloric undernutrition with an increased morbidity and mortality (30% of the dialysis patients) (Parker et al., 1983; Young et al., 1991). This leads to a rejection of protein restriction with, as a result, a proposed supply in the 1 to 1.2 g/kg/day range (Bergström, 1995 ; Cianciaruso et al., 1995 ; Qureshi et al., 1998 ; Antunes et al., 2010). However, it is still uncertain whether this policy is enough in order to equilibrate the N balance in these patients since there is a proportional relationship between the protein supply and the rate of N catabolism as it is estimated by the PCR (protein catabolism rate) (Movilli et al., 1993 ; Harty et al., 1994; Fouque et al., 2011a).
The protein-caloric undernutrition observed in dialysis patients is often linked to a deficient supply (Ikizler et al., 1995 ; Pollock et al., 1997, Kalantar-Zadeh, 2003), which is itself often linked to a depressed appetite (Bergström, 1995; Van Der Eijk & Farinelli, 1997). Moreover, seances of dialysis constitute in itself protein catabolism stimulation by means of an inflammatory response in contact with the membrane which induces the secretion of

hypercatabolic factors like interleukins (Valderrabano et al., 1996). The loss in glucose (25 g/seance) and in AAs (10-12 g/seance) can also decrease the protein anabolism capacity and thus led to an increased net proteolysis (Gutierrez et al., 1994; Ikizler et al., 1994). In practice, and in certain important undernutrition situations, it is necessary to provide a nutritional complement, especially AAs which are injected intravenously during the seance of dialysis. The dialysis fluid can be used also as a nutritional vehicle for supplementation of N (Chazot et al., 1997). The pre-dialytic parenteral nutrition seems to yield good results in order to preserve nutritional status (Cano et al., 1990), and it sounds to improve both morbidity and mortality on retrospective data (Capelli et al., 1994; Chertow et al., 1994).

Others studies showed that the catabolism rate of AAs and net protein synthesis could be affected by the speed of protein digestion (Boirie et al., 1997, Koopman et al., 2009). Thus, soluble proteins of milk are more quickly oxidized and lead to a less efficience protein synthesis than casein. It is more helpful to have slowly digested carbohydrate than rapid carbohydrate, and in the same view, it also would be helpful to select slowly degradated proteins (in particular plant proteins). This approach has not been sufficiently investigated in comparison with the quantitative approach.

In the elderly, the development of renal diseases is frequently linked to pathologies as diabete and/or cardiovascular diseases (Attman & Alaupovic, 1990; Parillo et al., 1988; Blicklé et al., 2007; Ng et al., 2011). Consequently, it is important to control the supply of both carbohydrates and lipids. In this view, it has been shown that diets enriched in fiber can improve blood glucose control and reduce serum cholesterol levels in diabetic patients. It has been also shown that the preservation of remaining nephron in nephrectomized rats is tightly dependent on the nature of the carbohydrate ingested. The kidney preservation could be, thus, improved by the supply of complex carbohydrates rather than simple carbohydrates (Lakshmanan et al., 1983; Kleinknecht et al., 1986).

Control of lipid supply and the balance in fatty acids is also important since CRF patients are frequently hyperlipidemic with an increase of the total amount of plasma cholesterol, triglycerides, phospholipides, LDL and VLDL and a decrease in HDL (Attman & Alaupovic, 1990; Gentile et al., 1995; Axelsson, 2010 ; Ng et al., 2011). In some animal models with a CRF, it has been shown that low-fat diets have protective effects on the progression of glomerular damages (Kher et al., 1985; Diamond & Karnovsky, 1987; D'Amico et al., 1992; Brown et al., 2000).

Furthermore, it is well known that diets for the CRF patients must be restricted in phosphorus and potassium and provide a calcium supplementation in order to help the fecal elimination of the phosphate (Gin & Rigalleau, 1995; Fouque et al., 2011b). Because of nutritional constraints inherent to the renal deficiency, it is particularly important to maintain the energetic balance of the patients and to provide a nutrition rich in protective factors, in particular, antioxidants to limit the severity of oxidative stress.

5. Role of fermentable carbohydrate in the dietetic of chronic renal failure: Experimental bases and discussion

There are synergistic actions between high fermentable carbohydrate diets and low protein diets, particularly as to their plasma urea lowering effects, and, hence progression of CRF. Although the primary determinant of the plasma urea concentration is the dietary protein level, feeding fermentable carbohydrate has also an important effect on this parameter (Younes et al., 1995a,b, 1996a, 1997; Bliss et al., 1996). Consequently, it is interesting to promote low protein diets, rich in various unavailable carbohydrates. This can be obtained by consuming a diet rich in plant products (cereal products, leguminous, vegetables and fruits). However, these diets are also particularly rich in potassium. Thus, to deal with this drawback, it is necessary to select foods rich in fermentable carbohydrate (resistant starch and oligosaccharides) to restrict the potassium supply.

Extra-renal urea excretion via the enteral route may be clinically relevant in patients with an impaired renal function. In CRF patients, the question of efficiency of the dietary protein restriction has seldom been considered according to the availability of fermentable carbohydrates. Consequently, it is necessary to carry out experiments in order to confirm these hypotheses and to determinate the optimal fermentable carbohydrate and protein supply for the protection of the renal function.

The selection of diets rich in slowly digested carbohydrates is particularly important in order to reduce the N catabolism because a part of AAs is metabolized for glucose production if the supply of carbohydrates is not optimal. In dialysis patients, catabolism is accelerated which theoretically increases the N demand. However, any increase of dietary N is expected to rise in parallel N catabolism and consequently precludes any significant improvement of the N balance. For this reason, it is important to increase the supply of the slowly digested carbohydrates in the diet of these patients which can contribute to decrease the hepatic gluconeogenesis from AAs. Therefore, in dialysis patients, it should be important that the fermentable carbohydrate would be provided together with a substential decrease of the protein level in the diet. This is possible because the increase of complex carbohydrate led to a better utilization of dietary N. It would also be important, in future, to explore the interest of slowly digested proteins.

The efficiency of fermentable carbohydrates to reinforce urea-lowering of a low-protein diet has been illustrated by experimental works in the rat (Younes et al., 1995b, 1996a, 1998, 2001). It appeared possible, using a diet rich in fermentable carbohydrates and low in protein, to drastically reduce the concentration of plasma urea, down to 0.75 mmol/L (Younes et al., 1996a). This urea lowering-effect of fermentable carbohydrates has been also observed in rat models of experimental renal failure (Younes et al., 1997, 1998, 2001) and in patients with CRF (Rampton et al.,1984; Bliss et al. 1996; Younes et al., 2006).

In nephrectomized rats, we have shown that feeding fermentable carbohydrates decreased the concentration of plasma urea from 32 mg/dL to 22 mg/dL, a 30% decrease. When, in addition, the dietary protein level was reduced from 18% to 10%, plasma urea was decreased from 56 mg/L to 22 mg/dL, a 60% decrease (Younes et al., 2001) (Fig. 3). Moreover, our results obtained in nephrectomized rats showed that the fermentable carbohydrates were all the more efficient to shift N excretion from the urinary route towards the fecal route because the protein level was low. Thus, we have shown that with a 18% protein level, fecal N represented 22% of total N excretion in rats fed fermentable carbohydrate diet vs. only 13% in rats in fiber-free conditions; whereas, with a lower protein level (10% casein diet) fecal N represented 40% of total N excretion (Fig. 5C) (Younes et al., 2001). As a result of this increase in fecal N excretion, the net effect of feeding fermentable carbohydrates with a dietary protein restriction was to decrease urinary N excretion from approximately 270 mg/day (18% casein, fiber-free diet) to approximately 100 mg/day (10% casein, fermentable carbohydrate diet); this represents a 63% decrease of urinary N (Fig. 5B) (Younes et al., 2001).

We have also compared the effects of fermentable carbohydrate intake in normal and nephrectomized rats: the data indicates that the hypertrophy of the remaining kidney (+40-50%) was effective in ensuring a relatively high rate of urea excretion, but it was not

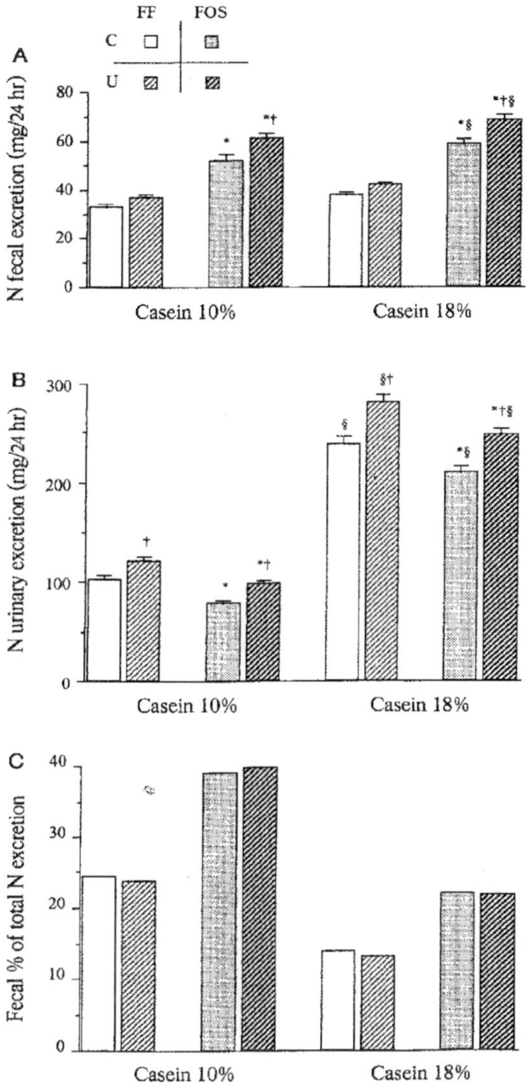

Fig. 5. Effects of dietary conditions on fecal and urinary N excretions and fecal percentage of total N excretion in control (C) or uremic (U) rats fed fiber-free (FF) or fructooligosaccharide (FOS) diets. * Significat difference (P<0.05) between groups of rats fed FF diets and groups of rats fed FOS diets. t Significat difference (P< 0.05) between groups of control rats and uremic rats. § Significat difference (P< 0.05) between groups of rats fed the moderately low protein level and those fed the moderately high protein level.

sufficient to counteract increased blood urea levels. Elevated blood urea had a minute influence on urea cycling and ammonia absorption in large intestine in rats fed the fiber-free diet. In contrast, a large increase in N fluxes through the large intestine was observed in nephrectomized rats fed fermentable carbohydrates (Fig. 2A,B). In these animals, a large part of urea taken up was reabsorbed as ammonia. This accelerated transfer of N in the large intestine results in a slightly higher fecal excretion in nephrectomized rats, when compared to normal rats (Fig. 5A). In turn, this led to a significant decrease of plasma urea, less pronounced in nephrectomized rats fed fermentable carbohydrate diet (-30%) than in normal rats (-45%) (Fig. 3). The urinary N excretion was also more effectively lowered by fermentable carbohydrates in normal rats (-30%) than in nephrectomized rats (-20%) (Fig 5B) (Younes et al., 2001).

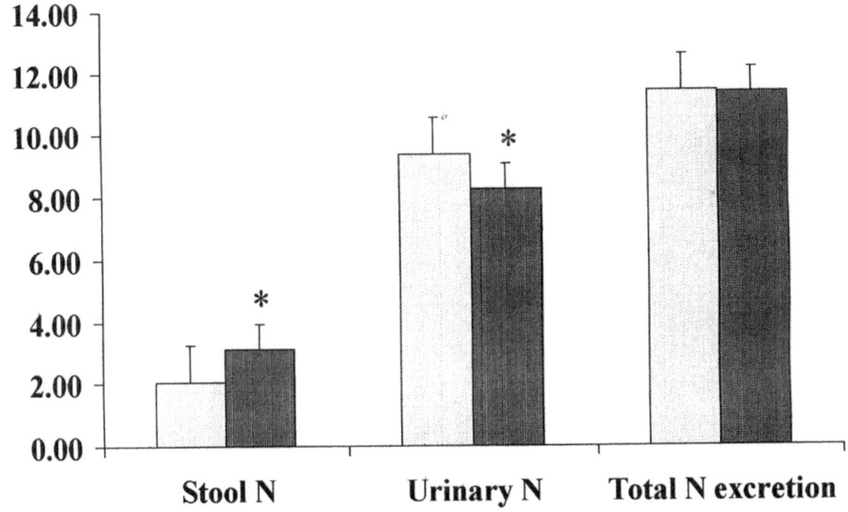

Fig. 6. Effects of dietary conditions on stool and urinary N excretions and the total N excretion in chronic renal failure patients consoming a fermentable carbohydrates (FC)-free diet or an enriched-FC diet. * Significat difference (P<0.05).

The question which arises is to know if the fermentable carbohydrates have the same effects on N metabolism in healthy men as in those with CRF. To our knowledge, this point has not been well documented. In CRF patients, supplementation with gum arabic or ispaghula (hemicellulose) has been shown to reduce serum urea N levels by 12% and 19%, respectively (Rampton et al., 1984; Bliss et al. 1996). In parallel, the total fecal N excretion, and particularly the bacteria fraction, was significantly increased with fermentable carbohydrates and accounted for 59% of the total increase in stool N contents (Stephen et al., 1995; Bliss et al., 1996). This suggests that the large intestine can partially compensate for the renal failure, provided that an appropriate supply of fermentable carbohydrate and protein is allowed. More recently, in a prospective study (Younes et al., 2006), the impact of fermentable carbohydrates (40 g/day) on uremia and N excretion ways was investigated during five weeks in CRF patients in presence of a controlled protein diet (0.8 g/kg/day). Patients were their own controls and treated by crossing over method after randomization (5 weeks with fermentable carbohydrates vs 5 weeks without fermentable carbohydrates). Feeding fermentable carbohydrates significantly increased the quantity of N excreted in stools from 2.1 ± 0.8 to 3.2 ± 1.1 g/day ($P < 0.01$) and decreased, in parallel, the urinary N excretion from 9.4 ± 1.7 to 8.3 ± 1.4 g/day ($P < 0.01$). The total N quantities excreted by the two ways were unchanged by the fermentable carbohydrates, which showed that the FC was efficient to shift N excretion from the urinary route toward the digestive route (Fig. 6).

In consequence to this increase of urea transfer into the colon, the plasma urea concentration was significantly decreased from 26.1 ± 8.7 to 20.2 ± 8.2 mmol/L ($P < 0.05$). In this short trial, we have not shown a significant difference in the concentration of plasma creatinine, nor in the creatinine clearance. Any changes in the nutritional status parameters (albumin, prealbumin) have been noted. However, the body weight was significantly increased (+ 600 g) when the diet of patients was enriched in fermentable carbohydrates.

6. Conclusion

In CRF, the plasma concentration of the end-products of protein catabolism, especially urea, is increased. Although most of the dietary attempts to treat this disease and to decrease the serum urea N involve a reduction of N intake, an additional manipulation of diet would be to add fermentable carbohydrates, which can increase N excretion in the feces. Our works and those of others have shown that a low protein diet remains beneficial and the combination of these two dietary changes brings about the greatest fecal urea excretion, together with a reduced urinary excretion. Of course, the colon could not substitute completely itself to the renal function. Reciprocally, when the digestive elimination route is disturbed, the consequences of renal failure are amplified.

In practice, it is recommended to increase fiber gradually by using a large variety of vegetal products to provide 35-40 g of fiber daily (24 g from cereals products, leguminous seeds, and other starchy foods; 8 g from vegetables; 2-4 g from fruits; 4 g from resistant starches, oligosaccharides and various hydrocolloids). Nevertheless, because intolerance seems to exist toward certain food, it is necessary to ensure that the recommended products are well tolerated by considering the supply of potassium, which is particularly present in fruits. Because of social and family environments, it is difficult to change dietary habits; thus, it is sometimes necessary to recommend preparations enriched with fermentable carbohydrates.

Finally, it is also important to indicate that a food rich in complex plant products could help facilitate the elimination of cholesterol and, hence, prevent the vascular complications caused by CRF. Moreover, plant products are rich in antioxidant micronutriments are very important in order to prevent lipid peroxidation and the production of free radicals, which is exaggerated in the CRF patients.

7. References

Addis T. (1948). *Glomerular Nephritis: Diagnosis and treatment,* in Addis (ed), Macmillan, New York, USA

Anderson JW, Baird P, Davis RH Jr, Ferreri S, Knudtson M, Koraym A, Waters V & Williams CL. (2009). Health benefits of dietary fiber. *Nutr Rev,* 67(4), pp. 188–205

Aparicio M, Cano NJ, Cupisti A, Ecder T, Fouque D, Garneata L, Liou HH, Lin S, Schober-Halstenberg HJ, Teplan V & Zakar G. 2009). Keto-acid therapy in predialysis chronic kidney disease patients: consensus statements. *J Ren Nutr,* 19(5 Suppl), pp. S33-5

Attman PO & Alaupovic P. (1990). Pathogenesis of hyperlipidemia in the nephrotic syndrome. *Am J Nephrol,* 10, pp. 78-84

Aufreiter S, Kim JH & O'Connor DL. (2011). Dietary oligosaccharides increase colonic weight and the amount but not concentration of bacterially synthesized folate in the colon of piglets. *J Nutr,* 141(3), pp. 366-72

Axelsson TG, Irving GF, Axelsson J. (2010). To eat or not to eat: dietary fat in uremia is the question. *Semin Dial.,* 23(4), pp. 383-8

Bauer-Marinovic M, Florian S, Müller-Schmehl K, Glatt H & Jacobasch G. (2006). Dietary resistant starch type 3 prevents tumor induction by 1,2-dimethylhydrazine and alters proliferation, apoptosis and dedifferentiation in rat colon. *Carcinogenesis,* 27(9), pp. 1849-59

Bender AE, Mohammadhia H & Alams K. (1979). Digestibility of legumes and available lysine content. *Qualitas Plantarum,* 29, 219-226

Bergström J. (1995). Why are dialysis patients malnourished ? *Am J Kidney Dis,* 26, pp. 229-241

Blicklé JF, Doucet J, Krummel T & Hannedouche T. (2007). Diabetic nephropathy in the elderly. *Diabetes Metab,* 33, 1, pp. S40-S55. Review

Bliss DZ, Stein TP, Schleifer CR & Settle RG. (1996). Supplementation with gum arabic fiber increases fecal nitrogen excretion and lowers serum urea nitrogen concentration in chronic renal failure patients consuming a low-protein diet. *Am J Clin Nutr,* 63, pp. 392-398

Bödeker D, Shen Y, Kemkowski J & Höller H (1992). Influence of short-chain fatty acids on ammonia absorption across the rumen wall in sheep. Experimental Physiology 77, pp. 369-376

Boirie Y, Dangin M, Gachon P, Vasson MP, Maubois JL & Beaufrère B. (1997) Slow and fast dietary proteins differently modulate postprandial protein accretion. Proc Natl Acad Sci 94, pp, 14930-14935, 1

Bown R, Gibson JA, Fenton JCB, Snedden W, Clark ML, Sladen GE: Ammonia and urea transport by the excluded human colon. Clin Sci Mole Med 48:279-287, 1975

Brenner BM. (1985). Nephron adaptation to renal injury or ablation. *Am J Physiol,* 249, pp. F324-F337

Brown SA, Brown CA, Crowell WA, Barsanti JA, Kang CW, Allen T, Cowell C, Finco DR. (2000). Effects of dietary poly-unsaturated fatty acid supplementation in early renal insufficiency in dogs. *J Lab Clin Med,* 135(3), pp. 275-86

Burkitt DP, Walker ARP & Painter NS. (1974). Dietary Fiber and disease. *JAMA,* 229, pp. 1068-1074

Canani RB, Costanzo MD, Leone L, Pedata M, Meli R & Calignano A. (2011). Potential beneficial effects of butyrate in intestinal and extraintestinal diseases. *World J Gastroenterol,* 17(12), pp.1519-28

Cano N, Labastie-coeyrehourq J, Lacombe P, Stroumza P, Costanzo-Dufetel J, Durbec JP, Coudray-Lucas C & Cynober L. (1990). Perdialytic parenteral nutrition with lipids and amino acids in malnourished hemodialysis patients. *Am J Clin Nutr,* 52, pp. 726-730

Capelli JP, Kushner H, Camiscioli TC, Chen SM & Torres MA. (1994). Effect of intradialytic parenteral nutrition on mortality rates in end-stage renal disease care. *Am J Kidney* Dis, 23, pp. 808-816.

Chazot C, Shamir E, Matias B, Laidlaw S & Kopple J. (1997). Dialytic nutrition: provision of amino acids in dialysate during hemodialysis. *Kidney Int,* 52, pp. 1663-1670

Chertow GM, Ling J, Lew NL, Lazarus JM & Lowrie EG. (1994). The association of intradialytic parenteral nutrition administration with survival in hemodialysis patients. *Am J Kidney Dis,* 24, pp. 912-920

Cianciaruso B, Brunori G, Kopple JD, Traverso G, Panarello G, Enia G, Strippoli P, De Vecchi A, Querques M, Viglino G, Vonesh E & Majorca R. (1995). Cross-sectional comparison of malnutrition in continuous ambulatory peritoneal dialysis and hemodialysis patients. *Am J Kidney Dis,* 26, pp. 475-486

Cummings JH & Mac Farlane GT. (1991). The control and consequences of bacterial fermentation in the human colon. *J Appl Bacteriol,* 70, pp. 443-459

Cummings JH, Mann JI, Nishida C & Vorster HH. (2009). Dietary fibre: an agreed definition. Lancet, 373, pp. 365-6

Cummings JH. (1984). Microbial digestion of complex carbohydrates in man. *Proc Nutr Soc,* 43, pp. 35-44

D'Amico G, Gentile MG, Manna G, Fellin G, Ciceri R, Cofano F, Petrini C, Lavarda F, Perolini S & Porrini M. (1992). Effect of vegetarian soy diet on hyperlipidemia in nephrotic syndrome. *Lancet,* 1, pp. 1131-1134

Demigné C & Rémésy C. (1979). Urea cycling and ammonia absorption in vivo in the digestive tract of the rat. Ann Biol Anim Biophys, 19(3B), pp. 929-935

Demigné C & Rémésy C. (1982). Influence of unrefined potato starch on cecal fermentations and volatiles fatty acid absorption in rats. *J Nutr,* 112, pp. 2227-34.

Diamond JR & Karnovsky MJ. (1987). Exacerbation of chronic aminonucleoside nephrosis by dietary cholesterol. *Kidney Int,* 2, pp. 671-677

Dobbins JW & Binder HJ. (1979). Effects of bile salts and fatty acids on the colonic absorption of oxalate. *Gastroenterology,* 70, pp. 1096-1100

Eastwood MA. (1992). The physiological effect of dietary fiber: an update. *Ann Rev Nutr,* 12, pp. 19-35

El Nahas AM & Coles GA. (1986). Dietary treatment of chronic renal failure: Ten unanswered questions. *Lancet,* 1, pp 597-560

Elia M & Cummings JH. (2007). Physiological aspects of energy metabolism and gastrointestinal effects of carbohydrates. *Eur J Clin Nutr,* 61 (Suppl 1), pp. S40-74.

FAO/WHO/UNU. (1985). Energy and protein requirements. In: technical report series 724. Geneva, World Health Organization, pp 1-206

Fouque D, Pelletier S, Guebre-Egziabher F. (2011b). Have recommended protein and phosphate intake recently changed in maintenance hemodialysis? J Ren Nutr., 21(1), pp. 35-8.

Fouque D, Pelletier S, Mafra D, Chauveau P. (2011a). Nutrition and chronic kidney disease. Kidney Int, 11 (in press)

Garneata L & Mircescu G. (2011). Nutritional intervention in uremia : myth or reality ? *J Renal Nutr,* 21, pp. 76-81

Gentile MG, Ciceri R, Manna GM, Delle Fave A, Zanoni C, Raschioni E, Combi S, Maiocchi V & D'Amico G. (1995). The role of fibre in treatment of secondary hyperlipidemia in nephrotic patients. *Eur J Clin Nutr,* 49, pp. S239-S241

Gibson TA, Park NJ, Sladen GE & Dawson AM. (1976). The roleof the colon in urea metabolism in man. *Clin Sci Mole Med,* 50, pp. 51-59

Gin H & Rigalleau V. (1995). Nutrition et insuffisance rénale. *Cah Nutr Diét,* 30, pp. 260-265

Giovannetti S. (1989). Low-protein diets for chronic renal failure, In : *Nutritional treatment of chronic renal failure,* Giovannetti S (ed), pp 179-190, Kluwer Academic Publishers, Boston, USA

Gretz N & Strauch M. (1986). Statistical problems in designing, conducting, and analyzing nutritional trials in patients with chronic renal failure. *Contr Nephrol,* 53, pp. 82-91

Gutierrez A, Alvestrand A, Bergström J, Beving H, Lantz B & Henderson L. (1994). Biocompatibility of hemodialysis menbranes: a study in healthy subjects. *Blood Purif,* 12, pp. 95-105

Harty JC, Boutlon H, Curwell J, Heelis N, Uttley L, Venning MC & Gokal R. (1994). The normalized protein catabolic rate is a flawed marker of nutrition in CAPD patients. *Kidney Int,* 45, pp. 103-109

Hatch M & Vaziri ND. (1994). Enhanced enteric excretion of urate in rats with chronic renal failure. *Clin Sci,* 86, pp. 511-516

Hostetter TH, Meyer TW, Rennke HG & Brenner BM. (1986). Chronic effects of dietary protein in the rat with intact and reduced renal mass. *Kidney Int,* 30, pp. 509-517

Ikizler TA, Flakoll PJ, Parker RA & Hakim RM. (1994). Amino acid and albumin losses during hemodialysis. *Kidney Int,* 46, pp. 830-837

Ikizler TA, Greene J, Wingard RL, Parker RA & Hakim RM. (1995). Spontaneous dietary protein intake during progression of chronic renal failure. *J Am Soc Nephrol,* 6, pp. 1386-1391

Jackson AA. (1995). Salvage of urea-nitrogen and protein requirements. *Proc Nutr Soc,* 54, pp. 535-547

Jahns F, Wilhelm A, Jablonowski N, Mothes H, Radeva M, Wölfert A, Greulich KO & Glei M. (2011). Butyrate suppresses mRNA increase of osteopontin and cyclooxygenase-2 in human colon tumor tissue. *Carcinogenesis,* 32(6), pp. 913-20

Jenkins DJ, Jenkins AL, Wolever TMS, Vuksan V, Rao AV, Thompson LU & Josse RG. (1994). Low glycemic index : lente carbohydrates and physiological effects of altered food frequency. *Am J Clin Nutr,* 59, pp. 706S-709S

Kalantar-Zadeh K, Ikizler TA, Block G, Avram MM & Kopple JD. (2003). Malnutrition-inflammation complex syndrome in dialysis patients: causes and consequences. *Am J Kidney Dis,* 42(5), pp. 864-81

Kennedy PM & Milligan LP. (1980). The degradation and utilization of endogenous urea in the gastrointestinal tract of ruminants: a review. *Can J Ani Sci,* 60, pp. 205-221

Kher V, Barcelli U, Weiss M, Pollak V. (1985). Effects of dietary linoleic acid enrichment on induction of immune complex nephritis in mice. *Nephron,* 39, pp. 261-266

Klahr S, Levey AS, Beck GJ, Caggiula AW, Hunsicker L, Kusek JW & Striker G. (1994). The effects of dietary protein restriction and blood-pressure control on the progression of chronic renal disease. Modification of Diet in Renal Disease Study Group. *N Engl J Med,* 330, pp. 877-884

Kleinknecht C, Laouari D, Hinglais N, Habib R, Dodu C, Lacour B, Broyer M: Role of amount and nature of carbohydrates in the course of experimental renal failure. Kidney Int 30:687-693, 1986

Koopman R, Crombach N, Gijsen AP, Walrand S, Fauquant J, Kies AK, Lemosquet S, Saris WH, Boirie Y & van Loon LJ. (2009). Ingestion of a protein hydrolysate is accompanied by an accelerated in vivo digestion and absorption rate when compared with its intact protein. *Am J Clin Nutr,* 90(1), pp. 106-15.

Lakshmanan FL, Howe JC & Barnes RE. (1983). Effect of dietary protein level and kind of carbohydrate on growth and selected pathological and biochemical parameters in male BHE rats. *Nutr Res,* 3, pp. 733-742

Langran M, Moran BJ, Murphy JL, Jackson AA. (1992). Adaptation to a diet low in protein: effect of complex carbohydrate upon urea kinetics in normal man. *Clin Sci*, 82, pp. 191-198

Levey AS, Adler S, Caggiula AW, England BK, Greene T, Hunsicker LG, Kusek JW, Rogers NL & Teschan PE. (1996a). Effects of dietary protein restriction on the progression of advanced renal disease in the Modification of Diet in Renal Disease Study. *Am J Kidney Dis*, 27, pp. 652-663

Levey AS, Adler S, Greene T, Hunsicker LG, Kusek JW, Rogers NL & Teschan PE. (1996b). Effects of dietary protein restriction on the progression of moderate renal disease in the Modification of Diet in Renal Disease Study. *J Am Soc Nephrol*, 7, pp. 2616-2626

Levey AS, Beck GJ, Bosch JP, Caggiula AW, Greene T, Hunsicker LG & Klahr S. (1996c). Short-term effects of protein intake, blood pressure, and antihypertensive therapy on glomerular filtration rate in the Modification of Diet in Renal Disease Study. *J Am Soc Nephrol*, 7, pp. 2097-2109

Levrat MA, Behr SR, Rémésy C & Demigné C. (1991). Effects of soybean fiber on cecal digestion in rats previously adapted to a fiber-free diet. *J Nutr*, 121, pp. 672-678

Levrat MA, Rémésy C & Demigné C (1991) Very acidic fermentations in the rat cecum during adaptation to a diet rich in amylase-resistant starch (crude potato starch). *J Nutr Biochem*, 2, pp. 31-36, 1991

Lin S. (2009). New research areas for keto acid/amino acid-supplemented protein diets. J Ren Nutr, 19 (5 Suppl), pp. S30-2

Luria SE. (1960). The bacterial protoplasma: composition and organisation, In : The bacteria. Gunsalus IC, Stainer RY (eds), pp. 1-34, Academic Press, New York

Macfarlane GT & Cummings JH. (1991). The colonic flora, fermentation, and large bowel digestive function, In: The Large Intestine: Physiology, Pathophysiology and Disease. Phillips SF, Pemberton JH, Shorter RG (eds), pp. 51-92, Mayo Foundation, Raven Press Ltd, New York

Macfarlane GT & Macfarlane LE. (2009). Acquisition, evolution and maintenance of the normal gut microbiota. *Dig Dis.*, 27 (Suppl 1), pp. 90-8.

Mackenzie HS & Brenner BM. (1998). Current strategies for retording progression of renal disease. *Am J Kidney Dis*, 31, pp. 161-170

Marsman KE & McBurney MI. (1996). Dietary fiber and short-chain acids affect cell proliferation and protein synthesis in isolated rat colonocytes. *J Nutr*, 126, 1429-1437

McCrary RF, Pitts TO & Puschett JB. (1981). Diabetic nephropathy: natural course, survivoship and therapy. *Am J Nephrol*, 1, pp. 206-218

Mitch WE. (1991). Dietary protein restriction in chronic renal failure: nutritional efficacy, compliance and progression of renal insufficiency. *J Am Soc Nephrol*, 2, pp. 823-831

Moran BJ & Jackson AA. (1990). 15N-urea metabolism in the functioning human colon: luminal hydrolysis and mucosal permeability. *Gut*, 31(4), pp. 454-7

Movilli E, Mombelloni S, Gaggiotti M & Malorca R. (1993). Effect of age on protein catabolic rate, morbidity and mortality in uremic patients with adequate dialysis. *Nephrol Dial Transplant*, 8, pp. 735-739

Ng KF, Aung HH & Rutledge JC. (2011). Role of triglyceride-rich lipoproteins in renal injury. *Contrib Nephrol*, 170, pp. 165-71

Parillo M, Riccardi G, Pacioni D, Iovine C, Contaldo F, Isernia C, De Marco F, Perrotti N & Rivellese A. (1988). Metabolic consequences of feeding a high-carbohydrate, high-fiber diet to diabetic patients with chronic kidney faillure. *Am J Clin Nutr,* 48, pp. 255-259

Parker TFI, Laird NM & Lowrie EG. (1983). Comparison of the study groups in the national cooperative dialysis study and a description of morbidity, mortality, and patient with drawal. *Kidney Int,* 23, pp. S42-S49

Pollock CA, Ibels LS, Zhu FY, Warnant M, Caterson RJ, Waugh DA & Mahony JF. (1997). Protein intake in renal disease. *J Am Soc Nephrol,* 8, pp. 777-783

Qureshi AR, Alvestrand A, Danielsson A, Divino-Filho JC, Outierrez A, Lindholm B & Bergström J. (1998). Factors predicting malnutrition in hemodialysis patients: A cross-sectional study. *Kidney Int,* 53, pp. 773-782

Rémésy C, Demigné C. (1989). Specific effects of fermentable carbohydrates on blood urea flux and ammonia absorption in the rat cecum. *J Nutr,* 119, pp. 560-565

Rémésy C, Moundras C, Morand C & Demigné C. (1997). Glutamine or glutamate release by the liver constitues a major mechanism for nitrogen salvage. *Am J Physiol,* 272, pp. G257-G264

Richards P. (1972). Nutritional potential on nitrogen recycling in man. *Am J Clin Nutr,* 25, pp. 615-625

Saunders RM & Betschart AA. (1980). The significance of protein as a component of dietary fiber. *Am J Clin Nutr,* 33, 960-961

Scheeman BA. (1978). Effect of plant fiber on lipase, trypsin and chymotrypsin activity. *J Food Sci,* 43, pp. 643

Stephen AM & Cummings JH. (1980). Mechanism of action of dietary fiber in the human colon. *Nature,* 284, pp. 283-284

Stephen AM & Cummings JH. (1980). The microbial contribution to human fecal mass. *J Med Microbiol,* 13, pp. 45-56

Stephen AM, Wiggins HS & Cummings JH. (1987). The effects of changing transit time on colonic microbial metabolism in man. *Gut,* 28, pp. 601-609

Stephen AM. (1987). Dietary fiber and colonic nitrogen metabolism. *Scand J Gastroenterol,* 22, pp. S110-S115

Tarini J & Wolever TM. (2010). The fermentable fibre inulin increases postprandial serum short-chain fatty acids and reduces free-fatty acids and ghrelin in healthy subjects. *Appl Physiol Nutr Metab,* 35(1), pp. 9-16.

Tessitore N, Venturi A, Adami S, Roncari C, Rugin C, Corgnati A, Bonucci E & Maschio G. (1987). Relationship between serum vitamin D metabolites and dietary intake of phosphate in patients with early renal failure. *Min Electr Metab,* 13, pp. 38-44

Tetens I, Livesey G & Eggum BO. (1996). Effects of type and level of dietary fiber supplements on nitrogen retention and excretion patterns. *Br J Nutr,* 75, pp. 461-469

Tom K, Young VR, Chapman T, Masud T, Akpele L & Maroni BJ. (1995). Long-term adaptive responses to dietary protein restriction in chronic renal failure. *Am J Physio,* 268, pp. E668-E677

Trinidad TP, Wolever TMS & Thompson LU. (1996). Effect of acetate and propionate on calcium absorption from the rectum and distal colon of humans. *Am J Clin Nutr,* 63, pp. 574-578

Turnbull GK, Lennard-Jones JE & Bartram CI. (1986). Failure of rectal expulsion as a cause of constipation : why fibre and laxatives sometimes fail. Lancet, 1, pp. 767-769

Valderrabano F, Perez-Garcia R & Junco E. (1996). How to prescribe optimal hemodialysis. *Nephrol Dial Transplant,* 2, 60-67, 1996

Van Der Eijk I & Farinelli MA. (1997). Taste testing in renal patients. *J Renal Nutr,* 7, pp. 3-9

Viallard V. (1984). Endogenous urea as a nitrogen source for microorganisms of the rabbit digestive tract. *Ann Nutr Metab,* 28, pp.151-155

Wrick KL, Robertson JB, Van Soat PJ, Lewis BA, Rivers JM, Roe DA & Hackler LR. (1983). The influence of dietary fiber source on human intestinal transit and stool out-put. *J Nutr,* 113, pp. 1464-79

Wrong OM, Vince AJ & Waterlow JC. (1985). The contribution of endogenous urea to fecal ammonia in man, determined by ^{15}N labelling of plasma urea. *Clin Sci,* 68, pp. 193-199

Younes H, Alphonse JC, Hadj-Abdelkader M & Rémésy C. (2001). Fermentable carbohydrate and digestive nitrogen excretion. *J Ren Nutr,* 11(3), pp.139-48

Younes H, Coudray C, Bellanger J, Demigné C, Rayssiguier Y & Rémésy C. (2001). Effects of tow fermentable carbohydrates (inulin and resistant starch) and their combination on calcium, and magnesium balance in rats. *Br J Nutr,* 86, pp. 479-485

Younes H, Demigné C, Behr S & Rémésy C. (1995a). Resistant starch exerts an uremia lowering effect by enhancing urea disposal in the large intestine. *Nutr Res,* 15, pp. 1199-1210

Younes H, Demigné C, Behr SR, Garleb KA & Rémésy C. (1996a). A blend of dietary fibers increases urea disposal in the large intestine and lowers urinary nitrogen excretion in rats fed a low protein diet. *J Nutr Biochem,* 7, pp. 474-480

Younes H, Demigné C, Rémésy C. (1996b). Acidic fermentation in the cecum increases absorption of calcium and magnesium in the large intestine of the rats. *Br J Nutr,* 75, pp. 301-314

Younes H, Egret N, Hadj-Abdelkader M, Rémésy C, Demigné C, Gueret C, Deteix P & Alphonse JC. (2006). Fermentable carbohydrate supplementation alters nitrogen excretion in chronic renal failure. *J Ren Nutr,* 16(1), pp. 67-74

Younes H, Garleb K, Behr S, Rémésy C & Demigné C. (1995b). Fermentable fibers or oligosaccharides reduce urinary nitrogen excretion by increasing urea disposal in the cecum. *J Nutr,* 125, pp. 1010-1016

Younes H, Garleb KA, Behr SR, Demigné C & Rémésy C. (1998). Dietary fiber stimulates the extra-renal route of nitrogen excretion in partially nephrectomized rats. *J Nutr Biochem,* 9, pp. 613-620

Younes H, Levrat MA, Demigné C & Rémésy C. (1995c). Resistant starch is more effective than cholestyramine as lipid-lowering agent in the rat. *Lipids,* 30, pp. 847-853

Younes H, Rémésy C, Behr S & Demigné C. (1997). Fermentable carbohydrate exerts a urea-lowering effect in normal and nephrectomized rats. *Am J Physiol,* 272, pp. G515-G521

Young GA, Kopple JD, Lindholm B, Vonesh EF, De Vecchi A, Scalamogna A, Castelnova C, Oreopoulos DG, Anderson GH & Bergström J. (1991). Nutritional assessment of continuous ambulatory peritoneal dialysis patients: an international study. *Am J Kidney Dis,* 17, pp. 462-471

Young GP, Gibson PR: Butyrate and the human cancer cell, in Cummings JH, Rombeau JL, Sakata T (eds): Physiological and Clinical Aspects of Short-chain fatty acids. U.K, Cambridge University Press, 1995, pp 319-336

6

Phosphorus and Calcium Metabolism Disorders Associated with Chronic Kidney Disease Stage III-IV (Systematic Review and Meta-Analysis)

L. Milovanova, Y. Milovanov and A. Plotnikova
I.M. Sechenov First Moscow State Medical University (MSMU)
Minsotszdravrazvitia of Russia, Moscow
Russia

1. Introduction

Kidneys play an important role in maintenance of the calcium and phosphorus balance. Renal failure is associated with disorders of all phases of the phosphorus and calcium turnover. The decrease of glomerular filtration rate (GFR) under 60 ml/min/1.73 m^2 is associated with phosphorus filtration rate decrease with further elevation of its serum level that results in parathyroid hormone (PTH) secretion stimulation. PTH suppresses phosphorus reabsorption; therefore, it returns its serum level to normal. However, when the GFR falls below the 30 ml/min/1.73 m^2 level, this mechanism becomes ineffective and persistent hyperphosphatemia develops. The latter enhances the PTH secretion. Hyperphosphatemia is associated with inhibition of 1α-hydroxylase effect in proximal renal tubules and the decrease of serum $1,25(OH)_2D_3$ (calcitriol) level. Calcitriol deficiency results in calcium absorption disorders in small intestine; as a result, hypocalcemia develops. Persistent hypocalcemia results in parathyroid glands hyperplasia (PTGH) that is associated with excessive PTH production and secretion. PTH hyper-production and hyperphosphatemia are the manifestations of secondary hyper-parathyroidism (SHPT). Hypocalcemia, vitamin D deficiency and hyperphosphatemia are the main factors responsible for secondary hyperparathyroidism. Hypocalcemia, vitamin D deficiency and hyperphosphatemia develop at the initial stage or renal dysfunction – Chronic Kidney Disease (CKD) III (GFR 60-30 ml/min/1.73 m^2); they progress with the increasing severity of renal failure (GFR 29-15 ml/min/1.73 m^2, CKD IV-V). Disorders of calcium and phosphorus balance associated with CKD result in bone diseases, generally called renal osteodystrophy. At the same time numerous cohort studies have broadened the focus of CKD-related mineral and bone disorders to include cardiovascular disease (which is the leading cause of death in patients at all stages of CKD). All three of these processes (abnormal mineral metabolism, abnormal bone and extra skeletal calcification) are closely interrelated and together make a major contribution to the morbidity and mortality of patients with CKD.

Since the publication of the 2003 K/DOQI guidelines for bone and mineral metabolism, there has been tremendous advancement in our understanding of mineral metabolism in CKD patients. Major modifications of K/DOQI bone guidelines are essential and should

reflect our improved understanding of calcium and phosphorus metabolism. At the same time there is a desperate need for randomized trials for better informed decision making and further optimization of care of CKD patients.
The aim of the review is to provide a literature summary concerning the diagnosis and treatment of mineral metabolism disorders in CKD, which will serve an action plan for clinicians.

2. Methods

Literature searches were made of 10 major databases, among which were: Medline, Pubmed, Embase, Cochrane Library and CINAHL. The search was carried out to capture all articles relevant to the topic of CKD and mineral metabolism, bone disorders, and vascular/valvular calcification/. This search encompassed original articles, systematic reviews and meta-analyses.

2.1 Agreed criteria for article inclusion have been

- Articles should be full-text. Brief publications and abstracts were not included.
- Research should be at least 10 patients in each group. The minimum mean duration of study was 6 months.
- Analyzed literature over 15 years.
- The article is detailed research protocol for assessing of its quality
- Patient examination and treatment protocol must meet K / DOQI guidelines protocol and KDIGO Clinical Practice for the Diagnosis, Evaluation, Prevention, and Treatment of Chronic Kidney Disease-Mineral and Bone Disorder (CKD-MBD) ---First of all articles included a high level of evidence:

- Randomized controlled trials
- Prospective nonrandomized without matching controlled trials
- Retrospective nonrandomized without matching controlled trials

Today, these are standard principles in dealing with the introduction into clinical practice of new diagnosis and treatment methods.

3. Pathogenesis of calcium and phosphorus turnover disorders in patients with CKD stages III-IV

3.1 Hyperphosphatemia

The serum level of phosphorus is based on the ratio of phosphorus absorption in gastro-intestinal tract, mobilization rate in bones (bones serve as calcium and phosphorus reservoirs) and renal excretion. Dietary consumption of phosphorus is about 1000-1200 mg; about 800 mg of this amount is being absorbed in intestines (phosphorus turnover pool). The turnover pool is subdivided into cell cytoplasm compartment (70%), bone compartment (29%) and serum (less than 1%). Phosphorus balance is maintained by kidneys. Usually, kidneys filter about 9 g of phosphorus; about 8 g (90%) are reabsorbed in proximal tubules. Reabsorption is mediated by three transporters: Na^+/Pi- co-transporters types I, II and III [Ermolenko, 2009; Lederer, 2011]. Transporters types I and II are located on the apical membranes of canalicular epithelium cells, while transporter type III is located on their basal membrane. Phosphorus reabsorption is associated with Na+ transport and depends on the number of Na^+/Pi- co-transporter molecules on the cell's membrane [Farrow E, 2010; Lederer, 2011; Quarles,2008].

High level of extracellular phosphorus is associated with suppression of $1\alpha OHD_3$-hydroxylase (enzyme mediating conversion of $25(OH)D_3$ to $1,25(OH)_2D_3$); low level of phosphorus results in opposite effect. The effect of extracellular phosphorus on enzyme's activity is independent of PTH or Na^+/Pi co-transporter. CKD can also result in hypophosphatemia associated with malabsorption, excessive use of phosphate-binding drugs, hyperventilation, vitamin D deficiency or long term glucocorticoid treatment. Chronic phosphate deficiency results in increased renal reabsorption mediated by formation of new Na^+/Pi co-transporter. It is associated with simultaneous $1,25(OH)_2D_3$ hyperproduction and increased plasma Ca2+ level . Increased intestinal absorption of Ca2+ and renal reabsorption result in suppression of PTH secretion and enhanced renal reabsorption of phosphorus. Therefore, the factors regulating phosphorus and calcium metabolism are interlinked. Calcitriol increases the phosphorus absorption through enhancement of its uptake by vesicles of enterocytes brush border [Hruska, 2008; Lederer, 2011]. Persistent hyperphosphatemia is found when GFR falls below 60 ml/min/1.73 m^2. Severe renal dysfunction (GFR under 30 ml/min/1.73 m^2) is associated with permanent hyperphosphatemia. CKD-associated phosphorus retention mediates hypocalcemia both through direct effect of hyperphosphatemia on plasma level of calcium, and indirectly - through an effect on parathyroid glands. The results of experiments demonstrate that hyperphosphatemia can stimulate secondary hyperparathyroidism; the process is unrelated to hypocalcemia and/or vitamin D3 deficiency. Therefore, in patients with CKD the plasma phosphorus level should be 2.7-4.6 mg/dl (0.87 - 1.49 mmol/l); and 3.5-5.5 mg/dl (1.13 - 1.78) in patients with CKD V [Fucumoto , 2008; Gutierrez , 2005; Hruska, 2008; Lederer, 2011; National kidney Foundation. K/DOQI Clinical Practice Guidelines for Bone Metabolism and Disease in Chronic Kidney Disease., 2003; KDIGO,2009].

3.2 Hypocalcemia

Dietary consumption of calcium in adults is 1.0 - 1.5 g/day. Most of this amount is absorbed in duodenum and proximal part of small intestine. Calcium absorption rate depends on its content in food and bone mineralization rate. Administration of calcium-based drugs with meals is associated with better absorption rate [Ermolenko, 2009; Fucumoto, 2008; National kidney Foundation. K/DOQI Clinical Practice Guidelines for Bone Metabolism and Disease in Chronic Kidney Disease, 2003; KDIGO, 2009]. Renal filtration rate is about 5-7 g/day; about 95-97.5% of calcium is reabsorbed in renal tubules. Bone tissue is the main calcium reservoir, containing up to 98% of total body calcium. In serum, about one-half of calcium is represented by free ions, while the rest of calcium is bound to plasma proteins (mainly with albumin) or to other cations. Plasma level of calcium ions regulates all its biological effects. CKD IV-V is associated with gastro-intestinal absorption disorders resulting in low calcium absorption that results in low plasma level of total calcium or calcium ions [Ermolenko, 2009; Fucumoto , 2008]. Meat and dairy products are the main sources of dietary calcium. Dietary calcium is protein-bound. Calcium is released in GIT by proteases. The Ca2+ absorption rate in duodenum depends on the level of calcium-binding protein - calbindin - in cytoplasm of the enterocytes. Active transport of Ca2+ ions is regulated by calcitriol that interacts with intra-cellular receptors, which controls the transcription of over 60 genes. These genes encode calbindin and Ca2+ pump proteins [Foley ,1998; Parfey ,2000; KDIGO,2009]. The factors influencing intestinal absorption of calcium are listed in Table 1.

Increase	Decrease
Vitamin D	Age
Low calcium uptake	High calcium uptake
High sodium uptake	Low sodium uptake
Phosphate deficiency	Glucocorticosteroids
Growth hormone	Phosphate loading
Estrogens	Thyroid hormones
Pregnancy, lactation	Metabolic acidosis
Furosemide	Thiazide diuretics

Table 1. Factors influencing intestinal absorption of calcium

In healthy patients Ca2+ excretion rate is 40-300 mg/day [Ermolenko, 2009; K/DOQI Clinical Practice Guidelines for Bone Metabolism and Disease in Chronic Kidney Disease, 2003; Quarles, 2008]. Hypophosphatemia results in decrease in plasma calcium ions level , both through direct binding and decreased renal production of $1,25(OH)_2D_3$. Calcium is the main regulator of PTH secretion. Even short-term hypocalcemia results in increased PTH secretion due to activation of Ca-receptors located on the surface of parathyroid gland. Persistent hypocalcemia results in increased level of PTH matrix RNA and pre-pro-PTH gene transcription that is associated with PTH hyperproduction and secondary hyperparathyroidism. The latter results in PTH hyper-production and hyper-secretion. In hypocalcemia PTH stimulates the production of $1,25(OH)_2D_3$ in kidneys that is associated with increased calcium absorption in gastro-intestinal tract [Fucumoto , 2008; Gutierrez, 2005]. In CKD IV-V the relationship of calcium level and PTH secretion is disordered, therefore, higher level of calcium ions is required to suppress the PTH production. Therefore, it is preferable to maintain the serum level of calcium ions within the ULN [Ermolenko, 2009 ; National kidney Foundation. K/DOQI Clinical Practice Guidelines for Bone Metabolism and Disease in Chronic Kidney Disease, 2003; KDIGO,2009, Patel,2009]. The calcium level in dialysis fluid for patients receiving haemo- and peritoneal dialysis should be 2.5 mEq/l (1.25 mmol/l). In patients with CKD IV-V the adenylate-cyclase of parathyroid glands is less sensitive to calcium inhibitory effect. Glucocorticoids suppress calcium absorption by inhibiting the transformation of $25OHD_3$ to $1,25(OH)_2D_3$; phosphates provide the same effect by forming insoluble complexes and oxalates [National kidney Foundation. K/DOQI Clinical Practice Guidelines for Bone Metabolism and Disease in Chronic Kidney Disease, 2003; KDIGO,2009].

3.3 PTH and calcitonin hyperproduction

3.3.1 PTH molecule (structure and effects)

PTH molecule contains 84 amino acid derivates (1-84) and contains short N-terminal fragment (PTH 1-34) and long C-terminal fragment (PTH 7-84). The molecular weight of PTH is 9425 Da. The gene mediating PTH synthesis is located on 11-th chromosome. Both whole PTH molecule and its N-terminal fragment possess biological effects [Block, 1998; Kestenbaum ,2005, Lederer, 2011].

PTH regulates the plasma level of Ca2+. Elevated Ca2+ plasma level suppresses the PTH synthesis [Block ,1998; Kestenbaum ,2005; Marchais,1999; Slinin, 2005]. This feedback enables the constant plasma level of Ca2+. PTH maintains constant Ca2+ plasma level through the following mechanisms:

- Stimulation of bone tissue resorption resulting in calcium passage to blood.
- Stimulation of renal reabsorption of calcium, resulting in lower excretion in urine.
- Increase of calcium absorption in small intestine (mediated by $1,25(OH)_2D_3$ synthesis stimulation).

Calcium level is regulated mainly by PTH-mediated effect on bone tissue; to a lesser extent it is regulated by effect on renal excretion of calcium. Long-term maintenance of calcium balance is mediated mainly by the PTH effect on $1,25(OH)_2D_3$ synthesis and, therefore, on the rate of calcium absorption in gastro-intestinal tract. The daily level of blood and bone tissue calcium turnover is about 500 mg. PTH is the main regulator of this turnover [Block ,2007; Quarles,2008].

PTH provides several direct and indirect effects on bone tissue. Persistent PTH level elevation results in bone tissue cells increase (primarily - of the osteoclasts) and intensive bone remodeling. The rate of PTH secretion by parathyroid glands depends on plasma level of Ca2+. Magnesium provides similar but less pronounced effect on PTH secretion. In fact, the physiological changes of magnesium level do not impact the PTH secretion; however, pronounced decrease of intra-cellular magnesium level results in increased PTH secretion [Block ,2007; Craver,2007; Lederer, 2011].

The effect of Ca2+ on PTH secretion is mediated through its interaction with Ca receptors (CaR) that are bound to G-proteins and have a large extracellular domain for binding to low-molecular weight ligands. Activation of receptors associated with high Ca2+ plasma level suppresses the PTH secretion. This inhibitory effect is mediated by secondary facilitators - inositol 1,4,5-triphosphate (IF3) and 1,2-diacylglycerine. CaR are found in parathyroid glands cells, in C-cells of the thyroid gland that secrete calcitonin, and also in brain and kidney cells. C-terminal fragments provide the anabolic effect on bone tissue [Ermolenko, 2009; Ketteler, 2011]. Normally, PTH and its fragments are excreted by kidneys and metabolized in cells of terminal tubules. Parathyroid gland produces both the complete PTH molecules, and their fragments. Complete molecules are subject to faster plasma elimination compared to C-terminal fragments. GFR decrease and metabolism disorders associated with CKD result in accumulation of C-terminal fragments in plasma. Intact PTH and its fragments can't be determined by I generation PTH tests; their results reflect the levels of inactive fragments. Recently, immuno-radiometry with double kit of antibodies to N-terminal and C-terminal epitopes has been introduced to measure the iPTH level. CKD IV-V is associated with iPTH level increase mostly due to hyper-secretion. iPTH hyper-secretion is promoted by Pi level elevation and decrease of serum Ca2+ level in extracellular fluid. iPTH interacts with membrane adenylatecyclase-bound receptor in proximal and distal renal tubules and causes phosphaturia, hypophosphatemia and enhances calcium reabsorption in distal renal tubules [Kestenbaum, 2005; Marchais, 1999; Lederer, 2011; Slinin, 2005]. Simultaneously, iPTH stimulates $1,25(OH)_2D_3$ synthesis in renal parenchyma. The decrease of bone tissue sensitivity to iPTH-mediated calcemia is found at initial GFR decrease (<85 ml/min/1.73 m^2). It does not regress during treatment. The same effect is found in many recipients of kidney grafts with decreased function (GFR under 70 ml/min/1.73 m^2) or in patients with acute renal failure. Acute renal failure is usually associated with hypocalcemia. It manifests during the oliguric stage and is present throughout the polyuric stage. Hypocalcemia regresses after the renal function normalization. Skeletal resistance to iPTH calcemic effect is associated with vitamin D3 deficiency and down-regulation of iPTH receptors. PTH effects osteogenesis through activation of osteoblasts while bone resorption is mediated through activation of osteoclasts.

However, osteoclasts have no PTH receptors, therefore, their stimulation is mediated by release of cytokines by osteoblasts. In experiments, the stimulation of osteoclast-mediated bone resorption by PTH was found in cell cultures containing both osteoclasts and osteoblasts [Block, 2007; Lederer, 2011; Marchais, 1999]. Cytokines IGF-1, IL-6, G-CSF mediate proliferation and differentiation of osteoclasts progenitor cells. Large multi-nuclear osteoclasts are formed. They start secreting organic acids and hydrolytic enzymes that dissolve the mineral matrix and organic substance of bone tissue. This process results in release of phosphorus, calcium and bicarbonate to extra-cellular fluid. Osteoblasts produce organic components (mostly – type I collagen); however, iPTH-mediated activation of resorption processes is more pronounced compared to activation of bone synthesis. As hypocalcemia develops, PTH removes calcium from bone tissue in order to maintain its constant level in extra-cellular fluid. Even mild elevation of iPTH level results in activation of mature osteoclasts and bone tissue resorption [Block , 1998; Kestenbaum ,2005; Lederer, 2011; Marchais,1999; Slinin, 2005].

3.3.2 Calcitonin

Calcitonin is secreted by the inter-follicular cells of thyroid gland. In 30% patients with terminal CKD elevated plasma level of calcitonin is found. Calcitonin provides phosphaturic effect by inhibiting the phosphates reabsorption in proximal convoluted tubules and enhances the activity of 1α-hydroxylase by stimulating the production of $1,25(OH)_2D_3$. Calcitonin decreases the Ca2+ serum and extra-cellular fluid levels, reduces the number of osteoclasts and suppresses their activity, and inhibits the process of osteolysis [Ermolenko, 2009; Lederer, 2011].

3.4 Vitamin D3 deficiency

Calcitriol (1,25-dihydroxycholecalciferol) is formed from vitamin D3 (cholecalciferol) as a result of hydroxylation (addition of the OH group) to position 25 (in liver) or to position 1 (in proximal convoluted tubules of kidneys); the hydroxylation process is mediated by α1-hydroxylase. In kidneys calcitriol induces Ca2+ and Pi reabsorption. In small intestine calcitriol enhances the production of calcium-binding protein that enhances Ca2+ absorption. In bone tissue calcitriol stimulates pre-osteoclasts proliferation and differentiation. Calcitriol induces the synthesis of organic bone matrix and regulates the process of bone tissue mineralization [Craver , 2007; Liu ,2006;Quarles,2008]. In patients with CKD III relative deficiency of $1,25(OH)_2D_3$ is found. When the GFR falls below 50 ml/min/1.73 m^2 (in children) or 30 ml/min/1.73 m^2 (in adults) relative deficiency is followed by absolute calcitriol deficiency [Craver , 2007; Liu ,2006; Zemchencov , 2009]. CKD progression is associated with the decrease of vitamin D receptors (VDR) and Ca-receptors of parathyroid gland that is associated with decreased sensitivity to effects of $1,25(OH)_2D_3$ and Ca2+. Patients with CKD IV-V have low $1,25(OH)_2D_3$ plasma level, associated with renal hydroxylation process disorders. Such patients develop $1,25(OH)_2D_3$ deficiency and are resistant to its effect. In patients with removed kidneys and patients receiving dialysis usually the plasma level of $1,25(OH)_2D_3$ can't be detected by standard analyses. Low plasma level of 25-hydroxy vitamin D [$25(OH)D_3$] is found in CKD patients with nephrotic proteinuria due to $25(OH)D_3$ losses with urine, in patients receiving peritoneal dialysis – due to PTH diffusion into peritoneal solution and in patients with low dietary uptake of vitamin D. Limited dietary uptake of phosphorus associated with decreased GFR in CKD patients results in elevated plasma $1,25(OH)_2D_3$ level and enhanced response of target organs to calcitriol effect. Calcitriol inhibits the activity of PTH through direct effect on PTH gene. It inhibits gene transcription and PTH synthesis and stimulates the sensitivity of calcium receptors in parathyroid cells. The results of experiments prove that calcitriol deficiency can initiate secondary hyperparathyroidism even without hypocalcemia. Calcitriol deficiency results in calcium intestinal absorption disorders and suppression of calcemia effect on iPTH. Hypocalcemia results in hyperparathyroidism [Ketteler,2011; Lederer, 2011; Liu ,2006; Zemchencov , 2009].

3.5 CKD-associated ectopic mineralization

Several authors consider CKD-associated hyperphosphatemia to be a special syndrome associated with specific bone remodeling, heterotopic mineralization and cardiovascular complications [Ermolenko, 2009; Hruska, 2008; National kidney Foundation. K/DOQI Clinical Practice Guidelines for Bone Metabolism and Disease in Chronic Kidney Disease, 2003, KDIGO,2009; Zemchencov, 2009].

In patients with CKD and hyperphosphatemia the rate of arterial hypertension and mean blood pressure levels are significantly higher compared to patients with normal plasma level of phosphorus. These conditions are associated with vascular adaptation system disorders; therefore, high blood pressure can result in significant mechanical loading and loss of arterial wall elasticity [London, 2000; Parfey, 2000]. Direct statistically significant correlation between high Ca × P index (over 70 mg^2/dl^2) and the rate of hypertrophic cardiomyopathy [Block ,1998; Kestenbaum ,2005; Marchais,1999; Slinin, 2005] has been demonstrated. Hypertrophic cardiomyopathy along with myocardial ischemia are the main reasons of congestive heart failure in patients with CKD. Moreover, high phosphorus levels promote non-atherosclerotic arterial calcification associated with vascular smooth muscles cells (VSMC) transformation into osteogenous phenotype [Lederer, 2011; Shanahan C, 1994].

CKD-associated hyperphosphatemia development is also associated with bone tissue remodeling. CKD patients have a broad spectrum of bone remodeling; however they have similar features - excessive bone tissue resorption compared to formation. The experimental data prove that hyperphosphatemia is associated with block of phosphate reservoir function of bone tissue [National kidney Foundation; K/DOQI Clinical Practice Guidelines for Bone Metabolism and Disease in Chronic Kidney Disease, 2003; Shanahan C,1994; Volgina, 2004]. However, the requirement of phosphorus in bone tissue increases. It results in phosphorus plasma level elevation. Soft tissues and blood vessels become new phosphorus reservoirs. Formation of phosphorus reservoirs in the walls of arteries result in their higher rigidity [Lederer, 2011; London,2000, National kidney Foundation. K/DOQI Clinical Practice Guidelines for Bone Metabolism and Disease in Chronic Kidney Disease, 2003; KDIGO,2009; Parfrey,2000; Zemchencov, 2009].

Recent studies have demonstrated that CKD patients with hyperphosphatemia (>6.5 mg/dl) have a higher risk of cardiovascular mortality compared to patients with lower phosphorus levels (<6.5 mg/dl). Therefore, maintenance of serum phosphorus level within <6.5 mg/dl limit seems to be an important therapeutic objective in these patients [Davies , 2003, 2005; National kidney Foundation. K/DOQI Clinical Practice Guidelines for Bone Metabolism and Disease in Chronic Kidney Disease, 2003; KDIGO,2009; Pletcher,2004; Wang,2006].

Two types of vascular calcification are typical for CKD: calcification of atherosclerotic neo-intimal plaques (intima calcification) and arterial tunica media calcification (media calcification) [London, 2000; Wang, 2006]. Both types of vascular calcification progress along with advancing CKD. Coronary arteries intimal calcification is the risk factor for of myocardial infarction [London, 2000; National kidney Foundation. K/DOQI Clinical Practice Guidelines for Bone Metabolism and Disease in Chronic Kidney Disease, 2003; KDIGO, 2009]. In CKD patients the calcification of media is characterized by extensive diffuse lesions (atherosclerosis of Moenkenberg). It results in coronary damage with acute coronary syndrome development, ectopic calcification of large arteries with pulse wave speed increase. It is manifested by increased systolic and pulse pressure and rapid left ventricle hypertrophy [Davies, 2005; London, 2000; Pletcher, 2004; Townsend, 2011; Wang, 2006]. Heart calcification is manifested mostly by coronary arteries and heart valves calcinosis. They result in mitral valve failure or stenosis, arrhythmias, congestive heart failure; however, diffuse myocardial calcification can develop [London, 2000; National kidney Foundation. K/DOQI Clinical Practice Guidelines for Bone Metabolism and Disease in Chronic Kidney Disease, 2003; KDIGO,2009].

Blood vessels calcification risk factors:

- Increased plasma levels of calcium and phosphorus
- $Ca^{2+} \times P^{5+}$ over 55 mg^2/dl^2 (5,5 $mmol^2/l^2$)
- Elevated plasma level of iPTH
- Fetuin A protein deficiency

Blood vessels calcification compromises the formation of arterio-venous fistula and complicates kidney transplantation.

Arteries of forearm, wrists, hands, lower extremities, abdominal cavity, thoracic cavity, pelvis and brain can undergo calcification [Ermolenko, 2009; National kidney Foundation. K/DOQI Clinical Practice Guidelines for Bone Metabolism and Disease in Chronic Kidney Disease, 2003, Zemchencov, 2009].

Some patients develop severe vascular calcification so that the arteries can't be pressed by the cuff during blood pressure measurement [London, 2000; National kidney Foundation. K/DOQI Clinical Practice Guidelines for Bone Metabolism and Disease in Chronic Kidney Disease, 2003; Townsend, 2011].

Electronic beam tomography is used to evaluate the calcium content in blood vessel walls [Davies ,2005; National kidney Foundation. K/DOQI Clinical Practice Guidelines for Bone Metabolism and Disease in Chronic Kidney Disease, 2003; KDIGO,2009; Wang, 2006].

The mechanisms of CKD-associated extra-osseous calcification are complicated and multi-factorial. It has been demonstrated that VSMC and other vascular cells (pericytes, fibroblasts) can transform into osteoblast-like cells that produce hydroxy-apatite - the main mineral of bone tissue. In case of hyperphosphatemia smooth muscles of blood vessels accumulate phosphorus, express the genes of bone proteins and turn into areas of calcification [Nishimura , 2011; Shanahan,1994; Wang, 2006].

Parathyroid gland hypertrophy in CKD patients contributes to severity of cardiovascular complications. It participates in development of myocardial fibrosis. iPTH elevates Ca2+ loading in cells and enhances the atherosclerotic changes. It also activates fibroblasts and provides direct impact on myocardium through myocardial cells metabolism disorders [Nishimura , 2011; Wang, 2006].

Myocardial fibrosis, coronary calcification and valves calcification promote the development and progression of systolic dysfunction and congestive heart failure. Left ventricle hypertrophy and increased Ca2+ level in myocardial cells result in diastolic dysfunction. These disorders are the main cause of cardiovascular mortality in CKD patients [London, 2000; Lederer, 2011; Nishimura , 2011; Pletcher,2004; Wang, 2006].

Hypoxia-induced 1-α factor (HIF1-α) and vascular endothelium growth factor are the main mediator of osteogenesis - angiogenesis interaction. It is considered that these factors induce vascular calcification through angiogenous signaling [Wang, 2006].
The initial stage of arterial media calcification is associated with elastin degradation. Matrix metalloproteinases (MMp-2 and MMP-9) destroy elastin with formation of soluble elastin peptides. The latter bind to laminin-elastin receptors (ELR) on the surface of smooth muscles cells. Excessive expression of growth factor β (TGF-β) contributes to elastin destruction also. It is known that it enhances VSMC calcification rate and plays an important role in proliferation of osteoblasts. VSMC osteogenous transformation is activated by consecutive signaling of ELR, TGF-β, and mitogen-activated proteinkinase. Calcification of media is associated with expression of several proteins related to osteogenesis: osteocalcin, osteopontin, matrix γ-GLA (carboxyglutamic acid) protein and osteoprotegrin [Isakova, 2008; KDIGO,2009; Wang, 2006; Zemchencov, 2009].

3.5.1 Relationship between osteogenesis and ectopic mineralization

The relationships between osteogenesis and blood vessels calcification has been established. New factors produced by kidneys and bone tissues have been identified recently. The morphogenetic proteins (FGF-23 and Klotho) regulate homeostasis of phosphates, vitamin D and bone tissue mineralization. The level FGF-23 (fibroblasts growth factor 23, produced mostly by osteocytes) is increased even at the pre-dialysis stage of CKD [Gutiérrez, 2009; Jean, 2009; Pande , 2006; Razzaque 2008, 2009; Zemchencov, 2009].
The role of circulating FGF-23 level increase at various CKD stages is being studied. It has been established that enhanced production of FGF-23 during CKD stages II-III contributes to adaptive increase of phosphorus excretion and decrease of calcitriol production [Boekel ,2008; Carpenter ,2005; Fang ,2001; Gutierrez ,2005, 2008; Kawata ,2007].
Later, when the CKD IV-V results in GFR decrease, the elevated FGF-23 level is not enough to prevent hyperphosphatemia and hyperparathyroidism. Prospective studies [Gutiérrez, 2009; Jean, 2009; Pande, 2006; Razzaque, 2009] demonstrate that elevated FGF-23 level in CKD patients at the stage of dialysis initiation is associated with mortality and vascular calcification independent of other risk factors or serum phosphorus and iPTH levels. Therefore, FGF-23 is the potential independent uremic toxin (Table 2).
There are 2 types of Klotho protein - trans-membraneous and extra-cellular (secreted). It is produced and secreted by the cells of proximal renal tubules; the trans-membraneous protein is also produced by the parathyroid gland cells [Makoto ,2009; Sitara,2006].
Makoto K demonstrated that trans-membraneous Klotho protein is a co-receptor of FGF-23 and therefore contributes to regulation of phosphorus, calcium and vitamin D turnover. Extra-cellular part of Klotho protein that is secreted to systemic circulation acts as an endocrine factor and encodes multiple growth factors, including insulin-like growth factor 1 and Wnt [Makoto, 2009].
In CKD patients the expression rate of Klotho protein is decreased; therefore, it is considered to be the factor of renal protection. It is obvious that phosphorus turnover regulation is an important link of CKD pathogenesis. Early correction of hyperphosphatemia by influencing the endocrine interactions of the bones-kidneys-parathyroid glands axis mediated by Klotho and FGF-23 improves the quality of life in CKD patients [Boekel ,2008; Carpenter ,2005; Fang ,2001; Gutiérrez, 2005, 2008, 2009; Jean,2009; Kawata ,2007; Pande , 2006; Razzaque 2008, 2009].
In CKD patients the FGF-23 serum level elevation precedes hyperphosphatemia; therefore, resistance to FGF-23 can be one of the early signs of CKD-related metabolic disorders. It is

considered that development of resistance to FGF-23 is associated with decreased renal expression of Klotho protein. Therefore, low rate of renal expression of Klotho protein can be a prediction of poor long-term outcome in dialysis patients [Makoto , 2009].

Authors	Study results
Razzaque M.S. [NDT 20094 24(1): 4-7]	Meta-analysis (10 studies). Most CKD patients demonstrated FGF-23 elevation prior to phosphorus level increase. In dialysis patients low level of trans-membraneous Klotho expression in renal cells was associated with poor cardiovascular prognosis
Gutierrez O.M. Nev Engl J Med 2008; 359(6): 584 - 592	10 044 CKD patients, stage V. FGF-23 plasma level increase at initial stage of dialysis was associated with a dose-related 1-year lethality increase. Lethality hazard ratio (OR = 5.7) was higher compared to hazard ratio for high phosphorus levels (OR = 1.2).
Jean G et al NDT 2009; 24(9); 2618-2620	219 CKD stage V patients. FGF-23 level elevation (median 2740 RU/ml) at initial stages of dialysis was associated with cardiovascular lethality not related to risk factors and plasma phosphorus levels
Gutierrez O.M. Circulation. 2009; 119(19): 2545-2552	162 CKD stage III-IV. Multivariate regressive analysis demonstrated correlation of serum FGF-23 elevation and left ventricle infarction (11% annual increase) or risk of coronaries calcification (2.4 fold increase)

Table 2. Relationship between elevated FGF-23 plasma level and poor CKD prognosis (results of prospective studies)

FGF-23 level decreases along with the decline of hyperphosphatemia; therefore, low phosphate diet and phosphate binders seems to be an appropriate treatment strategy beginning from early CKD stages. These measures prevent the cardiovascular complications and secondary hyperparathyroidism in CKD patients. CKD patients demonstrate fasting FGF-23 level elevation, even without hyperphosphatemia and hypocalcemia. It is not clear yet, which CKD stage is associated with initial FGF-23 serum level increase; however, it is considered that FGF-23 hyper-production precedes plasma phosphorus and iPTH levels increase [Gutiérrez,2009; Pande , 2006; Razzaque 2008, 2009].

In most clinical studies plasma phosphorus, calcium, FGF-23 and iPTH levels were measured in fasting conditions. However, at early CKD stages without hyperphosphatemia and hypocalcemia plasma FGF-23 and iPTH levels are increased after meals. Urine excretion rate of phosphorus increase after meals was found in 13 CKD patients with normal fasting phosphorus and calcium levels and in 21 healthy volunteers despite normal plasma levels of phosphorus and FGF-23. Increased postprandial urine excretion of calcium was found in both groups; in CKD patients it was associated with significant calcium level decrease and elevation of iPTH plasma level. Therefore, FGF-23 does not impact the postprandial phosphaturia both in healthy volunteers and in CKD patients; however, CKD patients developed postprandial transient calcuria associated with relative hypocalcemia. This effect might reflect early stages of secondary hyperparathyroidism development [Craver ,2007; Razzaque ,2008].

Recent studies demonstrate poor value of fasting iPTH evaluation in early diagnosing of secondary hyperparathyroidism; while assessment of FGF-23 plasma level (both fasting and postprandial) might be used as a sensitive screening test for secondary hyperparathyroidism development [Pande ,2006; Razzaque ,2009].

FGF-23 Elisa kit is used to evaluate FGF-23 serum level. Anti-Klotho polyclonal antibodies are used to evaluate Klotho levels in serum, spinal fluid, and urine. FGF-23/Klotho ratio in proximal renal tubules is assessed by immune-histochemical analysis [Gutiérrez,2009; Razzaque ,2009].

Therefore, in CKD patients phosphorus and calcium turnover disorders with hyperphosphatemia, vascular calcification, left ventricle hypertrophy are also mediated by newly discovered regulation mechanisms - Klotho and FGF-23. These effects are important risk factors of cardiovascular complications that are the cause of significant lethality rate in such patients.

3.5.2 Ectopic mineralization inhibitors

Calcification inhibitors deficiency is an important factor of arterial calcification development.

Matrix γ-Carboxyglutamic Acid Protein – MGP is a protein produced in bone tissue. It blocks the osteo-chondrocytous trans-differentiation of vascular smooth muscles cells into osteoblast-like cells. MGP also prevents the formation of crystallization areas in vascular tunica media and atherosclerotic plaques. It regulates the synthesis of skeletal matrix [Craver, 2007; London, 2000; National kidney Foundation. K/DOQI Clinical Practice Guidelines for Bone Metabolism and Disease in Chronic Kidney Disease, 2003; Zemchencov,2009].

Osteopontin – acidic protein that is being expressed in arterial calcification areas. It activates osteoblasts and inhibits hydroxyl-apatite formation. Osteopontin enters the crystallization loci and inhibits their formation [National kidney Foundation. K/DOQI Clinical Practice Guidelines for Bone Metabolism and Disease in Chronic Kidney Disease, 2003; Zemchencov,2009].

Osteoprotegrin – is expressed in atherosclerotic plaques and tunica media calcification loci. Osteoprotegrin inhibits the process of osteoclasts differentiation and the activity of bone alkaline phosphatase isoenzyme. Therefore, it hampers the process of tunica media and atherosclerotic plaques [Zemchencov,2009].

Protein a_2 Heremans-Schmid (Phetuin) – is a calcium-binding protein mostly produced in liver. Uremia is associated with significant decrease of this protein's level. Experimental studies demonstrated that phetuin A binding results in vascular calcification. It is stored in smooth muscles and prevents their transformation into osteoblast-like cells [Zemchencov,2009].

Pyrophosphates suppress the osteo-chondrogenous trans-differentiation of vascular smooth muscles cells and formation of hydroxyl-apatite crystals. They are synthesized from nucleotide-triphosphates; the synthesis process is mediated by nucleotide-pyrophosphatase. In CKD patients the levels of nucleotide-pyrophosphatase and pyrophosphates carrier in tunica media are decreased. IGF-1 and N3 fatty acids inhibit the differentiation of vascular smooth muscles cells into osteoblast-like cells and tunica media calcification also [Craver ,2007; National kidney Foundation. K/DOQI Clinical Practice Guidelines for Bone Metabolism and Disease in Chronic Kidney Disease, 2003; Zemchencov,2009].

3.5.3 Ectopic mineralization stimulators

Hyper-phosphatemia causes the induction of osteoblastic differentiation factors - Cbfa1/Runx2, osteocalcin and sodium-dependent phosphate co-transporter type III – Pit-1.

Pit-1 expression is stimulated by high levels of extra-cellular calcium. Matrix vesicles and bone matrix proteins are secreted into the peri-vascular space; further they are subject to mineralization [National kidney Foundation. K/DOQI Clinical Practice Guidelines for Bone Metabolism and Disease in Chronic Kidney Disease, 2003; KDIGO,2009; Zemchencov,2009].

3.6 Uremic toxins

Uremic toxins cause the expression of Cbfa1/Runx2, osteopontin, bone AP isoenzyme and osteoprotegrin independently of phosphorus levels. They enhance the secretion of bone morphogenesis protein (BMP-2) by vascular smooth muscles cells and stimulate their mineralization. As renal failure progresses, new factors are added to arterial calcification process [National kidney Foundation. K/DOQI Clinical Practice Guidelines for Bone Metabolism and Disease in Chronic Kidney Disease, 2003; KDIGO,2009; Moe , 2003; Sitara, 2003].

3.7 Oxidation stress and inflammation

Uremic intoxication is associated with oxidation stress and systemic inflammation. The latter one jeopardizes oxidation stress, typical for uremia. Formation of oxidants contributes to high oxidation rate of lipoproteins that enhance the transformation of vascular smooth muscle cells into osteoblast-like ones. VSMC osteoblastic transformation is stimulated by glucocorticosteroids, leptin and hyperglycemia [KDIGO,2009].

3.8 Vitamin D metabolism disorders

Vitamin D has been reported to contribute to regulation of VSMC activity and metabolism. Vascular smooth muscle cells express 1α-hydroxylase to convert $25(OH)D_3$ into $1,25(OH)_2D_3$; they also express vitamin D receptors (VDR). Calcitriol stimulates the VDR expression on smooth muscle cells. VDR is the factor of smooth muscles proliferation and differentiation. Depending on plasma levels, calcitriol can both stimulate and inhibit the proliferation of vascular smooth muscles cells. Calcitriol levels 10^{-7}–10^{-10} M stimulates vascular calcification in a dose-dependent way by increasing the ratio "nuclear factor receptor activator/ osteoprotegrin".

In CKD experimental models calcitriol analogues (paricalcitol and doxercalciferol) caused lesser vascular calcification compared to similar doses of calcitriol. Unlike calcitriol, paricalcitol didn't cause any increase of Cbfa1/Runx2 and osteocalcin expression rate. Doses of calcitriol and its analogues used in doses sufficient for iPTH hyper-production suppression prevented vascular calcification; however, higher doses of the drugs stimulated calcification [Craver ,2007; Finch,2010; National kidney Foundation. K/DOQI Clinical Practice Guidelines for Bone Metabolism and Disease in Chronic Kidney Disease, 2003; Zemchencov, 2009].

Study with 520 CKD patients (median follow-up 21 years) with mean GFR 30 ml/min/1,73 m^2 demonstrated that calcitriol treatment was associated with lethality rate decrease. Similar study demonstrated comparable results [National kidney Foundation. K/DOQI Clinical Practice Guidelines for Bone Metabolism and Disease in Chronic Kidney Disease, 2003].

Therefore, recent studies demonstrated that in CKD patients high doses of calcitriol and its analogues can stimulate vascular calcification, while their moderate doses provide a protective effect through type I collagen and promoter gene core-binding factor-α1 (Cbfa1) production inhibition. Collagen type I is the basis for calcium deposits, while Cbfa1 stimulates the production of type I collagen [Finch,2010; Moe , 2003; Sitara ,2003].

3.9 Clinical manifestations of soft tissues calcification

Metastatic calcification is found in patients with secondary hyperparathyroidism and with adynamic skeletal diseases susceptible to hypercalcemia due to inability of bone tissue to accept surplus calcium. Hyperphosphatemia with elevated $Ca^{2+} \times P^{5+}$ index (>55 mg^2/dl^2 or 4,5-5,5 $mmol^2/l^2$), dialysis-associated alkalosis and local tissue damage promote formation of calcium phosphate deposits in soft tissues [Craver ,2007; National kidney Foundation. K/DOQI Clinical Practice Guidelines for Bone Metabolism and Disease in Chronic Kidney Disease, 2003; KDIGO,2009; Zemchencov,2009].

Soft tissues and vascular calcifications contain hydroxyl-apatite crystals with Ca: Mg: P ratio similar to bone; amorphous micro-crystals of calcium, magnesium and phosphates ($CaMg_3(PO_4)_2$) are found in muscles, heart and lungs. It is considered that the variability of calcification depends on local tissue factors - hydrogen ions, magnesium, calcium and phosphorus levels. Formation of hydroxy-apatite crystals is associated with significant fibrosis; while formation of amorphous crystals doesn't result in fibrosis [Ermolenko, 2009; National kidney Foundation. K/DOQI Clinical Practice Guidelines for Bone Metabolism and Disease in Chronic Kidney Disease, 2003].

Formation of phosphorus and calcium salts deposits in skin results in severe itching that is resolved only after parathyroidectomy [National kidney Foundation. K/DOQI Clinical Practice Guidelines for Bone Metabolism and Disease in Chronic Kidney Disease, 2003, KDIGO,2009; Zemchencov,2009].

Skin calcification. Calcium salts deposits in skin are associated with formation of maculae and vesicles containing solid structures. Calcium salts crystals can be found at biopsy. After subtotal parathyroidectomy skin deposits of calcium salts undergo regression; therefore, secondary hyperparathyroidism is the leading factor of skin calcification [Craver, 2007; Zemchencov, 2009].

Formation of skin ulcers and tissue necrosis (calciphylaxis). This syndrome was described by Seyle in 1962; the author named it calciphylaxia. Recently, most authors prefer the name calcifying uremic arteriopathy. This clinical syndrome is characterized by progressing skin ischemia, affecting fingers of hands and feet, hips and ankles. It develops in patients receiving dialysis on a regular basis for 10 years and more. It is less frequent in patients receiving peritoneal dialysis. The syndrome is characterized by vascular calcification and sub-periosteum bone resorption. Painful erythematous subcutaneous vesicles or blue maculae are followed by ulceration or necrosis. Reynaud's syndrome can precede the affection of fingers of hands and feet. Ulcers develop slowly (for several months) or fast (within several weeks). Concomitant infections can result in fatal sepsis [National kidney Foundation. K/DOQI Clinical Practice Guidelines for Bone Metabolism and Disease in Chronic Kidney Disease, 2003, KDIGO,2009; Zemchencov,2009].

The treatment strategy is not established yet. Local treatment is ineffective; in most patients subtotal parathyroidectomy resulted in calciphylaxia regression, however, in some patients skin lesions persisted or even progressed.

Mineral metabolism disorders with secondary hyperparathyroidism and vascular calcification, local tissue lesions, obesity (especially in white females), vitamin C deficiency predispose to development of this syndrome. Vitamin C deficiency in CKD patients was reported to result in hyper coagulation; therefore vascular occlusions and tissue necrosis occur. However, administration of warfarin results in progression of skin lesions in these patients. Local tissue lesions at insulin, heparin or dextran administration sites are usual locations of ulceration or skin necrosis [Craver ,2007; National kidney Foundation. K/DOQI Clinical Practice Guidelines for Bone Metabolism and Disease in Chronic Kidney Disease, 2003; KDIGO,2009].

Calcification of eyes. Conjunctiva and corneal calcium deposits associated with vascular inflammation result in "red eyes" syndrome. This transient process recurs as new conjunctiva calcium deposits are formed [National kidney Foundation. K/DOQI Clinical Practice Guidelines for Bone Metabolism and Disease in Chronic Kidney Disease, 2003].

Conjunctiva deposits of calcium salts can be symptoms-free. In such cases they are found during ophthalmologic examination. Calcium salts deposits are represented by white plaques or small dot-like deposits on lateral or medial segments of the conjunctiva. They are also found on cornea or lateral/medial segments of eye border (band-like keratopathy). Calcium deposits in eye blood vessels result in local pH increase due to CO2 loss through the conjunctiva surface [Zemchencov,2009].

Visceral calcification. Usually calcium salts deposits are found in lungs, stomach, heart, skeletal muscles and kidneys. Usually calcifications can't be determined by standard X-ray; however, they are found during isotope scanning with ^{99m}Tc – pyrophosphate. Calcifications of lungs and heart can result in severe or fatal complications. Cases of pulmonary calcifications resulting in severe pulmonary fibrosis, pulmonary hypertension and left ventricle hypertrophy have been reported. Heart and lungs calcifications are one of the main causes of morbidity and mortality in dialysis patients [Craver ,2007; National kidney Foundation. K/DOQI Clinical Practice Guidelines for Bone Metabolism and Disease in Chronic Kidney Disease, 2003 , Zemchencov, 2009; Huang Chou-Long, 2010].

High level of dietary vitamin C that is being metabolized into oxalates can result in calcium oxalate deposits formation in soft tissues, heart, mitral and aortal valves, resulting in cardiomyopathy and fatal heart failure [National kidney Foundation. K/DOQI Clinical Practice Guidelines for Bone Metabolism and Disease in Chronic Kidney Disease, 2003;KDIGO,2009].

Peri-articular calcification. Calcium salts deposits formation in peri-articular space results in limited mobility and tendovaginitis. Affected joints contain transparent synovial with normal viscosity and cell counts [Darry ,2008; Masuyama,2006; National kidney Foundation. K/DOQI Clinical Practice Guidelines for Bone Metabolism and Disease in Chronic Kidney Disease, 2003;KDIGO,2009]. This acute condition is called calcifying peri-arthritis. Uric acid salts are also found in the peri-articular tissues (secondary gout). This condition is often associated with chondro-calcinosis. Pseudo-gout is diagnosed when pyro-phosphate crystals are found in synovial cells. The study including 135 dialysis patients demonstrated the increase of peri-articular calcification rate from 9 to 42% from dialysis year 1 to dialysis year 8 [Zemchencov,2009].

Some dialysis patients develop large tumor-like formations in the peri-articular regions. They contain encapsulated lime fluid and soft calcium-based substance. Usually these formations are painless; however, their size can limit the mobility of the joint. Tumor-like calcium deposits can regress if serum phosphorus is adequately controlled by phosphorus binders or after subtotal parathyroidectomy [Craver ,2007; National kidney Foundation. K/DOQI Clinical Practice Guidelines for Bone Metabolism and Disease in Chronic Kidney Disease, 2003; Zemchencov,2009].

4. Prevention and treatment of CKD associated phosphorus and calcium metabolism disorders

4.1 Diet and phosphate binders

Low phosphate diet and/or phosphate binders are considered to be an important therapeutic approach targeted to prevent life-threatening complications in CKD patients. According to K/DOQI Practical Clinical Recommendations, daily phosphorus uptake should be limited to 800-1000 mg (adjusted by requirement in protein) in CKD III-IV patients with serum phosphorus level over 4.6 mg/dl (1.49 mmol/l) and over 5.5 mg/dl (1.78 mmol/l) in dialysis patients or in patients with plasma iPTH level exceeding normal limits established for corresponding CKD stages [Craver ,2007; National kidney Foundation. K/DOQI Clinical Practice Guidelines for Bone Metabolism and Disease in Chronic Kidney Disease, 2003]. If dietary phosphorus limitations are insufficient to control phosphorus and iPTH levels, phosphate binders are recommended [Moore, 2010; Wang, 2006]. Long-term administration of calcium-based phosphate binders can result in hypercalcemia. Calcium carbonate - associated hypercalcemia is found 3.5 fold more frequent compared to calcium acetate associated hypercalcemia because calcium carbonate interacts with phosphorus at pH 5.0, when its dissolution rate is decreased [Ketteler,2011; Zemchencov,2009]. Calcium - based phosphate binders decrease the serum phosphorus level effectively and can be used for initial phosphate-binding treatment. Total daily dose of elementary dietary calcium should be within 1.5 g/day [National kidney Foundation. K/DOQI Clinical Practice Guidelines for Bone Metabolism and Disease in Chronic Kidney Disease, 2003]. Calcium based phosphate binders should not be used in dialysis patients with hypercalcemia (adjusted total serum calcium level over 10.2 mg/dl or 2.54 mmol/l) and in patients with plasma PTH level under 130 pg/ml (14.4 pmol/l) as measured by 2 consequent analyses [Craver, 2007; Moore, 2010;KDIGO,2009]. Calcium-free phosphate binders should be used in these patients. At present, sevelamer hydrochloride (renagel) is widely used in clinical setting for binding of dietary phosphates. Renagel is synthetic calcium- and hydroxyl-aluminum free drug. It is not absorbed in gastro-intestinal tract. The drug decreases plasma levels of iPTH, phosphorus and Ca×P index; it also corrects the dyslipidemia [Craver ,2007;KDIGO,2009]. The drug administration does not result in calciemia, therefore its combinations with active vitamin D analogues are safe. Renagel is effective for control of vascular and soft tissues calcification. Renagel is indicated for to patients with elevated serum phosphorus level and total adjusted calcium level over 5.5 and 10.2 mg/dl, respectively, and iPTH level decrease under 130 pg/ml and metastatic calcification [Craver ,2007; KDIGO,2009]. Long-term Renagel administration can result in decrease of furosemide's diuretic effect and hypochloremic acidosis associated with bicarbonates loss [Craver ,2007; Block ,2010; Reddy ,2009]. Table 3 represents the pattern of sevelamer hydrochloride dosage choice based on serum phosphorus level.

Serum phosphorus level	Sevelamer hydrochloride dosage (800 mg tablets)
6–7,5 mg/dl (1,94–2,42 mmol/l)	1 tablet × 3 times per day
> 7,5 mg/dl (2,42 mmol/l)	2 tablets × 3 times per day

Table 3. Sevelamer hydrochloride dosage choice based on serum phosphorus level

Equivalent doses of sevelamer hydrochloride (calculated in mg/kg) are used for transfer from calcium-based phosphate binders. Sevelamer hydrochloride dosage is 800 tablet per

one meal [National kidney Foundation. K/DOQI Clinical Practice Guidelines for Bone Metabolism and Disease in Chronic Kidney Disease, 2003; KDIGO,2009]. In USA and Europe lactane (Fosrenol) carbonate is used for phosphate binding in gastro-intestinal tract. 500, 750 and 1000 mg Fosrenol tablets are available. Treatment course continues until normal phosphorus level is reached (1.13 - 1.78 mmol/l; 3.5 - 5.5 mg/dl). Maximum daily dosage - 3750 mg (for short-term treatment - 5-7 days). However, lactane is subject to partial absorption and can accumulate in bone tissue [Craver ,2007; Moore, 2010]. At present sevelamer carbonate and Zerenex phosphate binder, containing inorganic iron compounds are being studied. Preliminary data indicate similar efficacy to calcium salts [Craver ,2007; National kidney Foundation. K/DOQI Clinical Practice Guidelines for Bone Metabolism and Disease in Chronic Kidney Disease, 2003; Volgina, 2004].
In patients receiving peritoneal dialysis phosphorus elimination rate can be increased by replacement of cellulose acetate membranes by poly-sulfone membranes or by switching to hemodiafiltration with higher phosphorus clearance compared to dialysis. Enhanced blood flow in the hemodialysis apparatus results in increased creatinine clearance; however, it does not change the phosphorus elimination rate. On the other hand, dialysis prolongation (transfer from 3 times per week regimen to daily dialysis) results in 30% decrease of the pre-dialysis serum phosphorus level and enables reduction of phosphate binders administration frequency [Craver ,2007; National kidney Foundation. K/DOQI Clinical Practice Guidelines for Bone Metabolism and Disease in Chronic Kidney Disease, 2003]. In patients receiving peritoneal dialysis frequent exchange of dialysis solution in peritoneal cavity results in higher creatinine and phosphorus clearance. Total adjusted plasma calcium level should be maintained within normal limits (8.4 - 9.5 mg/dl or 2.1 - 2.37 mmol/l) [1]. In dialysis patients receiving calcium-based phosphate binders and active vitamin D metabolites dose reduction or drug withdrawal is recommended when the total adjusted calcium serum level exceeds 10.2 mg/dl (2.54 mmol/l). Dosages should be suspended until total adjusted serum calcium level returns to normal. If these measures are ineffective, dialysis fluid with low calcium level (1.5 - 2.9 mEq/l) should be used for 3-4 weeks. Phosphorus-calcium ratio should be kept under 55 mg^2/dl^2. This can be achieved through serum phosphorus level maintenance within the target limits [Craver ,2007; National kidney Foundation. K/DOQI Clinical Practice Guidelines for Bone Metabolism and Disease in Chronic Kidney Disease, 2003, Volgina, 2004].
Hyperphosphatemia control enables FGF-23 level decrease in CKD patients. Elevated FGF-23 serum level is associated with higher mortality rate in patients with terminal CKD. The possibility of using neutralizing antibodies for excessive FGF-23 production control is under discussion. However, the clinical benefit of this method is not clear yet [Yamazaki ,2008].
Hypocalcemia treatment should include oral calcium salts - e.g., calcium carbonate and/or vitamin D active metabolites [Craver ,2007; National kidney Foundation. K/DOQI Clinical Practice Guidelines for Bone Metabolism and Disease in Chronic Kidney Disease, 2003].

4.2 Vitamin D active metabolites

When iPTH plasma level exceeds the target limits established for corresponding CKD stage and the $25(OH)D_3$ level is under 30 ng/ml, treatment with vitamin D2 should be initiated. It is considered, that at early CKD stages ergocalciferol is safer compared to calciferol [Craver, 2007; Moore,2010; National kidney Foundation. K/DOQI Clinical Practice Guidelines for Bone Metabolism and Disease in Chronic Kidney Disease, 2003, Volgina, 2004]. Dose adjustment should be based on the rate of $25(OH)D_3$ deficiency. If the $25(OH)D_3$ level is under 15 ng/ml (37 nmol/l), 50 000 IU/week × 4 weeks ergocalciferol dosage regimen should be used; later the 50 000 IU/month × 4 months regimen is used. If 25(OH)D_3 serum level is 20-30 ng/ml (50-75 nmol/l), 50 000 IU × 1 month treatment regimen should be used for 6 months [Craver ,2007; National kidney Foundation. K/DOQI Clinical Practice Guidelines for Bone Metabolism and Disease in Chronic Kidney Disease, 2003; KDIGO,2009]. Treatment with vitamin D is recommended for patients with pre-dialysis stages of CKD with a normal 25(OH)D_3 levels (over 30 ng/ml or 75 nmol/l) and decreased plasma level of as adjusted total calcium, elevated serum iPTH level and normal serum phosphorus level. Active vitamin D metabolites (calcitriol, alpha-caclidol or doxecalciferol) are more effective for iPTH synthesis and secretion suppression [Craver ,2007; National kidney Foundation. K/DOQI Clinical Practice Guidelines for Bone Metabolism and Disease in Chronic Kidney Disease, 2003; KDIGO,2009; Volgina, 2004]. Lower initial dosages are recommended (see Table 4).

iPTH plasma level, pg/ml [pmol/l]	Serum level		Calcitriol or alpha-calcidol, orally	Doxecalciferol, orally
	Ca, mg/dl [mmol/l]	P, mg/dl [mmol/l]		
> 70 [7,7] (CKD III) or > 110 [12,1] (CKD IV)	< 9,5 [2,37]	< 4,6 [1,49]	0,25 mcg/day	2,5 mcg 3 times per week

Table 4. Serum iPTH, adjusted total calcium and phosphorus levels requiring vitamin D active metabolites. Initial doses for patients with CKD stages III - IV

Calcitriol dosage should be within 0.5 mcg/day, except for cases, when the adjusted total calcium level increase is under 0.2-0.3 mg/dl/month. [Craver ,2007; Moore,2010; National kidney Foundation. K/DOQI Clinical Practice Guidelines for Bone Metabolism and Disease in Chronic Kidney Disease, 2003 KDIGO, 2009;]. Treatment with active vitamin D metabolites should be conducted only in patients with adjusted total calcium serum level under 9.5 mg/dl (2.37 mmol/l) and serum phosphorus level under 4,6 mg/dl (1.49 mmol/l) [National kidney Foundation. K/DOQI Clinical Practice Guidelines for Bone Metabolism and Disease in Chronic Kidney Disease, 2003; KDIGO,2009; Zemchencov,2009]. Patients receiving hemodialysis or peritoneal dialysis with serum iPTH level over 300 pg/ml (33.0 pmol/l) should receive active vitamin D metabolites (e.g., calcitriol, alpha-calciferol, paricalcitol, doxecalciferol, see Table 5) in order to decrease serum iPTH level up to target level 130–300 pg/ml (14,4–33,0 pmol/l) [Craver ,2007; National kidney Foundation. K/DOQI Clinical Practice Guidelines for Bone Metabolism and Disease in Chronic Kidney Disease, 2003, KDIGO,2009; Volgina, 2004].

In patients receiving peritoneal dialysis oral calcitriol or doxecalciferol dosages are 0.5-1.0 and 2.5-5.0 mcg 2-3 times per week, respectively [Craver ,2007; National kidney Foundation. K/DOQI Clinical Practice Guidelines for Bone Metabolism and Disease in Chronic Kidney Disease, 2003;KDIGO,2009]. Alternative regimen of oral calcitriol is 0.25 mcg daily [National kidney Foundation. K/DOQI Clinical Practice Guidelines for Bone Metabolism and Disease in Chronic Kidney Disease, 2003; KDIGO,2009]. During the initial stage of active vitamin D metabolites or during the dosage increase period serum phosphorus and calcium levels should be monitored each 2 weeks throughout the first month; monthly monitoring is recommended later [Craver ,2007; National kidney Foundation. K/DOQI Clinical Practice Guidelines for Bone Metabolism and Disease in Chronic Kidney Disease, 2003;KDIGO,2009].

iPTH, pg/ml [pmol/l]	Ca, mg/dl [mmol/l]	P, mg/dl [mmol/l]	Ca-P	Calcitriol	Paricalcitol	Doxecalciferol
300–600 [33–66]	< 9,5 [2,37]	< 5,5 [1,78]	< 55	0,5–1,5 mcg, i/v 0,5–1,5 mcg orally	2,0–5,0 mcg, i/v	5 mcg, orally 2 mcg, i/v
600–1000 [66–110]	< 9,5 [2,37]	< 5,5 [1,78]	< 55	1,0–3,0 mcg, i/v 1,0–4,0 mcg, orally	6,0–10,0 mcg, i/v	5–10 mcg, orally 2–4 mcg, i/v
> 1000 [110]	<10 [2,5]	< 5,5 [1,78]	< 55	3,0–5,0 mcg, i/v 3,0–7,0 mcg, orally	10,0–15,0 mcg, i/v	10–20 mcg, orally 4–8 mcg, i/v

Table 5. Recommended initial doses of active vitamin D metabolites - based on iPTH, phosphorus and calcium serum levels and CaxP index in patients receiving dialysis

In most patients effective suppression of iPTH secretion results in recovery of parathyroid glands hyperplasia [National kidney Foundation. K/DOQI Clinical Practice Guidelines for Bone Metabolism and Disease in Chronic Kidney Disease, 2003]. High concentrations of $1,25(OH)_2D_3$ stimulate apoptosis of parathyroid gland cells [Craver ,2007; Moore,2010]. This effect is used for "drug parathyroidectomy", when $1,25(OH)_2D_3$ is injected into the hyperplasic parathyroid glands [National kidney Foundation. K/DOQI Clinical Practice Guidelines for Bone Metabolism and Disease in Chronic Kidney Disease, 2003, Volgina, 2004]. Paricalcitol, or $1,25(OH)_2D_2$ is effective for iPTH suppression. Paricalcitol is selective active vitamin D metabolite with modified lateral chain (D2) and A ring (19-nor). Paricalcitol (Zemplar) selectively induces VDR (S-VDRA) gene expression in parathyroid glands, suppresses iPTH secretion without activation of intestinal VDR. The drug has no effect on bone resorption, therefore, it causes hypercalcemia less frequently compared to non-selective active vitamin D metabolites. Unlike calcimimetics, paricalcitol possesses significant pleyotropic effects that provide the decrease of cardiovascular complications risk and inhibit CKD progress (anti-proteinuria effect). The anti-proteinuria effect of paricalcitol has been demonstrated in 3 double blind randomized placebo-controlled studies enrolling 220 patients with CKD III-IV and hyperparathyroidism [Ermolenko, 2009]. By the end of week 24, proteinuria level decrease was demonstrated in 51% of patients receiving paricalcitol and in 25% of patients from placebo group (p 0.004). PTH level 30% decrease was found in 91% of patients receiving paricalcitol compared to 13% of patients in placebo group (p<0,001). Decreased level of intact PTH <110 pg/ml was found in 75% of patients from paricalcitol group and in 12% of patients from placebo group [KDIGO,2009]. Our study that enrolled 50 CKD III-IV patients with systemic diseases (35 patients - lupus erythematous, 15 patients - different types of vasculites) had similar results. Patients were randomized in 2 groups; calcitriol 0.35 mcg/day was used in Group 1, paricalcitol 1 mcg/day - in Group 2. Prior to treatment, proteinuria levels were 1.2 +/- 0.6 g/day in Group 1 and 1.3 +/- 0.4 in Group 2; iPTH levels were 75 +/- 17.4 pg/mal and 80 +/- 16.6 pg/ml, respectively. Calcinosis/atherosclerosis of carotids was found in 27.3% of patients in Group 1 and in 33.3% of patients in Group 2. Calcitriol and paricalcitol were generally well tolerated. As a result, iPTH plasma levels reached normal levels after 3 months of treatment in patients with elevated iPTH levels at baseline. In patients receiving paricalcitol, proteinuria level decrease occurred faster ($p<0.05$) and the arterial hypertension decrease by the end of Month 3 was more pronounced ($p<0.01$) compared to patients receiving calcitriol. In 4 of 12 patients from Group 2 with diagnosed atherosclerosis/calcinosis, no episodes of hypercalcemia or signs of atherosclerosis/calcinosis were reported. Hypercalcemia episodes were reported in 27.3% of patients receiving calcitriol; progressing of atherosclerosis/ calcinosis diagnosed at baseline was reported in 3 patients [Milovanova, 2011].

Paricalcitol is manufactured as 1, 2 and 4 mcg capsules or 1 ml (5 mcg) ampoules. Capsules are indicated for treatment and prophylaxis of secondary hyperparathyroidism associated with CKD III, IV and V; ampoules are indicated to patients with CKD V. In patients receiving peritoneal dialysis, the drug should be administered through slow intravenous injections (minimum duration - 30 seconds) in order to minimize the infusion-associated pains. Recommended initial dose of paricalcitol is 0.04 - 0.1 mcg/kg. Paricalcitol dose choice depends on baseline iPTH level: initial dose (mcg) = iPTH (pg/ml)/80. The drug is administered as bolus injections; within at least 1 day after dialysis. Paricalcitol capsules are administered once per day, every day or 3 times per week [KDIGO,2009]. The results of 3 prospective randomized multicenter studies demonstrate that paricalcitol effectively suppresses iPTH secretion, decreases the activity of bone AP isoenzyme and decreases the plasma level of osteocalcin. These effects are indicative of bone resorption rate decrease [Moore, 2010].

In patients with CKD III-IV with iPTH plasma level over 70 pg/ml (7.7 pmol/l) and 110 pg/ml (12.1 pmol/l) receiving low phosphorus diet, paricalcitol, calcitriol, alpha-calcidol or doxecalciferol are recommended for treatment and prophylaxis of bone disease (see Table 5) [KDIGO,2009]. In patients with CKD V and iPTH plasma level over 300 pg/ml (33.0 pmol/l) with renal osteodystrophy paricalcitol, calcitriol, doxecalciferol and alpha-calcidol are recommended to suppress the excessive iPTH secretion and normalize the elevated metabolic profile of bone tissue [Craver, 2007;KDIGO,2009; Slinin,2005].

5. Summary

Phosphorus metabolism disorders play an important role in CKD pathogenesis. Therefore, early control of hyperphosphatemia is required to improve the quality of life in CKD patients. Numerous cohort studies have shown associations between disorders of mineral metabolism, cardiovascular disease and mortality. These observational studies have broadened the focus of CKD-related mineral and bone disorders to include cardiovascular disease (which is the leading cause of death in patients at all stages of CKD). All three of these processes (abnormal mineral metabolism, abnormal bone and extra skeletal calcification) are closely interrelated and together make a major contribution to the morbidity and mortality of patients with CKD. Mechanisms of CKD-associated extra-osseal calcification are complicated and multi-factorial. Recently, new mediators of osteogenesis-angiogenesis interactions have been identified - they are hypoxia - induced factor 1-α (HIF1-α) and vascular endothelium growth factor (VEGF). These factors induce vascular calcification through angiogenous signaling. New factors produced by kidneys and bone tissue have been identified. They are morphogenetic proteins (FGF-23 and Klotho) that contribute to phosphorus and vitamin D turnover and bone mineralization regulation. It has been suggested that resistance to FGF-23 is one of the early manifestations of CKD-associated metabolic disorders. This effect is mediated through decreased renal expression of Klotho. It has been reported that calcitriol and paricalcitol increase the rate of Klotho expression in kidneys. The possibility to use anti-FGF neutralizing antibodies to control FGF-23 hyperproduction is under discussion. However, further studies are required to evaluate their effects related to the system of complicated interactions between bone tissue, kidneys and parathyroid glands.

5.1 Recommendations for further research

Further research is needed to determine the reference values of corrected total serum calcium levels, depending on age, sex and race of patients with CKD and dialysis patients. Also, research is needed to determine the adequate calcium intake, the timing of the therapy with calcium and used calcium supplement drugs.

Very interesting is the new vitamin D metabolites testing, which are less likely to cause hypercalcemia. The ideal aim of such trials is to reduce serum IPTG levels with an insignificant change in serum calcium concentration. It would be useful to evaluate the relationship between serum IPTG levels and histological stage of hyperparathyroid bone disease in relation to the degree of renal failure progression.

Regulation of the IPTG level is a complex task. Need to find an acceptable balance between adequate levels of IPTG, accompanied by no bone lesions, and prevention of accelerated calcinosis / atherosclerosis

It is neededto carry out long-term studies evaluating the efficacy, side effects and impact on morbidity and mortality of various phosphate-binding drugs. Although the recently completed studies have demonstrated the benefits of sevelamer compared with calcium phosphate binders in prevention of aortic and coronary artery calcification progression in patients with CKD stage 4, research evaluating a positive impact on cardiovascular morbidity and mortality in dialysis patients is needed.

The next perspectives of controlled clinical trials in nephrology are associated primarily with the cooperation of medical, educational and scientific centers, including online, on the basis of professional social organizations. This interaction can intensify the integration of nephrologists in international clinical research, to organize the original clinical research on common standards(Good Clinical Practice, Good Research Practice), involving the maximum number of nephrology, outpatient and inpatient treatment centers.

6. References

Block, G.; Hulbert-Shearon, T.; Levin, N. et al. (1998). Association of serum phosphorus and calcium x phosphateproduct with mortality risk in chronic hemodialysis patients: a national study. Am. J. Kidney Dis.,31, 1998, pp. 607–617

Block, G.; Raggi, P.; Bellasi, A. et al. (2007). Mortality effect of coronary calcification and phosphate binder choice in incident hemodialysis patients. Kidney Int., 71, 2007, pp. 438–441

Block, G.; Brillhart, S.; Persky, M. et al. (2010). Efficacy and safety of SBR759, a new iron-based phosphate binder. Kidney Int.; 77, 2010,pp. 897-901

Boekel, G. (2008). Tumor producing fibroblast growth factor 23 localized by two-staged venous sampling. Eur. J. Endocrinol., 158, 2008, pp.431–437

Carpenter, T. (2005). Fibroblast growth factor 7: an inhibitor of phosphate transport derived from oncogenic osteomalacia-causing tumors. J. Clin. Endocrinol. Metab., 90, 2005, pp. 1012–1020

Craver, L.; Marco M.P.; Martinez I. et al. (2007). Mineral metabolism parameters throughout chronic kidney disease stages 1–5--achievement of K/DOQI target ranges. Nephrol. Dial. Transplant., 22, 2007,pp. 1171–1176

Darry, L. (2008). Endocrine function of bone in mineral metabolism. Clin. Invest., 118(12),2008, pp. 3820-3828

Davies, M.; Lund, R. & Hruska, K. (2003). BMP-7 is an efficacious treatment of vascular calcification in a murine model of atherosclerosis and chronic renal failure. J. Am. Soc. Nephrol., 14, 2003, pp. 1559–1567

Davies, M.; Lund, R.; Mathew S. et al. (2005). Low turnover osteodystrophy and vascular calcification are amenable to skeletal anabolism in an animal model of chronic kidney disease and the metabolic syndrome. J. Am. Soc. Nephrol., 16, 2005, pp.917–928

Ermolenko, V.(2009). Chronic renal failure. Nephrology: national leadership. Ed. NA Mukhina. M. GEOTAR Media.,2009, pp. 579-629

Fang, M.; Glackin, C.; Sadhu, A. et al. (2001).Transcriptional regulation of alpha 2(I) collagen gene expression by fibroblast growth factor-2 in MC3T3-E1 osteoblast-like cells. J. Cell. Biochem., 80, 2001,pp. 550–559.

Farrow, E & White,K(2010). Recent Advances in Renal Phosphate Handling.Published in final edited form as: Nat Rev Nephrol.; 6(4), 2010 April, pp.207–217. Published online 2010 February 23. doi: 10.1038/nrneph.2010.17

Finch, J., Tokumoto, M., Nakamura, H.et al.(2010) Effect of paricalcitol and cinacalcet on serum phosphate, FGF-23, and bone in rats with chronic kidney disease. Am J Physiol Renal Physiol., June; 298(6),2010,: pp.1315–1322.

Foley, R.; Parfrey, P. & Sarnak, M.J.(1998). Clinical epidemiology of cardiovascular disease in chronic renal disease. Am. J. Kidney Dis., 32, 1998, pp. 112–119

Fucumoto, S. (2008). Physiological regulationand Disorders of Phosphate metabolism – Pivotal Role of Fibroblast Growth factor-23. Inter. Med., 47, 2008, pp. 337-343

Go, A.; Chertow, G.; Fan, D. et al.(2004).Chronic kidney disease and the risks of death, cardiovascular events, and hospitalization. New. Engl. J. Med., 351,2004,pp.1296–1305

Gutierrez, O.; Isacova, T.; Rhee, E. et al. (2005). Fibroblast Growth factor-23 Mitigates Hyperphosphatemia But Accentuates Calcitriol Deficiency in chronic Kidney Disease. Kidney Int., 16,2005, pp. 2205-2215

Gutiérrez, O.; Mannstadt, M.; Isakova, T. et al. (2008). Fibroblast growth factor 23 and mortality among patients undergoing hemodialysis. New Engl. J. Med., 359,2008, pp. 584–592

Gutiérrez, O.(2009).Fibroblast Growth Factor 23 and Left Ventricular Hypertrophy in Chronic Kidney Disease. Circulation.; 119,2009,pp. 2545-2552

Hruska, K. ; Mathew, S.; Lund, R. et al. (2008) Hyperphosphatemia of Chronic Kidney Disease. Kidney Int., 74(2),2008, pp. 148–157

Huang Chou-Long (2010). Regulation of ion channels by secreted Klotho: mechanisms and implications. Kidney Int.; 77, 2010, pp. 855-860

Isakova, T. & Gutierrez, O. (2008).Postprandial Mineral Metabolism and Secondary Hyperparathyroidism in early CKD. J. Am. Soc. Nephrol., 19(3), 2008, pp. 615-623

Jean, G. (2009) High levels of serum FGF-23 are associated with increased mortality in long haemodialysis patients. N.D.T., 24(9),2009, pp. 2792-2796

Kawata, T. (2007). Parathyroid hormone regulates fibroblast growth factor-23 in a mouse model of primary hyperparathyroidism. J. Am. Soc. Nephrol., 18, 2007, pp. 2683–2688

Kestenbaum, B.; Sampson, J.; Rudser, K. et al. (2005). Serum phosphate levels and mortality risk among people with chronic kidney disease. J. Am. Soc. Nephrol.,16, 2005, pp.520–528

Ketteler,M.(2011). Phosphate Metabolism in CKD Stages 3–5: Dietary and Pharmacological Control

Int J Nephrol. Published online 2011 May 23. doi: 10.4061/2011/970245

KDIGO Clinical Practice for the Diagnosis, Evaluation, Prevention, and Treatment of Chronic Kidney Disease-Mineral and Bone Disorder (CKD-MBD)(2009). Kidney International, Vol 76, suppl 113,august 2009.

Lederer, E. & Levi, M. (2011). What is New in Phosphate homeostasis? Advances in Chronic Kidney Disease, vol.18, No 2, 2011, pp. 254-260

Liu, S.; Tang, W.; Zhou, J. et al. (2006). Fibroblast Growth Factor 23. Is a Counter-Regulatory Phosphaturic Hormone for Vitamin D. J. Am. Soc. Nephrol.,17, 2006,pp.1305–1315

London, G.(2000). Cardiovascular risk in end-stage renal disease:vascular aspects. Nephrol. Dial. Transplant.,15(Suppl 5), 2000,pp. 97-104

Marchais, S.; Metivier, F.; Guerin, A. et al. (1999). Association of hyperphosphataemia with haemodynamic disturbances in end-stage renal disease. Nephrol. Dial. Transplant.,14, 1999,pp. 2178–2183

Makoto, K. (2009). Klotho in chronic kidney disease—What's new? Nephrol. Dial. Transplant., 24(6),2009, pp. 1705-1708

Masuyama, R. (2006). Vitamin D receptor in chondrocytes promotes osteoclastogenesis and regulates FGF23 production in osteoblasts. J. Clin. Invest., 116, 2006, pp.3150–3159

Milovanova, L.; Milovanov, Y.& Kozlovsky, L.(2011). Phosphorus-calcium metabolism disordersin chronic kidney disease stages III-V. Klin. nefrol., 1,2011,pp. 58-68

Moe, S.; Duan, D.; Doehle, B. et al.(2003). Uremia induces the osteoblast differentiation factor Cbfa1 in human blood vessels. Kidney Int.,63,2003,pp.1003–1011

Moore, C. & Pai, A. (2010). Optimizing pharmacotherapy in chronic kidney disease. Advances in Chronic Kidney Disease, vol.17, No 5,2010, pp. 768-778

National kidney Foundation. K/DOQI Clinical Practice Guidelines for Bone Metabolism and Disease in Chronic Kidney Disease. (2003). Am. J. Kidney Dis., (suppl. 3), 42, 2003,pp.1-201.

Nishimura, M.; Tsukamoto, K.; Tamaki, N.et al. (2011). Risk stratification for cardiac death in hemodialysis patients without obstructive coronary artery disease. Kidney Int., 79, 2011,pp. 363-371

Pande, S.; Ritter, C.; Rothstein, M. et al. (2006). FGF-23 and sFRP-4 in chronic kidney disease and post-renal transplantation. Nephron Physiol., 104, 2006, pp. 23–32

Parfey, P.(2000). Cardiac disease in dialysis patients: diagnosis, burden of disease, prognosis, risk factors and management. Nephrol. Dial. Transplant., 5(Suppl 5),2000,pp. 58-68.

Patel, T.& Singh, A.(2009) Kidney Disease Outcomes Quality Initiative (K/DOQI GUIDELINES) for Bone and Mineral Metabolism: Emerging Questions. Semin Nephrol., March; 29(2),2009, pp.105–112.

Pletcher, M.; Tice, J.; Pignone, M. et al.(2004). Using the Coronary Artery Calcium Score to Predict Coronary Heart Disease Events: A Systematic Review and Meta-analysis. Arch. Int. Med.,2004, pp. 1285–1292

Quarles,L(2008) Endocrine functions of bone in mineral metabolism regulation.J Clin Invest. December 1; 118(12),2008,pp.3820–3828. Published online 2008 December 1. doi: 10.1172/JCI36479

Correction in J Clin Invest. 2009 February 2; 119(2): 421.

Razzaque, M.(2008). FGF23-mediated regulation of systemic phosphate homeostasis Klotho an essential player? Am. J. Physiol. Renal Physiol., 19(11), 2008, pp. 1-27

Razzaque, M.(2009). Does FGF23 toxicity influence the outcome of chronic kidney disease? Nephrol. Dial. Transplant., 24(1),2009, pp. 4-7

Reddy, V.; Symes, F.; Sethi, N. (2009). Dietitian-Led Education Program to Improve Phosphate Control in a Single-Center Hemodialysis Population., 4(19),2009, pp. 314-320

Shanahan, C.; Cary, N.; Metcalfe, J. et al. (1994). High expression of genes for calcification-regulating proteins in human atherosclerotic placques. J. Clin. Invest., 93, 1994,pp. 2393–2402

Sitara, D.(2004). Homozygous ablation of fibroblast growth factor-23 results in hyperphosphatemia and impaired skeletogenesis, and reverses hypophosphatemia in Phex-deficient mice. Matrix Biol., 23, 2004,pp.421–432

Sitara, D.(2006). Genetic ablation of vitamin D activation pathway reverses biochemical and skeletal anomalies in Fgf-23-null animals. Am. J. Pathol., 169, 2006, pp. 2161–2170

Slinin, Y.; Foley, R. & Collins, A. (2005). Calcium, Phosphorus, Parathyroid Hormone, and Cardiovascular Disease in Hemodialysis Patients: The USRDS Waves 1, 3, and 4 Study. J. Am. Soc. Nephrol., 16, 2005, pp.1788–1793

Townsend R. & Sica, D.(2011). Hypertension in Chronic Kidney Disease- Views from Waterfront. Advances in Chronic Kidney Disease, vol.18, No 1,2011, pp. 234-245

Volgina, G.(2004). Secondary hyperparathyroidism in chronic renal failure. Vitamin D active metabolites treatment. Nefrol. dial., 2 (6), 2004,pp. 116-127

Wang, L.; Jerosch-Herold, M.; Jacobs, J. et al.(2006). Coronary Artery Calcification and Myocardial Perfusion in Asymptomatic Adults: The MESA (Multi-Ethnic Study of Atherosclerosis). J. Am. Coll. Cardiol.,48, 2006, pp.: 1018–1026

Yamazaki, Y. (2008). Anti-FGF23 neutralizing antibodies show the physiological role and structural features of FGF23. J. Bone Miner. Res., 23,2008, pp. 1509–1518

Zemcencov, A. ; Gerasimchuk, R.(2009). Vitamin D receptor activators and vascular calcification (literature review). Nefrol. dial., 4 (11),2009, pp. 276-292

Recent Trials in Hypertension

Samra Abouchacra[1] and Hormaz Dastoor[2]
[1]*Tawam Hospital*
[2]*Mafraq Hospital*
United Arab Emirates

1. Introduction

There are numerous trials in hypertension many of which have focused on cardiovascular (CV) outcomes (death, non-fatal Myocardial Infarction, stroke, congestive heart failure). These trials have influenced our clinical practice in terms of setting out guidelines in the treatment of Hypertension. However, the last three years have seen newer trials emerge which we feel will influence the new upcoming guidelines.

Making sense of these trials and applying their conclusions into clinical practice remains a formidable challenge to physicians. In this chapter we will not only review landmark trials, but also attempt to analyse them and suggest recommendations to be applied in daily practice. The trials will be evaluated according to the following three major categories:

1. **Trials in Patients with Essential Hypertension (Hypertension Trials)**
2. **Trials in patients with renal disease and renal outcomes (Renal Trials)**
   a. Non-Diabetic
   b. Diabetic
3. **Trials in patients with high cardiovascular risk and focusing on cardiovascular outcomes. (Cardiovascular Trials)**

2. Hypertension trials

All physicians are faced with the dilemma of which drug is the best choice for patients with essential hypertension. By best choice we mean, the drug that is most economical, has a high safety profile and improves cardiovascular mortality. Our drug choice has been influenced over time by various published trials that will be reviewed. However, it is important to start first by evaluating a trial looking at lifestyle modification in essential hypertension.

TOHP Trial (Trial of Hypertension Prevention) (1) and its long-term follow-up **TOHP-2**(2) were the main studies on lifestyle modification. This randomized, placebo controlled trial of 2812 patients demonstrated that weight loss is the most effective lifestyle modification, reducing SBP and DBP on average by 2.9/2.3 mm Hg for every 4 kilogram weight loss. Dietary sodium restriction reduced BP by 2/1 mm Hg for every 44-meq/ day decreasing salt intake. All other arms, reductions in calcium or magnesium, fish oil and stress management failed to achieve sustained blood pressure improvement. Though non-pharmacologic measures lead to modest BP effects, it nevertheless has great clinical significance. This was also shown in large trials such as ALLHAT and VALUE, where even small differences of -4/-3 mm Hg were associated with significant reduction in stroke (23%), coronary heart disease (15%) and mortality (14%).

As monotherapy most of the drugs produce effective response in about 30 percent of cases (3,4). However there is wide inter-patient and inter-racial variability. Black patients for instance, respond better to CCBs and diuretics, whereas white patients have better response to ACE/ARBs and Beta-blockers. This variability may be related to low renin-high volume conditions in the former and high renin-low volume in the latter. Hence results of individual trials are not generalizable and apply only to the specific study population.

TOMHS Trial (Treatment of Mild Hypertension Study) attempted to evaluate the response of 5 major first line drugs in a predominant white population (5). The efficacy of the drugs was essentially similar although the CCB group (Amlodipine) had the highest percentage of patients responding to monotherapy.

ALLHAT Trial (Antihypertensive and Lipid Lowering to prevent Heart Attack Trial) is a randomised prospective trial of 45,000 patients with hypertension and one additional risk factor for coronary heart disease (6). ALLHAT compared primary (fatal coronary heart disease and non fatal myocardial infarction) and secondary (congestive heart failure, stroke etc.) cardiovascular outcomes among those randomly assigned chlorthalidone (12.5-25 mg/day) to one of three other arms: CCB (Amlodipine), ACEI (Lisinopril) and alpha adregenic blocker (Doxazosin). The initial mean untreated and treated blood pressures were similar (156/89 and 145/83). The Doxazosin arm was prematurely terminated due to increased risk of heart failure compared to diuretics. It should be noted that though the Doxazosin arm was stopped in February 2000, the primary end point, reduction in cardiovascular mortality from myocardial infarction was not different between two groups. This occurred despite the thiazide diuretic groups having a SBP 3 mm Hg lower than the alpha-blocker group.

The incidence of primary outcome (fatal coronary heart disease and non fatal myocardial infarction) was similar for all three agents. The CCB arm compared to diuretic had a higher rate of heart failure but other secondary outcomes were similar. The ACEI arm compared to diuretic had higher combined cardiovascular outcomes, stroke and heart failure. Blacks and non-diabetics in the ACEI arm had higher rates of these unfavourable outcomes. The higher risk of heart failure seen with Amlodipine and Lisinopril was greatest in the first year. This was attributed mainly to better blood pressure control in the diuretic arm. The risk was greatly attenuated after the first year when blood pressures were similar. The mean increase in fasting glucose in non-diabetics was higher in diuretic arm versus ACEI or CCB. The ALLHAT Trial showed that in patients with hypertension and high risk for cardiovascular disease, diuretics (chlorthalidone), CCB (Amlodipine) and ACEI (Lisinopril) had same protection from fatal coronary heart disease and nonfatal myocardial infarction. Amlodipine was not associated with excessive cardiac deaths as suggested by INSIGHT trial though the higher rate of congestive heart failure is consistent with other trials (7).

ANBP2 Trial (Second Australian National Blood Pressure) compared an ACEI (Lisinopril) with diuretic (Hydrochlorothiazide) in elderly hypertensive patients (8). The ANBP2 trial was a prospective trial of 6000 participants. The primary outcome was all cardiovascular events. These included coronary events (myocardial infarction, sudden death from cardiac events), cardiovascular events (heart failure, vascular cause of death) and cerebrovascular (stroke or transient ischemic episode). At the end of the study both arms had similar reductions of blood pressure of 26/12 mm Hg. Approximately 65 percent of patients in both arms needed monotherapy while the rest needed two or more agents. The ACEI arm had better cardiovascular outcomes as compared to the diuretic arm. While fatal events were the same in both arms, the incidence of non-fatal cardiovascular events was less in the ACEI arm. This was in contradiction to the ALLHAT trial that showed that diuretics were more effective in cardiovascular outcomes.

Stop-Hypertension 2 Trial comparing ACEI (Lisinopril) vs. dihydropyridine CCB (DHP-CCB) in this case Felodipine or Isradipinevs. Beta-blocker and /or diuretic, found no difference in cardiovascular end points (9). **NORDIL Trial (Nordic Diltiazem Trial)** comparing CCB (Diltiazem) combined with either a diuretic or Beta-blockers or both showed no cardiovascular outcome differences between the three groups at similar level of blood pressure control (10). The conclusion of Stop-Hypertension 2 study and NORDIL study show that CCBs are equally effective in cardiovascular outcome trials of low- medium risk patients.

MRC Trial (Medical Research Council Trial) (11) found no difference in cardiovascular outcomes between thiazide diuretic and Propanolol, but there was a significant increased risk of stroke in the Propanolol arm. This trial was predominantly in middle aged men with mean diastolic pressure 99-109 mm Hg. A subsequent MRC trial (12) comparing Atenolol to Hydrochlorothiazide plus Amiloride suggested Beta-blockers did not reduce cardiovascular mortality or coronary events but did reduce the incidence of cerebrovascular incidents, while diuretics reduced all of these endpoints.

In the **ACCOMPLISH trial (Avoiding Cardiovascular Events Through Combination Therapy in Patients Living With Systolic Hypertension)**, 11,500 patients with hypertension and mean baseline BP 145/80, who are at high risk of cardiovascular events, were randomly assigned to a combination therapy with Benazepril plus either Amlodipine or hydrochlorthiazide (12.5 to 25 mg/day) (13). At 36 months, the trial was terminated early. Benazepril- Amlodipine therapy was associated with significant reductions in the primary composite end point of fatal or non fatal cardiovascular events (9.6 versus 11.8 percent) and the secondary end point of cardiovascular death or non fatal MI or stroke (5.0 versus 6.3 percent). The mean blood pressure was slightly (about 1mm Hg) lower in the Benazepril-Amlodipine arm (132/73 versus 133/74), a difference that was too small to account for the large difference in outcomes. In a subset of 573 patients with 24 hour Ambulatory BP monitoring there was a non-significantly higher BP (1.3/0.3 mm Hg) in the Benazepril-Amlodipine group. The benefits seen in the Benazepril-Amlodipine arm appear to be independent of blood pressure lowering. The study also cannot distinguish benefit from Benazepril-Amlodipine and harm from Benazepril-hydrochlorthiazide arms.

2.1 Choice of antihypertensive medications in essential hypertension

The 2007 American heart Association and 2007 European Society of Hypertension (14) and European Heart Association (15) concluded that it is the amount of Blood Pressure reduction and not the class of drug used which determines the reduction in Cardiovascular risk in patients with Hypertension.

The initial choice recommended by the Joint National Commission 7(JNC7) for uncomplicated essential hypertension is thiazide diuretics (16) If thiazides fail to control blood pressure then ACEI/ARBs, CCBs or BB can be added. The use of these drugs is guided by cost or comorbid conditions for specific therapies. Post-ACCOMPLISH trial, since most patients with mild hypertension end up using more than one drug, either long acting ACE inhibitor/ARB or dihydropyridine calcium channel blocker could be recommended as first line therapy. Those with moderate to severe hypertension (Stage II) as defined by JNC7 having blood pressures greater than 20/10 mm Hg above goal should be considered initially for dual therapy. The combination of long acting ACEI/ARB with a dihydropyridine CCB would probably be the therapy of choice given the favourable results in the ACCOMPLISH trial.

Trial	Population Studied	Intervention	Outcome	Comments
TOHP Trial (Hypertension Prevention)	placebo controlled trial of 2812 hypertensive patients	Lifestyle modification on BP control.	Weight loss most effective Calcium, Magnesium, fish oil – no effect. Small BP differences (-4/-3 mm Hg) associated with significant reduction in stroke (23%), coronary disease (15%) & mortality (14%).	
TOMHS Trial (Treatment of Mild Hypertension)	predominant white population	Efficacy of 5 major first line drugs on BP control	Efficacy similar But Amlodipine had highest percentage of responders to monotherapy	
ALLHAT Trial (Antihypertensive and Lipid Lowering to prevent Heart Attack)	45,000 patients with hypertension and one additional coronary disease risk factor	Randomly assigned chlorthalidone (12.5-25 mg/day) to one of three other arms: CCB (Amlodipine), ACEI (Lisinopril) and alpha adregenic blocker (Doxazosin)	Primary outcome (fatal coronary disease, non fatal myocardial infarction) similar for all three agents. **Doxazosin arm prematurely terminated due to increased risk of heart failure vs diuretics a) CCB vs diuretic - higher rate of heart failure but other secondary CV outcomes similar b) ACEI vs diuretic- higher combined cardiovascular outcomes, stroke and heart failure *a) & b) attributed to better BP control in diuretic arm*	For hypertensives at high risk for cardiovascular disease, diuretics, CCB and ACEI offer similar in protection vs fatal coronary disease & nonfatal myocardial infarction
ANBP2 Trial (Second Australian National Blood Pressure)	Prospective trial of 6000 elderly hypertensive patients	ACEI (Lisinopril) vs diuretic (Hydrochlorothiazide)	Primary outcome: all cardiovascular events (myocardial infarction, sudden death from cardiac events)- ACEI arm had better outcomes vs diuretic Fatal events same in both arms, but non-fatal cardiovascular events were less in ACEI arm	

Stop-Hypertension 2 Trial	Low-medium CV risk hypertensive patients	ACEI (Lisinopril) vs. dihydropyridine CCB Felodipine or Isradipine vs Beta-blocker and /or diuretic	No difference in cardiovascular end points	CCBs equally effective in cardiovascular outcome
NORDIL Trial (Nordic Diltiazem Trial)	Low-medium CV risk hypertensive patients.	Comparing CCB (Diltiazem) combined with either diuretic or Beta-blockers or both.	No cardiovascular outcome differences	CCBs equally effective in cardiovascular outcome
MRC Trial (Medical Research Council Trial)	Middle aged men with mean diastolic BP 99-109.	Thiazide diuretic vs Propanolol. Second MRC trial comparing Atenolol to Hydrochlorothiazide plus Amiloride	No difference in cardiovascular outcomes but significant increased stroke risk in Propanolol arm Beta-blockers did not reduce cardiovascular mortality or coronary events but reduced cerebrovascular incidents, while diuretics reduced all these endpoints	
ACCOMPLISH trial (Avoiding Cardiovascular Events Through Combination Therapy in Patients Living With Systolic Hypertension	11,500 patients with hypertension and baseline BP 145/80, high risk of cardiovascular events	Benazepril plus either Amlodipine or hydrochlorthiazide (12.5 to 25 mg/day).	Terminated early Benazepril- Amlodipine showed significant reductions in primary composite end point (fatal or non fatal cardiovascular events) and secondary end point (cardiovascular death or non fatal MI or stroke)	Cannot distinguish benefit from Benazepril-Amlodipine vs. harm from Benazepril-hydrochlorthiazide

Table 1. Summary of Trials in Patients with Essential Hypertension

3. Renal trials

Renal outcome trials can be divided into those pertaining to patients with diabetic versus non- diabetic kidney disease. In the latter, the focus has been on short-term reduction of proteinuria and long term delay in progression of kidney disease. On the other hand, in diabetic kidney disease trials have focused on reduction of protein excretion as a surrogate end point since it correlates directly with the rate of decline in renal function.

a. Non- Diabetic kidney disease:

Most trials on reduction of proteinuria have focused on ACEI. This class of drugs has been known to reduce intraglomerular pressure mainly by inhibition of Angiotensin II- mediated efferent arteriole vasoconstriction. In addition, ACEI alter the permaselective properties of

the glomerular basement membrane and have antifibrotic effects that are thought to further reduce proteinuria.
How do other drugs compare with ACEI in proteinuria reduction?
In a trial (17) comparing non-dihydropyridine CCBs (Verapamil and Diltiazem) versus dihydropyridine CCBs (Amlodipine and Nifedipine), the former were found to have a significant (30%) reduction in proteinuria while the latter had no decrease or even an increase in protein excretion. It is postulated that DHP CCBs cause afferent arteriole dilatation allowing more of the aortic pressure to be transmitted to the glomerulus. Hence despite lowering of systemic blood pressure the intraglomerular pressure (IGP) remains elevated without significant decrease in proteinuria. Similarly Beta-blockers, diuretics, alpha-blockers have no effect on reducing IGP and hence proteinuria (18,19,20). Studies have also examined the comparative effectiveness of Angiotensin II receptor blockers (21). In one study of patients with IgA nephropathy Enalapril and Irbesartan had similar effects on proteinuria (22). The antiprotenuric effect of ACEI and A2RBs increases when used at supramaximal doses. For instance, Temlisartan 80 mg when used twice vs. once daily had significantly greater decline in proteinuria and progression of kidney disease, despite similar BP reduction. Additionally, combination therapy with ACEI and A2RBs has shown significant beneficial effect on proteinuria and kidney disease progression, more so when used in maximal or submaximal doses than maximum dose of either drug alone (23). This meta-analysis comparing combination therapy at submaximal doses to either agent alone at maximal doses confirmed these findings with greater reduction in proteinuria.
While the above trials focused on reduction of proteinuria, other trials in non-diabetics have shown benefits of ACEI in reducing progression to chronic kidney disease.
Though, the **ALLHAT Trial** (24) of more than 44,000 hypertensive patients failed to show superiority of ACEI, DHP-CCBs and alpha-blockers over a thiazide diuretic with respect to cardiovascular outcomes. In post hoc analysis neither ACEI nor CCB was superior to thiazide diuretic with respect to renal outcomes. This trial was contradictory to other primary renal outcome trials that showed benefit of ACEI over other drug classes. Some of the factors responsible for this controversy will be explored.The ALLHAT did not select patients with renal disease as an inclusion criterion, since it was not mainly a renal outcome trial. Blood pressure was also lower in thiazide arm as compared to the other arms hence equivalency of blood pressure was not achieved. Furthermore, no urine tests were performed even though renal outcomes were studied thus failing to identify those who were at highest risk for progression and most likely to derive benefit from ACEI i.e. patients with proteinuric diabetic kidney disease. Hence, in the ALLHAT trial little or no attention was paid to kidney function, consequently the results of ALLHAT regarding renal outcomes remain unresolved.
REIN Trial (Ramipril Efficacy in Nephropathy) of non-diabetic chronic kidney disease patients treated with Ramipril or placebo plus other medications to a target diastolic pressure less than 90 mm Hg. At same level of blood pressure control, the Ramipril group had a significant decrease in rate of decline of GFR (25). The disparity was predominantly so significant in groups excreting > 3 grams/day, necessitating premature termination of the study in favour of the Ramipril group. As a follow-up to this study patients excreting > 3grams/day on Ramipril were continued on same drug, but those on placebo were also switched to Ramipril. Analysis of this follow-up revealed that patients assigned as well as those shifted to Ramipril, had significant attenuation in the rate of deterioration of renal

function compared to the conventional therapy group. Longer follow-up at 5 years showed that some patients in the Ramipril group actually had an increase in GFR. Further analysis also revealed that Ramipril was efficious in patients with less severe proteinuria (>1 gram but < 3 grams/day) and also decreased the rate of decline in GFR in all tertiles of GFR (low: 11-33 ml/min/1.73m2, middle: 33-51 ml/min/1.73 m2, high: 51-101 ml/min/1.73m2).In the REIN 2 Trial (26), DHP CCB's were once again found to be non efficacious in patients with chronic kidney disease. In this trial patients on Ramipril (up to 5 mg) were randomly assigned to conventional (DBP<90) or intensive BP control (DBP<80) groups. Felodipine was added for intensive blood pressure control. After 19 months there was no significant difference in proteinuria, decline in GFR or progression to ESRD in the intensive Felodipine treated group despite lower blood pressure.

MDRD Trial (Modification of Diet in Renal Disease) compared two groups: one with usual blood pressure control (target 140/90) and one with aggressive control (target 125/75) over a three-year period. The achieved blood pressures were 130/80 and 125/75 respectively. The patients were further subdivided into 3 groups by severity of proteinuria, i.e.: < 1 gram, 1-3 grams and > 3 grams of protein excretion per day. More than half the patients were treated with ACEI and the mean GFR of the approximately 600 patients was 39 ml/min (27). The patients with <1 gram/day proteinuria had the slowest decline in GFR of the three groups (approximately 3 ml/year). No difference was seen in the low blood pressure group. Patients in 1-3 gram/day group had a more rapid deterioration in GFR with mild benefit in lower BP group. Those in >3 gram/day group had the fastest rate of loss in GFR but at the same time there was a substantial attenuation in rate of GFR decline in the low blood pressure group. This study showed that the greater the proteinuria, the faster is the decline in GFR. However with blood pressure control the rate of decline in GFR can be attenuated. While this trial did not evaluate the efficacy of ACEI, the Benazepril Trial did. 600 patients with chronic kidney disease (diabetic and non diabetic but not hypertensive nephrosclerosis) on treatment for blood pressure control were randomised to either Benazepril or placebo (28). The Benazepril group had significantly lower proteinuria, greater reduction in blood pressure, less doubling of serum creatinine and progression to dialysis. Though the drug was compared to placebo, it did show the efficacy of ACEI.

The role of combination ACEI with A2RB's was addressed in the COOPERATE Trial (Combination Treatment of Angiotensin II receptor blocker and Angiotensin converting enzyme inhibitor in non diabetic renal disease) where Losartan 100mg/day, Trandolapril 3mg/day or a combination of the two were compared (29). All the three arms of the trial had the same blood pressure reduction. However the largest decrease in proteinuria was seen in the combination group (77 percent) versus Losartan (42 percent) or Trandolapril (44 percent). The composite end point of doubling serum creatinine or progression to ESRD was less with combination (11 percent) therapy than either Losartan (23 percent) or Trandolapril (23 percent). In the COOPERATE trial, those who could not tolerate maximum doses of combination therapy were treated with sub-maximal doses. Even then the antiprotenuric effects were greater than with either of the single agents. This was further verified in another trial (30) comparing Losartan 50 mg/day, Benzalapril 10 mg/day, Losartan (25mg/day) plus Benzalapril 5 mg/day. Although similar blood pressure lowering was observed, combination therapy at half the dose resulted in significantly lower proteinuria than either drug alone.

Non-Diabetic Trial	Population Studied	Intervention	Outcome	Comments
REIN Trial (Ramipril Efficacy in Nephropathy)	Non-diabetic chronic kidney disease patients	Ramipril or placebo	Ramipril group had significant decrease in rate of GFR decline especially significant in groups excreting > 3 g/d but also in less severe proteinuria DHP CCB's non efficacious	ACEi significant attenuation in rate of deterioration of renal function
MDRD Trial (Modification of Diet in Renal Disease)		Usual (140/90) vs aggressive BP control (125/75)	The greater the proteinuria, the faster is the decline in GFR With BP control rate of GFR decline attenuated	
Benazepril Trial	600 patients with chronic kidney disease (diabetic and non diabetic but not hypertensive nephrosclerosis)	Benazepril or placebo	Benazepril significantly lower proteinuria, greater reduction in BP, less doubling of serum creatinine and progression to dialysis	Trial demonstrates efficacy of ACEI
COOPERATE Trial (Combination Treatment of Angiotensin II receptor blocker & Angiotensin converting enzyme inhibitor in non diabetic renal disease)	Non-diabetic renal disease	Losartan Trandolapril or a combination	Doubling serum creatinine or progression to ESRD was less with combination than either Losartan or Trandolapril Even with sub-maximal doses of combination therapy, antiprotenuric effects greater than with either of the single agents	Largest decrease in proteinuria seen in combination group

Table 2. A. Summary of Trials in patients with renal disease and renal outcomes (Renal Trials). NON-DIABETIC

b. Trials in Diabetic kidney disease:
These are divided into three major groups.

i. Prevention of Incipient Diabetic Nephropathy- BENEDICT Trial
ii. Trials on microalbuminuric Diabetic Nephropathy- HOPE, IRMA, MARVAAL Trials
iii. Trials on overt Diabetic nephropathy-IDNT, RENAAL, DETAIL, AVOID, ONTARGET Trials

i. Prevention of Incipient Diabetic Nephropathy

BENEDICT Trial (Bergamo Diabetic Nephrogenic Trial) is a prospective (31), randomised trial in 1209 hypertensive patients with type 2 diabetes mellitus and normal urine albumin excretion whose aim was to prevent the progression to microalbuminuria. Patients were randomised to a 3-year trial of non DHP CCB (Verapamil 240 mg/day), ACEI (Trandolapril 2 mg/day), combination (Verapamil 180 mg/day and Trandolapril 2mg/day) and placebo. The primary outcome was the development of persistent microalbuminuria, which occurred at a rate of 11.9% in Verapamil only group, 6 %in Trandolapril group, 5.7 % in the combination group and 10% in the placebo. The study showed that Verapamil was similar to placebo and the use of ACEI was effective in reducing the incidence of microalbuminuria whereas the addition of non DHP CCB did not decrease the risk of its development. It can be concluded that ACEIs are the medication of choice in reducing microalbuminuria in diabetic nonmoalbuminuric hypertensive patients.

ii. Trials on microalbuminuric Diabetic Nephropathy

PRIME Trial (Program for Irbesartan Mortality and Morbidity Evaluation) consisted of two large trials comparing IDNT (Irbesartan in Diabetic Nephropathy Trial) (32,33,34) and IRMA (Irbesartan in Patients with Type 2 Diabetes and Microalbuminuria), which evaluated the renal and cardiovascular effects of Irbesartan on hypertensive patients with diabetes (40). In particular, these two large trials addressed the question of whether ARB can prevent the development of clinical proteinuria (IRMA) or delay the progression of nephropathy (IDNT) in type2 diabetes. The latter will be discussed with the trials on overt nephropathy.

IRMA Trial (Irbesartan in Patients with Type 2 Diabetes and Microalbuminuria Study Group), a multicentre, randomized, double-blind, placebo-controlled trial, evaluated the effect of Irbesartan in preventing the onset of clinical proteinuria in patients with type 2 diabetes, hypertension and microalbuminuria (35). A total of 590 patients were randomized to receive therapy with Irbesartan 150 mg, Irbesartan300 mg, or placebo. Additional antihypertensive agents (excluding ACE-I, ARB, and Dihydropyridine calcium-channel blockers) were allowed in each arm of the study to achieve the target BP of<135/85 mmHg. The primary end point of the study was the onset of overt nephropathy, defined as the occurrence of a urinary albumin excretion rate >200 µg/min and at least 30%higher than baseline. Secondary outcomes were the regression to normoalbuminuria and changes in albuminuria and renal function.

The mean duration of follow-up was 2 yr. The average BP during the course of the study was 143/83 mmHg in the 150-mg group, 141/83 mmHg in the 300-mg group, and 144/83 mmHg in the placebo group. Although the difference in systolic pressure between the Irbesartan 300-mg group and the placebo group was only 3mmHg, it was statistically significant. With respect to the primary end point, Irbesartan 150and 300 mg showed a reduction of 44 and 68%, respectively versus placebo. Moreover, albuminuria was reduced by 38% in the 300-mg group, 24% in the150-mg group, and remained unchanged in the usual care group. In this last group, the reduction in BP from 153/90 to 144/83mmHg resulted in stabilization of albuminuria. In addition, regression to normoalbuminuria was more frequent in the patients who were treated with the higher dose of Irbesartan (17, 12, and 10.5/100 patient-years in the 300-mg, 150-mg, and placebo group, respectively). On the basis of these data, Irbesartan seems to be much more effective in preventing the development of clinical proteinuria and in favouring the regression to normoalbuminuria than conventional therapy. The renoprotective, dose-dependent effect of Irbesartan seems to be independent of its BP-lowering effect, even though the 3-mmHg difference in systolic pressure may have played a role. Similar findings were shown in other trials as discussed below.

HOPE Trial (Heart Outcomes and Prevention Evaluation) and MICRO-HOPE (Microalbuminuria and Renal Outcomes) Trial retrospectively analysed changes of proteinuria over4.5 yrs., and compared Ramipril's effects to placebo in9297 participants, including 3577 with diabetes and 1956 with microalbuminuria. In particular, one of every three participants with diabetes developed new microalbuminuria, and one of five diabetic participants with microalbuminuria developed overt nephropathy (36,37). We know little about the development of new microalbuminuria in type 2 diabetes; these data indicate that it develops ata surprisingly high rate. Assuming a constant rate of appearance of new overt nephropathy over time, the **HOPE** study also confirms that approximately 50% of microalbuminuric people with type2 diabetes will develop overt nephropathy in 10 years (38). ACE inhibition was shown to be effective in reducing the progression of albuminuria in all participants including the subgroups with and without diabetes mellitus.

MARVAL Trial (Microalbuminuria Reduction with Valsartan) compared Valsartan 80mg/day versus Amlodipine 5 mg/day in type 2 diabetic microalbuminuric patients (39). A target BP of 135/85 mm Hg was aimed for by double dosing after four weeks followed by addition of bendrofluazide and Doxazosinas needed. The primary end point of percentage reduction in proteinuria was 44 percent with Valsartan and 8 percent with Amlodipine. For the same level of attained BP, Valsartan lowered albuminuria more effectively than Amlodipine in patients with type 2 diabetes and microalbuminuria, including the subgroup with baseline normotension. This indicates BP-independent antiprotenuric effect of Valsartan. Moreover, more patients reverted to normoalbuminuria with Valsartan.

Recommendations clinical pearl The above three studies clearly show that blocking of the Renin Angiotensin Aldosterone System (RAAS) with ACEI or ARBs in patient with type II diabetes mellitus reduces the risk of progression of microalbuminuria to overt proteinuria and may even revert it back to normoalbuminuria, both in hypertensive and normotensive patients.

iii. Trials on overt Diabetic nephropathy

For patients who already have overt nephropathy, trials in type 1 and type 2 diabetics show benefits of ACEI and ARBs in reducing progression to end stage renal disease (ESRD) as will be discussed. In Type 1 DM the largest trials (40,41) were in patients who already had overt nephropathy with serum creatinine less than 2.5 mg/dl who were randomised to either Captopril or placebo. After four years there was significant decrease in rate of decline in renal function in the Captopril arm versus placebo. This rate was reduced from 1.4 mg/dl in the placebo group to 0.6 mg/dl in the Captopril group. The beneficial effect was seen mainly in patients whose initial serum creatinine was greater than 1.5 mg/dl, while no benefit was seen with lower baseline serum creatinine likely because the rate of progression was very slow in this group (0.1-0.2 mg/dl/year). The beneficial effect of Captopril was seen in both normotensive and hypertensive patients. However, it has been suggested that reducing BP to less than 120/75 regardless of the agent may slow progression of kidney disease (42).

In another study (43) of 301 patients with overt nephropathy of whom 271 were hypertensive and 30 were normotensive, the remission rates (defined as proteinuria less 300 mg/day) and regression rates (defined as rate of decline in GFR< 1 ml/min/year) were significantly greater in the lower blood pressure groups. The main antihypertensive drugs were ACEI in about 179 patients. The lower blood pressure group (mean arterial pressure 93 mm Hg) had remission and regression rates of 58 and 42 percent while the higher blood pressure group (mean arterial pressure 113 mm Hg) had rates of only 17 and 7 percent, after a mean follow up of 7 years. Thus aggressive blood pressure control in patients with overt nephropathy will induce greater remission and regression rates, especially when ACEI are used.

In Type 2 diabetics with overt nephropathy much of the prevailing evidence is with ARBs. Similar to the trials described above, control of blood pressure is essential to limit progression to ESRD however the optimal lower limit is not defined. **The UKPDS Trial (United Kingdom Prospective Diabetes Study)** showed that every 10 mm Hg decrease in systolic blood pressure reduced diabetic complications by 12 percent, with the lowest risk below 120 mm Hg (43). However in the IDNT Trial (Irbesartan Diabetic Nephropathy Trial) lowering SBP less than 120 mm Hg was associated with increased risk of all cause cardiovascular mortality (33,34). However in the group with increased cardiovascular mortality there was a higher incidence of underlying heart disease and heart failure. Moreover, the number of patients was too low to determine if the effect of low blood pressure was independent of prior cardiac disease. The two major trials which have clearly shown the benefits of ARBs in patients with proven nephropathy due to Type 2 DM will be reviewed.

The IDNT Trial (Irbesartan Diabetic Nephropathy Trial) of 1715 patients with diabetic nephropathy who were randomly assigned to Irbesartan 300 mg/day versus Amlodipine 10 mg/day versus placebo (33,34). After 30 months of follow up, the composite end points of development of ESRD or death from any cause were 23% and 20 % lower with Irbesartan than Amlodipine and placebo respectively. The rates for doubling serum creatinine were also 37% and 30 % lower for Irbesartan than Amlodipine and placebo respectively (33,34,35).

The RENAAL Trial (Reductions of endpoints in NIDDM with the Angiotensin II Antagonist Losartan) of 1513 patients with type 2 diabetic nephropathy, in which patients were assigned Losartan (50-100 mg/day) versus placebo with additional drugs added for further blood pressure control (except ACEI). The composite end points of doubling serum creatinine or ESRD were 25% and 28 % lower with Losartan than placebo (44). Both the above studies underline the positive effect of ARBs on progression of diabetic nephropathy.

The DETAIL Trial is the only study which offered head to head comparisons between ACEI and ARBs for diabetic nephropathy in type 2 diabetics (45). Temlisartan versus Enalapril were compared in patients with albuminuria (defined as micro and macroalbuminuria). After five years of follow-up there was a smaller but non-significant decline in GFR with Enalapril versus Temlisartan (14.9 ml/min versus 17.9 ml/min per 1.73 m2). Both arms had similar secondary end points of urine albumin excretion, doubling serum creatinine, progression to ESRD and cardiovascular events.

Combination ACEI and ARBs in diabetic proteinuric kidney disease have not been studied in large trials. Nevertheless, three small studies (46,47,48) have shown benefit of combination therapy over either ACEI or ARBs (the latter two used at either maximal or sub-maximal dose).

While diuretics are not known to have antiprotenuric effects despite lowering blood pressure, Aldosterone antagonists either used alone or in combination with ACEI or ARBs have been shown to reduce proteinuria. In a trial of 59 patients with Type 2 diabetes and nephropathy on ACE or A2RBs, the addition of Spironolactone 50 mg/day versus placebo was associated with a 40% reduction in proteinuria and 7/3 mm Hg decrease in BP (49). Eplernone 50 mg/day when added to ACEI in patients with type 2 diabetes was associated with a significant 40% reduction in proteinuria compared to placebo (50). While no long term studies have shown a benefit of Aldosterone blockers in reducing the rate of loss of GFR, their antiprotenuric and BP lowering effects would be expected to translate into nephroprotection.

GEMINI Trial (Metabolic Effects of Carvedilol vs. Metoprolol in Patients with Type 2 Diabetes Mellitus and Hypertension)1200 participants with type 2 diabetes mellitus showed that when Carvedilol was added to blockers of RAAS improvements not only in glycaemic control but also in risk of developing microalbuminuria were seen. These were markedly reduced over Metoprololat similar levels of blood pressure control. (51). It was also noted that those without microalbuminuria had a 7/4 mm Hg greater reduction in blood pressure as compared to those with microalbuminuria (52). This observation supports previous data of a blunted vascular response associated with microalbuminuria. It also suggests that not all have the same detrimental effect on diabetes and the risk of its development.

The **AVOID Trial (Aliskerin in the Evaluation of Proteinuria in Diabetes)** of 599 patients with Type 2 diabetes and nephropathy, evaluated the renoprotective effects of dual blockade of the renin angiotensin aldosterone system (RAAS) by adding treatment with Aliskerin (maximum dose 300 mg daily), an oral direct renin inhibitor, to treatment with the maximal recommended dose of Losartan (100 mg daily) (53). At 6 months the primary end point of reduction in albumin- creatinine ratio was a mean of 20% in Aliskerin group versus placebo with over 50% reduction in 25% of patients in Aliskerin group versus 12.5% in placebo. This was despite a small difference in BP between the two groups (systolic 2mm Hg/ diastolic 1 mm Hg) favouring Aliskerin. Clinical pearl This suggests Aliskerin may have renoprotective effects that are independent of blood pressure lowering effects in hypertensive patients with type 2 diabetes and nephropathy who are already receiving the recommended therapy.

The ONTARGET trial (The Ongoing Telmisartan alone and in combination with Ramipril Global Endpoint Trial), in which 25,620 patients with vascular disease or diabetes were randomized to the ACE inhibitor Ramipril, ARB Telmisartanor the combination of the two drugs (54). The primary renal outcome was a composite of dialysis, doubling of serum creatinine and death. The number of events of primary composite outcomes was similar for Ramipril and Temlisartan but was increased with combination therapy. Although the combination therapy reduced proteinuria more than either single therapy, overall it worsened major renal outcomes.

Finally, the controversial meta-analysis by Casas (55) will be discussed. This included thirteen trials with 37,089 subjects. Casas concluded that drugs which inhibit the Renin Angiotensin Aldosterone system (RAAS) provide only marginal benefit for nondiabetic kidney disease and no benefit in diabetic renal disease. The authors state that if there is a benefit of ACEI or ARBs in diabetics, it is simply due to better blood pressure control, which was 2 to 7 mm Hg lower in the ACEI groups. When their analysis was limited to studies with no evident blood pressure difference, no benefit was identified. Similar findings were noted in the ABCD trial (Appropriate Blood Pressure Control Trial) in patients with microalbuminuria and mean baseline GFR of 84 ml/min. No difference in renal outcomes at 5 years was observed between ACEI and calcium channel blockers when their BP was lowered to below 130/80 mm Hg (56).

Trial Diabetic	**Population Studied**	**Intervention**	**Outcome**	**Comments**
BENEDICT Trial (Bergamo Diabetic Nephrogenic Trial)	1209 hypertensive patients with type 2 diabetes mellitus and normal urine albumin excretion	Non DHP CCB Verapamil vs ACEI Trandolapril vs combination vs placebo	Primary outcome: Development of persistent microalbuminuria. Verapamil similar to placebo ACEI effective in reducing incidence of microalbuminuria	ACEIs are of choice in reducing microalbuminuria in diabetic nonmo-albuminuric hypertensive patients
PRIME	Consisted of	Whether ARB can		

Trial(Program for Irbesartan Mortality and Morbidity Evaluation)	two large trials on type 2 diabetics: IDNT (Irbesartan in Diabetic Nephropathy Trial) IRMA (Irbesartan in Patients with Type 2 Diabetes & Microalbuminuria)	prevent development of clinical proteinuria (IRMA) or delay progression of nephropathy (IDNT)		
IRMA Trial (Irbesartan in Patients with Type 2 Diabetes and Microalbuminuria Study Group)	**Patients with Type 2 Diabetes and Microalbuminuria.**	Irbesartan 150 mg or Irbesartan 300 mg vs placebo	Primary end point: Onset of overt nephropathy- Irbesartan 150and 300 mg showed a reduction vs placebo Secondary outcomes: Regression to normoalbuminuria and changes in albuminuria & renal function- Regression more frequent with higher Irbesartan dose	Irbesartan more effective in preventing development of clinical proteinuria and regression to normoalbuminuria than conventional therapy
HOPE Trial (Heart Outcomes and Prevention Evaluation) and MICRO-HOPE (Micro-albuminuria and Renal Outcomes) Trial	9297 participants, including 3577 with diabetes and 1956 with Microalbuminuria	Follow changes of proteinuria and compare Ramipril's vs placebo	Approximately 50% of microalbuminuric people with type2 diabetes will develop overt nephropathy in 10 years ACE inhibition effective in reducing progression of albuminuria in all, including subgroups with and without diabetes mellitus	
MARVAL Trial (Microalbuminuria Reduction with Valsartan)	Patients with type 2 diabetes and microalbuminuria	Valsartan vs Amlodipine	Primary end point: reduction in proteinuria- Valsartan more effective including subgroup with baseline normotension & more patients reverted to normo-albuminuria	BP-independent antiprotenuric effect of Valsartan

Trials on Overt Diabetic Nephropathy	Type 1 DM with overt nephropathy & serum creatinine < 2.5 mg/dl 301 Patients with overt nephropathy, 271 hypertensive & 30 normotensive	Randomised to either Captopril or placebo Normal vs lower BP groups Main antihypertensive drugs were ACEI in 179 patients	Significant decrease in rate of decline in renal function in the Captopril arm Beneficial effect of Captopril in both normotensive & hypertensive patients Significantly greater nephropathy remission & regression rates in lower BP group	Aggressive BP control in patients with overt nephropathy will induce greater remission & regression rates, especially when ACEI are used
The UKPDS Trial (United Kingdom Prospective Diabetes Study)		Showed that every 10 mm Hg decrease in systolic BP reduced diabetic complications by 12 %, with lowest risk below 120 mm Hg		
IDNT Trial(Irbesartan Diabetic Nephropathy Trial	1715 patients with diabetic nephropathy	Irbesartan vs Amlodipine vs placebo	Composite end points: development of ESRD or death from any cause- lower with Irbesartan than Amlodipine and placebo Doubling serum creatinine lower for Irbesartan.	Positive effect of ARBs on progression of diabetic nephropathy Of note: lowering SBP < 120 mm Hg associated with increased risk of all cause cardiovascular mortality. However this group had higher incidence of underlying heart disease & heart failure and number of patients was too low to determine if lower BP effect was independent of prior cardiac disease
RENAAL Trial (Reductions of endpoints in NIDDM with	Type 2 diabetic nephropathy	Effect of Losartan (50-100 mg/day) vs placebo	Composite end points of doubling serum creatinine or ESRD: lower with Losartan	Positive effect of ARBs on progression of diabetic nephropathy

the Angiotensin II Antagonist Losartan)				
DETAIL Trial	Type 2 diabetics with diabetic nephropathy (micro and macro albuminuria)	Temlisartan vs Enalapril on diabetic nephropathy progression	A smaller but non-significant decline in GFR with Enalapril vs Temlisartan Similar secondary end points of urine albumin excretion, doubling serum creatinine, progression to ESRD & cardiovascular events	
GEMINI Trial(Metabolic Effects of Carvedilol vs. Metoprolol in Patients with Type 2 Diabetes Mellitus and Hypertension)	1200 participants with type 2 diabetes mellitus	Carvedilol vs Metoprolol was added to RAAS blockers	Improvements in glycaemic control & risk of developing microalbuminuria with carvedilol vs Metoprolol	Confirms blunted vascular response associated with microalbuminuria Suggests that not all beta Blockers have same detrimental effect on diabetes & risk of its development
AVOID Trial (Aliskerin in the Evaluation of Proteinuria in Diabetes)	599 patients with Type 2 diabetes and nephropathy	dual blockade: adding Aliskerin to maximal dose of Losartan vs placebo	Primary end point: reduction albumin- creatinine ratio- 20% in Aliskerin group vs 12.5% in placebo despite a small difference in BP	Aliskerin may have renoprotective effects independent of BP lowering
ONTARGET trial (The Ongoing Telmisartan alone and in combination with Ramipril Global Endpoint Trial),	25,620 patients with vascular disease or diabetes	ACE inhibitor Ramipril vs ARB Telmisartan vs combination	Primary renal outcome: composite of dialysis, doubling of serum creatinine & death: similar for Ramipril and Temlisartan but was increased with combination therapy Although combination therapy reduced proteinuria more than either single therapy, overall it worsened major renal outcomes	
Meta-analysis by Casas	Thirteen trials 37,089 subjects		Drugs which inhibit RAAS provide only marginal benefit for nondiabetic kidney disease & no benefit in diabetic renal disease When analysis was limited to studies with no BP difference, no benefit was identified	

ABCD trial (Appropriate Blood Pressure Control Trial)	Patients with microalbuminuria & mean baseline GFR 84 ml/min	Comparison of ACEI & CCB	No difference in renal outcome when BP lowered < 130/80 mmHg	

Table 2. B. Summary of Trials in patients with renal disease and renal outcomes (Renal Trials). DIABETIC

4. Cardiovascular trials

While it has been suggested that ACEI/ARBs are beneficial in individuals with cardiovascular disease, it is the achieved blood pressure rather than the specific drug that may be responsible for the benefits. Also, while the JNC 7 recommends a target blood pressure of less than 140/90, the data cited below also suggest that as in CKD (chronic kidney disease), a blood pressure target of less than 130/80 may be appropriate.

In the **HOPE Trial (Heart Outcomes Prevention Evaluation)** (57,58) patients with high cardiovascular risk (without acute MI, LV dysfunction or heart failure) were randomly assigned to Ramipril 5-10 mg/day or placebo. The trial was terminated prematurely after 4.5 years because of significant benefits in the Ramipril arm with only14% reaching the primary end point (any cardiovascular event: CVA, MI, Cardiovascular death) versus 17.8 percent in the placebo group. A reduction was also seen in stroke events despite a mean BP of 135/76, which was only 3.3/1.4 mm Hg less than placebo (59). However, although the benefits were thought to be independent of BP control, an analysis of a subset of 38 patients who underwent ambulatory blood pressure monitoring showed a significant drop in night time blood pressure.

The **EUROPA Trial (European Trial on Reduction of cardiac Events with Perindopril in Stable Coronary Artery Disease)** was similar to the HOPE but patients in this trial had lower cardiovascular risk as evidenced by lower prevalence of hypertension, diabetes or peripheral vascular disease as well as lower cardiovascular mortality in the placebo group. The mean blood pressure at entry was 137/82 mm Hg. In this study patients were given Perindopril (8 mg once a day) or placebo and were followed for a mean of 4.2 years with primary end point of MI, cardiac arrest or cardiovascular death. A significant reduction in primary end point was noted in favour of the Perindopril group vs. Placebo (8 versus 10). However Perindopril therapy was associated with a blood pressure that was 5/2 mm Hg lower than placebo (60). Hence from both of these trials it can be concluded that the benefits of ACEI may be due to lowering of blood pressure and not to intrinsic property of the ACEI.

The two trials comparing ACEIs and CCBs were the VALUE and CAMELOT Trials.

The **VALUE Trial (Valsartan Antihypertensive Long-term use evaluation)** evaluated Valsartan versus Amlodipine in 15,000 hypertensive patients with mean blood pressure 155/88 mm Hg. Initial findings noted fewer Myocardial Infarctions and strokes within the Amlodipine arm, however further analysis showed significant differences in blood pressure in favour of Amlodipine group. The structure of the trial was so designed to gradually introduce diuretics in the Valsartan arm over several months. Until this was achieved, a higher blood pressure in the Valsartan group produced higher event rates that subsequently disappeared as blood pressure control improved. A post hoc attempt to control for this difference with matched blood pressure pairings of Amlodipine and Valsartan groups showed no difference in cardiac events, MI, stroke or mortality (61).

This study once again suggested that the main determinant of cardiovascular event was blood pressure response.

The **CAMELOT Trial (**Comparison of Enalapril vs. Amlodipine to Limit Occurrences of Thrombosis) compared Amlodipine (10 mg per day) and Enalapril (20 mg per day) versus placebo in reducing cardiovascular endpoints in patients with known coronary disease (62). The main outcomes were non-fatal MI, cardiac arrest and other cardiovascular events, which occurred at a rate of 23 % in placebo, 16.6% in Amlodipine and 20.2 % in the Enalapril group. Blood pressure increased by 0.7/0.6 mm Hg in placebo group and decreased by 4.8/2.5 mm Hg and 4.9/2.4 mm Hg in the Amlodipine and Enalapril groups respectively. Though there were equivalent hard endpoint events (all-cause mortality, non fatal MI, stroke) in both Amlodipine and Enalaprilarms, the soft endpoint events such as angina pectoris were significantly reduced by Amlodipine, hence reducing the total in favour of Amlodipine. While Amlodipine is known to have anti-anginal effect it is not the case with Enalapril. Also there were differences in pharmacodynamics of the drugs as Enalapril once a day has a half life of 11 hours while that of Amlodipine is 50 hours. Hence, since Enalapril was taken in the mornings, the blood pressure readings during the day will have severely underestimated the rise in night time BP in the Enalapril arm compared to Amlodipine.

The role of CCBs in patients with high cardiovascular risk was further evaluated in the four trials outlined below. The INSIGHT Trial **(Intervention as a Goal in Hypertension Treatment)** of 6000 high risk patients defined as having Hypertension plus at least one additional cardiovascular risk factor, compared CCB (Nifedipine) to Hydrochlorothiazide plus Amiloride (63). In this study total cardiovascular outcome (cardiovascular death, myocardial infarction, congestive heart failure, stroke) were the same in both groups, however the Nifedipine arm showed higher risk of fatal myocardial infarction and non fatal heart failure.

The **INVEST Trial** (The International verapamil-Trandolapril Study Hypertensive patients with known coronary artery disease compared Verapamil (maximum dose 180 mg twice daily) and Atenolol (maximum dose 50 mg twice daily) in reducing cardiovascular mortality and morbidity. Trandanopril and/or Thiazides were added for additional blood pressure control as needed. There was no difference in primary outcomes of death, non fatal myocardial infarction or nonfatal stroke (64). Hence, while DHP-CCBs (Nifedipine) were shown to increase cardiovascular mortality, non DHP-CCBs (Verapamil) have not shown such adverse outcomes. It has been shown that the peak and trough concentrations and variability in blood pressure with short acting Nifedipineare likely responsible factors for the increased cardiovascular mortality. This was further evaluated by the **ACTION Trial** (A Coronary Disease Trial Investigating Outcomes with Nifedipine GITS) comparing long acting Nifedipine (60 mg once a day) to placebo in patients with chronic stable angina (65). Most patients were treated with other anti-anginal therapy including Beta-blockers, aspirin and lipid lowering drugs and had a mean BP of 137/80.The primary end point was survival free of major cardiovascular events. At a follow up of 4.9 years, the mean blood pressure was significantly lower in the long acting Nifedipine group however despite this, it did not reduce primary end points or all cause mortality. The lack of benefit despite lowering of blood pressure may be due to lower cardiovascular risk of the patient population studied.

The **ASCOT Trial (The Anglo-Scandinavian Cardiac Outcomes Trial)** was designed to compare the incidence of adverse cardiovascular outcomes with Amlodipine 5 mg versus

Atenolol 50 mg in patients with hypertension and at least three other risk factors for Coronary Heart Disease. The combined primary outcome was fatal coronary events and nonfatal MI. Surprisingly, the trial was stopped prematurely due to worse outcomes in the Atenolol treated group (66, 67). Possible reasons for the difference in outcomes include lower blood pressure in Amlodipine group as well as once daily usage of Atenolol despite pharmokinetics favouring twice daily use as in the INVEST trial. It was estimated that the difference in blood pressure accounts for at least half the variance in outcomes. Therefore in summary, the ASCOT trial which included patients with no active cardiovascular disease, there was a difference in outcomes between Amlodipine and Atenolol partially attributed to BP differences between the two groups. In INVEST trial no such **difference was observed though it was in a different population.**

In the NAVIGATOR Trial (Valsartan in Impaired Glucose Tolerance Outcomes Research) in patients with Impaired Glucose Tolerance, over 9300 patients who had or were at risk of cardiovascular disease were randomly assigned to Valsartan (up to 160 mg/day) or placebo (68). The mean baseline BP was 140/83 mm Hg in both arms. At a median of 6.5 years there was no difference in the rate of cardiovascular events, despite significant lower blood pressure with Valsartan (132/78 mm HG, 2.8/1.4 mm Hg lower than placebo).

In the **ACCORD BP Trial (Action to Control Cardiovascular Risk in Diabetes)** of Goal Systolic Pressure less than 120 mm Hg in Type 2 Diabetes, 4733 patients were randomly assigned to a goal systolic blood pressure of less than 120 or less than 140 mm Hg (69). The mean baseline BP was 139/76 mm Hg at year one and thereafter, the average systolic pressures were 119 and 134 mm Hg in the two groups. At a mean follow up of 4.7 years, there was no significant difference between the groups in the primary outcome of cardiovascular death or non-fatal MI or stroke (1.9 versus 2.1 percent). The annual rate of all cause mortality was non-significantly higher with intensive therapy (1.28 versus 1.19 percent). Serious adverse events occurred in a higher proportion (3.3 versus 1.3 percent) in the intensive therapy arm. However, a prespecified secondary outcome, the annual rate of stroke, was significantly lower with intensive therapy (0.32 versus 0.53 percent). The conclusion of the ACCORD Trial, for those who meet the entry criteria (type 2 Diabetes Mellitus plus either cardiovascular disease or at least two additional risk factors for cardiovascular disease), the authors and reviewers of this topic suggest that the risks and burdens of aiming for a systolic pressure of less than 120 mm Hg plus the lack of experience of almost all physicians in attaining such a goal may be too great a burden to achieve the small reduction in stroke that may be attained (absolute benefit 1 in 89 patients at five years).

The **ONTARGET Trial** randomly assigned over 25,000 patients with atherosclerotic disease to Ramipril, Temlisartan, or both (54). There was a progressive reduction in stroke risk at attained systolic pressures of 121 compared to 130 mmHg or higher; in contrast, there was an increase in myocardial infarction risk at attained systolic pressures below 126 mmHg and cardiovascular mortality was unchanged or increased at attained systolic pressures below 130 mmHg expand.

The **PROGRESS Trial (Preventing Strokes by Lowering Blood Pressure in patients with Cerebral Ischemia)** compared Perindopril with or without adding Indapamide (a thiazide diuretic) to placebo in patients with a prior stroke (70). There was a progressive trend toward lower rates of recurrent stroke at lower systolic pressures down to below 120 mmHg in Perindopril group as compared to placebo. However as this was a placebo controlled trial the benefits of a particular anti hypertensive group of drugs were not studied.

Trials	Population Studied	Intervention	Outcome	Comments
HOPE Trial (Heart Outcomes Prevention Evaluation)	Patients with high cardiovascular risk (without acute MI, LV dysfunction or heart failure)	Randomly assigned to Ramipril 5-10 mg/day or placebo	Terminated prematurely because of significant benefits in Ramipril arm only14% reaching primary end point (any cardiovascular event: CVA, MI, Cardiovascular death) vs17.8% in placebo A reduction in stroke was also seen with Ramipril	Although benefits were thought to be independent of BP control, an analysis of subset who underwent ABPM showed a significant drop in night time BP
EUROPA Trial (European Trial on Reduction of cardiac Events with Perindopril in Stable Coronary Artery Disease)	Similar to HOPE but patients with lower cardiovascular risk	Perindopril (8 mg once a day) vs placebo	Primary end point: MI, cardiac arrest or cardiovascular death- significant reduction in favour of Perindopril Perindopril associated with (5/2 mmHg) lower BP	Benefits of ACEI may be due to BP lowering and not to intrinsic property of the ACEI
VALUE Trial (Valsartan Antihypertensive Long -term use evaluation)	15,000 hypertensive patients	Valsartan vs Amlodipine	Initial findings fewer Myocardial Infarctions and strokes in Amlodipine arm, however there were significant differences in BP in favour of Amlodipine A post hoc attempt to control for this difference with matched BP pairings of Amlodipine and Valsartan groups showed no difference in cardiac events, MI, stroke or mortality	Suggests that main Determinant of cardiovascular event is BP response
CAMELOT Trial (Comparison of Enalapril vs. Amlodipine to Limit Occurrences of Thrombosis)	Patients with known coronary disease	Compared Amlodipine (10 mg per day) and Enalapril (20 mg per day) vs placebo in reducing cardiovascular endpoints	Equivalent hard endpoint events (all-cause mortality, non fatal MI, stroke) in both Amlodipine and Enalapril arms Soft endpoint events such as angina pectoris were significantly reduced by Amlodipine, hence reducing the total in favour of Amlodipine	Amlodipine has anti-anginal properties Differences exist in pharmacodynamics of the drugs (Enalapril half life shorter than Amlodipine 11 vs 50 hrs)
The INSIGHT Trial **(Intervention as a Goal in**	6000 high risk patients defined as having	CCB (Nifedipine) to Hydrochlorothiazide plus Amiloride	Cardiovascular outcome (cardiovascular death, myocardial infarction, congestive heart failure,	

Hypertension Treatment)	Hypertension plus at least one additional cardiovascular risk factor		stroke) were same However Nifedipine arm showed higher risk of fatal myocardial infarction & non fatal heart failure	
The INVEST Trial (The International verapamil-Trandolapril Study)	Hypertensive patients with known coronary artery disease	Compared Verapamil and Atenolol in reducing cardiovascular mortality & morbidity Trandanopril and/or Thiazides added for BP control as needed	No difference in primary outcomes of death, non fatal myocardial infarction or nonfatal stroke	In contrast to outcomes with Nifedipine suggesting that peak / trough concentrations and variability in BP with short acting Nifedipine might be responsible for increased cardiovascular mortality
ACTION Trial (A Coronary Disease Trial Investigating Outcomes with Nifedipine GITS)	Patients with chronic stable angina	long acting Nifedipine (60 mg once a day) vs placebo	Primary end point: survival free of major cardiovascular events Mean BP significantly lower in long acting Nifedipine group however despite this, it did not reduce primary end points or all cause mortality	May be due to lower cardiovascular risk of the patients
ASCOT Trial (The Anglo-Scandinavian Cardiac Outcomes Trial)	Patients with hypertension and at least three other risk factors for Coronary Heart Disease	Amlodipine 5 mg vs Atenolol 50 mg	Primary outcome: fatal coronary events and nonfatal MI Stopped prematurely due to worse outcomes in Atenolol group	Reasons for difference in outcomes include lower BP in Amlodipine group and once daily usage of Atenolol despite pharmokinetics favouring twice daily use
NAVIGATOR Trial (Valsartan in Impaired Glucose Tolerance Outcomes Research	Over 9300 patients with Impaired Glucose Tolerance at risk of cardiovascular disease	Randomly assigned to Valsartan or placebo	No difference in rate of cardiovascular events, despite significant lower BP with Valsartan	
ACCORD BP Trial (Action to Control Cardiovascular Risk in Diabetes)	4733 patients type 2 Diabetes Mellitus plus either cardiovascular	Randomly assigned to goal systolic BP < 120 vs <140 mm Hg	No significant difference in primary outcome of cardiovascular death or non-fatal MI or stroke	

	disease or at least two additional risk factors		All cause mortality was non-significantly higher with intensive therapy Higher rate of serious adverse events in intensive therapy arm but secondary outcome: annual stroke rate was significantly lower	
ONTARGET Trial	Over 25,000 patients with atherosclerotic disease	Randomly assigned to Ramipril, Temlisartan, or both	Reduction in stroke risk at systolic BP 121 vs 130 mmHg or higher An increase in myocardial infarction risk at systolic BP < 126 mmHg Cardiovascular mortality unchanged or increased at systolic BP < 130 mmHg	
PROGRESS Trial (Preventing Strokes by Lowering Blood Pressure in patients with Cerebral Ischemia)	Patients with a prior stroke	Perindopril with or without Indapamide (thiazide diuretic) vs placebo	Trend toward lower rates of recurrent stroke at lower systolic BP (down to < 120 mmHg) in Perindopril group	As this was placebo controlled trial, benefits of a particular anti hypertensive group of drugs were not studied

Table 3. Summary of Cardiovascular Trials

"Reconciling the evidence"

Some controversies still exist in hypertension trials. For example, though it is established unequivocally that hypertension is a risk factor for chronic kidney disease and cardiovascular disease, the superiority of individual drug classes over others, with regards to these outcomes remains unclear. Landmark trials, such as the ALLHAT (Antihypertensive and Lipid Lowering to Prevent Heart Attack Trial) (6) lie at the heart of this controversy. Their finding of no superiority for Angiotensin converting enzyme inhibitors (ACEI) with respect to ESRD outcome is in clear contradiction to the multitude of outcome trials in CKD patients where the role of ACEI has been established.

Further confusion in comparing outcomes from various trials arises because of variability in their design, patient demographics, underlying cardiovascular risk factors as well as the studied primary outcomes. This leads to tremendous variability in studies addressing the supremacy or lack of, for a specific drug class. For instance, the LIFE trial (Lorsartan Intervention for End Points) (71) demonstrated lower CV outcomes for patients with LVH treated with Losartan versus Atenolol despite equivalent blood pressure (BP) control. Conversely, in VALUE (Valsartan Antihypertensive Long Term Use Evaluation)(72) Valsartan did not show benefit in cardiovascular mortality as compared to Amlodipine for the same level of blood pressure control. However, there was significant difference in the blood pressure between the two groups favouring the Amlodipine arm. These studies show

how the conduct of different trials can lead to contrasting findings with respect to superiority of one drug over the other and the care needed to evaluate them.

Controversies further arise when trials designed to study cardiac outcomes are used to evaluate renal outcomes. One example is the ALLHAT trial (6), which showed that diuretics were superior to ACEI with regards to renal outcomes, even though it was primarily designed to study cardiac and not renal outcomes. This is in contrast to most studies with primary renal outcomes which showed that administration of ACEI or Angiotensin receptor blockers (ARBs) was associated with lower urine protein excretion, slower doubling of serum creatinine and lower rate of decline of GFR and hence progression to End Stage Renal Disease (ESRD). However these renal outcome trials were not designed or powered to evaluate cardiovascular events. Therefore it is important to carefully scrutinize trials to identify the primary outcome they were intended to and thus are powered to assess.

Possible explanations for the adverse outcomes seen with ACEI in ALLHAT include the following:

The diuretic arm had better control of blood pressure. During The first two years there was a significantly better BP control of at least 4 mm Hg in the diuretic arm.

The ACEI may be handicapped by the unfavourable use of Beta-blockers as add- on therapy in a significant number of black patients.

In the ALLHAT trial Beta-blockers were used as a second line agent in all four groups. Specifically, only 18 percent of the ACEI group received a diuretic and mainly in the last year or two. This led to a 4-5 mm Hg higher blood pressure in the ACEI arm likely accounting for greater CV outcomes.

The ALLHAT trial hence concluded that diuretics are similar if not superior to ACEI and CCBs with regards to cardiovascular protection and mortality. However the increased incidence of diabetes mellitus noted with diuretic use is not without significant clinical consequences. Notably, the effect of diabetes on CV event rates is not apparent until a minimum of 6 years and becomes progressively more pronounced. It eventually results in increased cardiovascular event rate at 15 years, which is similar to that seen in pre-existing diabetes. This was shown in **SHEP trial** (Systolic Hypertension in Elderly Program) where new onset diabetes was associated with a high risk of CV events, similar to its incidence in patients with diabetes at the beginning of the study (73). Hence, because of the short observation period of ALLHAT of only 12.5 years, diuretic-linked new onset diabetes, would be expected to result in increased CV events had the follow- up been extended.

Possible explanations for the contrasting findings between the ALLHAT and ANBP2 trials include:

1. Different patient demographics, with a predominant white population as compared to high proportion of black patients in ALLHAT trial who were in fact older. As stated previously white patients have shown better response to ACEI's than diuretics.
2. The patient population were different, ALLHAT included patients with one additional cardiovascular risk factor.
3. In ANBP2 trial the antihypertensive agent (Lisinopril or Hydrochlorothiazide) and dose were chosen by the physician. The possible high dose use of Hydrochlorothiazide with its associated adverse cardiovascular side effects may have contributed to adverse outcomes.
4. Primary outcomes for ALLHAT and ANBP2 were different. While in ALLHAT the primary outcome was death from coronary causes or nonfatal myocardial infarction, in ANBP2 it was all fatal and nonfatal cardiovascular events. Once again this highlights how differences between ALLHAT and ANBP2 trials in design, demographics and outcomes can influence the results of the study.

Though, the **ALLHAT Trial** (24) of more than 44,000 hypertensive patients failed to show superiority of ACEI, DHP-CCBs and alpha blockers over a thiazide diuretic with respect to cardiovascular outcomes. In post hoc analysis, neither ACEI nor CCB was superior to thiazide diuretic with respect to renal outcomes. This trial was contradictory to other primary renal outcome trials that showed benefit of ACEI over other drug classes. Some of the factors responsible for this controversy will be explored. The ALLHAT did not select patients with renal disease as an inclusion criterion, since it was not mainly a renal outcome trial. Blood pressure was also lower in thiazide arm as compared to the other arms hence equivalency of blood pressure was not achieved. Furthermore, no urine tests were performed even though renal outcomes were studied thus failing to identify those who were at highest risk for progression and most likely to derive benefit from ACEI i.e. patients with proteinuric diabetic kidney disease. Hence, in the ALLHAT trial little or no attention was paid to kidney function, consequently the results of ALLHAT regarding renal outcomes remain unresolved.

In addition, the Casas meta-analysis was heavily weighted on the ALLHAT (non renal outcome trial) and little or no attention was paid to IDNT, RENAAL, AASK and REIN trials, the latter studies upon which our current guidelines are based. Hence, this analysis correctly concludes that these agents benefit non-diabetic renal disease and, mistakenly deduces that ACEI/A2RBs are non beneficial in diabetic proteinuric kidney disease. This partially flawed trial may result in physicians using less effective antihypertensive drugs in patients with kidney disease. Any attempt to reconcile the renal outcomes in ALLHAT, a cardiovascular outcomes trial, with those from IDNT, RENAAL, REIN, AASK and other renal trials fails because of different patient populations, designs and outcomes. Though less expensive antihypertensive drugs are desirable for BP control, they are less effective for renoprotection in chronic kidney disease and should therefore be used as adjuncts. Moreover, the average GFR of the studies selected was equivalent to Stage 2 CKD, and was much higher than in those studies that showed benefit of ACEI and ARBs.

Clinical pearls

It can be concluded that ACEIs are the medication of choice in reducing microalbuminuria in diabetic hypertensive patients. Studies clearly show that blocking of the Renin Angiotensin Aldosterone System (RAAS) with ACEI or ARBs in patient with type II diabetes mellitus reduces the risk of progression of microalbuminuria to overt proteinuria and may even revert it back to normoalbuminuria, both in hypertensive and normotensive patients. It is also likely that Aliskerin may have additional renoprotective effects, independent of blood pressure lowering, in hypertensive patients with type2 diabetes and nephropathy who are already receiving the recommended therapy.

Recommendations on choice of antihypertensive agents

The choice of antihypertensive agents in diabetic patients is based upon their ability to prevent adverse cardiovascular events and to slow progression of renal disease, if present.

The two major studies which would influence the choice of therapy are the ALLHAT and ACCOMPLISH trials. To summarize again, in the ALLHAT trial, the benefits from diuretics compared to other classes, may have been related to the lower attained blood pressures. Another factor which was not addressed was the detrimental effects of thiazides on glucose metabolism. In the ACCOMPLISH trial, on the other hand, the combination of an ACE inhibitor and CCB provided better cardiovascular protection as compared to ACE inhibitor with thiazide.

While long acting ACEI or ARB would be the drug of choice in diabetic patients with hypertension and microalbuminuria, we would also recommend adding a long acting dihydropyridine calcium channel blocker as combination therapy for uncontrolled hypertension, given the results of ACCOMPLISH trial. If a Beta-blocker is given, Carvedilol may be the drug of choice because of potential benefits on glycemic control and lower rate of development of microalbuminuria compared to Metoprolol. A loop diuretic is likely to be necessary in patients with renal disease or heart failure.

Recommendations on target/goal blood pressure

Based on the trials described above including ACCORD BP trial, we recommend, a goal blood pressure of less than 140/90 mmHg in patients with diabetes. A goal blood pressure of less than 130/80 mmHg is recommended for patients with diabetic nephropathy and proteinuria (defined as 500 mg/day or more). These recommendations differ from the pre-ACCORD era when a goal of less than 130/80 mmHg was recommended for all diabetic patients.

Goal BP recommendations

While the guidelines suggested by European Society of Hypertension/European Society of Cardiology and American Heart Association recommend a blood pressure less than 130/80 for patients with atherosclerotic cardiovascular disease, the recent ACCORD trial along with ONTARGET and PROGRESS raise some concerns with this target.

We recommend antihypertensive therapy to lower the blood pressure to less than 140/90 mmHg in all patients. An attempt to lower the systolic pressure below 130 to 135 mmHg should be undertaken, if it can be achieved without producing significant side effects, though this has not been well defined. The risks of aiming for a goal systolic pressure of less than 120 mmHg may be too great a burden to achieve the small reduction in stroke that may be attained (absolute benefit 1 in 89 patients at five years). However, such a goal may be considered in highly motivated patients who would accept more aggressive antihypertensive therapy to further reduce their risk of stroke.

5. References

[1] Whelton PK, He J, Appel LJ, et al: Primary Prevention of Hypertension: Clinical and Public Health advisory from the National High Blood Pressure Education Program. JAMA 2002; 288: 1882.

[2] He J, Whelton PK, Appel LJ, et al: Long term weight loss and dietary sodium reduction on incidence of hypertension. Hypertension 2000;35: 544

[3] Turnball F: Effects of different blood pressure lowering regimens on cardiovascular events: Results of Prospectively designed overviews of randomised trials. Lancet 2003; 362: 1527

[4] Materson BJ, Reda DJ, Cushman WC, et al: Single drug therapy for hypertension in men. A comparison of six antihypertensive agents with placebo. N Engl J Med1994;330:1689

[5] Neaton JD, Grimm RH, PrineasRJet al: Treatment of Mild Hypertension study: Final results. JAMA 1993;270:713

[6] Major outcomes in high risk hypertensive patients randomised to Angiotensin converting enzyme inhibitor or calcium channel blocker vs. diuretic: The Antihypertensive and Lipid Lowering Treatment to Prevent Heart Attack Trial (ALLHAT). JAMA 2002; 288: 2981

[7] Pahor M, Psaty BM, Alderman MH, et al. Health Outcomes associated with calcium antagonists compared with other first line antihypertensive therapies. A Meta analysis of randomised controlled trials. Lancet 2000; 356: 1949.

[8] Wing LM, Reid CM, Ryan P, et al: A comparison of outcomes with Angiotensin converting enzyme inhibitors and diuretics for hypertension in the elderly. N Engl J Med 2003; 348:583.

[9] Hansson L, Lindholm LH, Ekbom T, et al: Randomised trial of old and new antihypertensive drugs in elderly patients: cardiovascular mortality and morbidity the Swedish Trial in Old patients with Hypertension-2 study. Lancet 1999; 354: 1751

[10] Hansson L, Hedner T, Lung- Johansen P, et al: NORDIL Study Group. Randomised trial of effects of calcium antagonists compared with diuretics and Beta blockers on cardiovascular mortality and morbidity in hypertension: the Nordic Diltiazem (NORDIL) study. Lancet 2000; 356:359

[11] MRC trial of treatment of mild hypertension: principal results. Medical Research Council Working Party. Br Med J (Clin Res Ed) 1985;291:97

[12] Medical Research Council trial of treatment of hypertension in older adults: principal results. MRC Working Party. BMJ 1992; 304:405

[13] Jamerson K, Weber MA, Bakris GL, et al: ACCOMPLISH Trial Investigators. Benazepril plus Amlodipine or hydrochlorothiazide for hypertension in high-risk patients. N Engl J Med. 2008; 359(23):2417.

[14] Rosendorff C, Black HR, Cannon CP, et al. Treatment of hypertension in the prevention and management of ischemic heart disease: a scientific statement from the American Heart Association Council for High Blood Pressure Research and the Councils on Clinical Cardiology and Epidemiology and Prevention. Circulation 2007; 115:2761.

[15] Mancia G, De Backer G, Dominiczak A, et al. 2007 Guidelines for the management of arterial hypertension: The Task Force for the Management of Arterial Hypertension of the European Society of Hypertension (ESH) and of the European Society of Cardiology (ESC). Eur Heart J 2007; 28:1462.

[16] Chobian AV, Bakris GL, Black HR, et al. The Seventh Report of the Joint National Committee on Prevention, detection, Evaluation, and Treatment of High Blood Pressure: the JNC 7 report. JAMA 2003; 289:2560.

[17] Bakris GL, Weir MR, Secic M, et al: Differential effects of calcium antagonists subclasses on markers of nephropathy progression. Kidney Int 2004; 65: 1991.

[18] Gansevoort RT, Sluiter WJ, Hemmelder MH, et al: Antiproteinuric effects of blood pressure lowering agents. A Meta analysis of comparative trials. Nephrol Dial Transplant 1995; 10: 1963.

[19] Apperloo AJ, de Zeeuw D, Sluiter HE et al: Differential effects of Enalapril and Atenolol on proteinuria and renal haemodynamics in non diabetic renal disease. BMJ 1991; 303: 821.

[20] Rosenberg ME, Hostetter TH. Comparative effects of antihypertensives on proteinuria. Angiotensive converting enzyme inhibitor versus alpha 1 antagonist. Am J Kidney Dis 1991; 18: 472.

[21] Hilgers KF, Mann JF. ACE inhibitors versus AT (1) receptor antagonists in patients with chronic renal disease. J Am SocNephrol 2002; 13: 1100.

[22] Remuzzi A, Perico N, Sangalli F et al: ACE inhibition and AnG II receptor blockade improve glomerular size selectivity in IgA nephropathy. Am J Physiol 1999; 276: F457.

[23] Aranda P, Segura J, RuilopeLM, et al: Long term renoprotective effects of standard versus high dose Temlisartan in hypertensive nondiabetic nephropathies. Am J Kidney Dis 2005; 46:1074.

[24] Rahman M, Pressel S, Davis BR, et al: Renal outcomes in high risk hypertensive patients treated with and Angiotensin converting enzyme inhibitor or calcium

channel blocker vs. a diuretic: a report from the Antihypertensive and Lipid Lowering Treatment to Prevent Heart Attack Trial (ALLHAT). Arch Intern Med 2005; 165: 936.
[25] Randomised placebo controlled trial of effect of Ramipril on decline in glomerular filtration rate and risk of terminal renal failure in proteinuric, non diabetic nephropathy. The GISEN Group (GruppoItaliano di StudiEpidemiologici in Nfrologia). Lancet 1997; 349: 1857.
[26] Ruggenenti P, Perna A, Loriga G, et al: Blood pressure control for renoprotection in patients with non diabetic chronic renal disease (REIN-2): multicenter, randomised, controlled trial. Lancet 2005;365: 939.
[27] Klahr S, Levey AS, Beck GJ, et al: The effects of dietary protein restriction and blood pressure control on the progression of chronic renal disease. N Engl J med 1994; 330:877.
[28] Maschio G, Alberti D, Janin G, et al: Effect of Angiotensin converting enzyme inhibitor Benazepril on the progression of chronic renal insufficiency. N Engl J Med 1996; 334:939.
[29] Nakao N, Yoshimura A, Morita H, et al: Combination treatment of Angiotensin II receptor blocker and Angiotensin converting enzyme inhibitor in non diabetic renal disease (COOPERATE): A randomised control trial. Lancet 2003; 361: 117.
[30] Rutkowski P, Tylicki L, Renke M, et al: Low dose dual blockade of the renin Angiotensin system in patients with primary glomerulonephritis. Am J Kidney Dis 2004; 43:260.
[31] Remuzzi G, Macia M, Ruggenenti P, et al: Prevention and treatment of diabetic renal disease in type 2 diabetes: the BENEDICT study. J AM SocNephrol 2006; 17 (Suppl2): S90.
[32] Ravera M, RattoE,Vettoretti S, et al: Prevention and treatment of diabetic nephropathy: The program for Irbesartan Mortality and Morbidity Evaluation. J Am SocNephrol 2005;16: 48.
[33] Berl T, Hunsicker LG, Lewis JB, et al: Impact of achieved blood pressure on cardiovascular outcomes in the Irbersartan diabetic Nephropathy trial. J Am SocNephrol 2005; 16: 2170.
[34] Pohl MA, Blumenthal S, Cordonnier DJ, et al: Independent and additive impact of blood pressure control and Angiotensin II receptor blockade on renal outcomes in the Ibersartan diabetic nephropathy trial. J Am SocNeprol 2005; 16: 3027.
[35] Lewis EJ, Hunsicker LJ, Clarke WR, et al: Renoprotective effect of the Angiotensin receptor antagonist irbersartan in patients with nephropathy due to type 2 diabetes. N Engl J Med 2001; 345: 851.
[36] Parving HH, Lehnert H, Brochner-Mortensen J, et al: Irbesartan in Patients with Type 2 Diabetes and Microalbuminuria Study Group: The effect of irbesartan on the development of diabetic nephropathy in patients with type 2 diabetes. N Engl J Med 2001;345: 870
[37] Heart Outcomes Prevention Evaluation Study Investigators: Effects of Ramipril on cardiovascular and microvascular outcomes in people with diabetes mellitus: results of the HOPE study and MICRO-HOPE sub study. Heart Outcomes Prevention Evaluation Study Investigators. Lancet 2000; 355: 253.
[38] Gerstein HC: HOPE and MICRO-HOPE. Reduction of cardiovascular events and microvascular complications in diabetes with ACE inhibitor treatment. Diabetes Metab Res Rev 2002; Supp3:S82.

[39] Viberti G, Wheeldon NM; for the MARVAL Study Investigators: Microalbuminuria reduction with Valsartan in patients with type 2 diabetes mellitus: Blood pressure independent effect. Circulation 2002: 106 : 672

[40] Lewis EJ, Hunsicker LG, Bain RP et al: The effect of Angiotensin converting enzyme inhibition on diabetic nephropathy. N Engl J Med 1993; 329: 1456.

[41] Herbert LA, Bain RP, Verme D, et al: Remission of nephrotic range proteinuria in Type I Diabetes. Kidney Int 1994; 46:1688.

[42] Hovind P, Rossing P, Tarnow L, et al: Remission and regression in the nephropathy of type 1 diabetes when blood pressure is controlled aggressively. Kidney Int 2001; 60: 277.

[43] Adler AI, Stratton IM, Neil HA et al: Association of systolic blood pressure with microvascular and macrovascular complications of type 2 diabetes (UKPDS 36): prospective observational study. BMJ 2000; 321: 421.

[44] Brenner BM, Cooper ME, de Zeeuw D, et al: Effects of losartan on renal and cardiovascular outcomes in patients with type 2 diabetes and nephropathy. N Engl J Med 2001;345:861-9

[45] Barnett AH, Bain SC, Bouter P, et al: Angiotensin receptor blockade versus converting enzyme inhibition in type 2 diabetes and nephropathy. N Engl J Med; 351: 1952.

[46] Jacobsen P, Andersen S, Rossing K, et al: Dual blockade of the renin Angiotensin system versus maximal recommended dose of ACE inhibition in diabetic nephropathy. Kidney Int 2003; 63: 1874.

[47] Morgensen CE, Neldam S, Tikkanen I, et al: Randomised controlled trial of dual blockade of renin Angiotensin system in patients with hypertension, microalbuminuria, and non insulin dependent diabetes: the Candersartan and Lisinopril Microalbuminuria (CALM) study. BMJ 2000; 321: 1440.

[48] Song JH, Cha SH, Lee HJ, et al: Effect of low dose dual blockade of renin Angiotensin system on urinary TGF-Beta in Type 2 diabetic patients with advanced kidney disease. Nephrol Dial Transplant 2006; 21: 683.

[49] Vanden, Meiracker AH, Baggen RG, et al: Spironolactone in type 2 diabetic nephropathy: effects of proteinuria, blood pressure and renal function. J Hypertens 2006; 24: 2285.

[50] Epstein M, Williams GH, Weinberger M, et al: Selective aldosterone blockade with eplerenone reduces microalbuminuria in patients with type 2 diabetes. Clin J Am SocNephrol 2006; 1: 940.

[51] Bakris GL, Fonseca V, Kathole RE, et al: Metabolic effects of Carveldiol vs. metoprolol in patients with type 2 diabetes mellitus and hypertension. JAMA 2004; 292: 2227.

[52] Bakris GL, Fonseca V, Katholi RE, et al: Differential effects of Beta blockers on albuminuria in patients with type 2 diabetes. Hypertension 2005; 46: 335.

[53] Parving HH, Persson F, Lewis JB, et al. Aliskiren combined with Losartan in type 2 diabetes and nephropathy. N Engl J Med 2008; 358:2433.

[54] ONTARGET Investigators: Yusuf S, Teo KK, et al. Temlisartan, Ramipril, or both in patients at high risk for vascular events. N Engl J Med 2008; 358:1547.

[55] Casas JP, Chua W, Luokogeorgakis, et al: Effects of inhibitors of renin Angiotensin system and other antihypertensive drugs on renal outcomes: systematic review and meta- analysis. Lancet 2005; 366:2026.

[56] Villarosa IP, Bakris GL: The Appropriate Blood Pressure Control in Diabetes (ABCD) Trial. J Hum Hypertens 1998;12: 653.

[57] Yusuf S, Sleight P, Pogue J, et al: Effects of Angiotensin converting enzyme inhibitor, Ramipril , on cardiovascular events in high risk patients. The Heart Outcomes Prevention Evaluation Study Investigators. N Engl J Med 2000; 342: 145.

[58] Dagenais GR, Yusuf S, Bourassa MG, et al: Effects of Ramipril on coronary events in high risk persons: results of the heart Outcomes Prevention Evaluation Study. Circulation 2001; 104: 522.

[59] Bosch J, Yusuf S, Pogue J, et al: Use of Ramipril in preventing stroke: double blind randomised trial. BMJ 2002; 324: 699.

[60] Daly CA, Fox KM, Remme WJ, et al: The effect of Perindopril on cardiovascular morbidity and mortality in patients with diabetes in the EUROPA study: results from the PERSUADE sub study. Eur Heart J 2005; 26: 1369.

[61] Weber MA, Julius S, Kjeldsen SE, et al: Blood pressure dependent and independent effects of antihypertensive treatment on clinical events in the Value trial. Lancet 2004; 363: 2049.

[62] NissenSE,Tuzcu EM, Libby P, et al: Effect of antihypertensive agents on cardiovascular events in patients with coronary disease and normal blood pressure: the CAMELOT study: a randomised controlled trial. JAMA 2004; 292: 2217.

[63] Brown MJ, Palmer CR, Castaigne A, et al: Morbidity and Mortality in patients randomised to double blind treatment with a long acting calcium channel blocker or diuretic in the International Nifedipine GITS study: Intervention as a Goal in Hypertension Treatment (INSIGHT). Lancet 2000; 356:366.

[64] Pepine CJ, Handberg EM, Cooper-DeHoffRM, et al: A calcium antagonist versus a non-calcium antagonist hypertension treatment strategy for patients with coronary artery disease. The International Verapamil- Trandolapril Study (INVEST): a randomised controlled trial. JAMA 2003; 290: 2805.

[65] Poole-Wilson PP, Lubsen PJ, Kirwan BA, et al: Effect of long acting Nifedipine on mortality and cardiovascular morbidity in patients with stable angina requiring treatment (ACTION trial): randomised controlled trial. Lancet 2004; 364: 849.

[66] Dahlof B, Sever PS, Poulter NR, et al: Prevention of cardiovascular events with an antihypertensive regimen of Amlodipine adding Perindopril as required versus Atenolol adding Bendroflumethiazide as required, in the Anglo- Scandinavian Cardiac outcomes trial- Blood Pressure Lowering Arm (ASCOT-BPLA): a multicenter randomised controlled trial. Lancet 2005; 366: 895

[67] Poulter NR, Wedel H, Dahlof B, et al: Role of blood pressure and other variables in the differential cardiovascular event rates noted in the Anglo Scandinavian Cardiac Outcomes Trial-Blood Pressure Lowering Arm (ASCOT-BPLA). Lancet 2005; 366: 907.

[68] NAVIGATOR Study Group, McMurray JJ, Holman RR, et al. Effect of Valsartan on the incidence of diabetes and cardiovascular events. N Engl J Med 2010; 362: 1477.

[69] ACCORD Study Group, Cushman WC, Evans GW, et al. Effects of intensive blood-pressure control in type 2 diabetes mellitus. N Engl J Med 2010; 362:1575.

[70] PROGRESS Collaborative Group. Randomised trial of a perindopril=based blood - pressure -lowering regimen among 6,105 individuals with previous stroke or transient ischaemic attack. Lancet 2001; 358:1033.

[71] Brenner BM, Cooper ME, de Zeeuw D, et al: Effects of Losartan on renal and cardiovascular outcomes in patients with type 2 diabetes and nephropathy. N Engl J Med; 345: 861.

[72] Parving HH, Hommel E, Jensen BR. Long-term beneficial effect of ACE inhibition on diabetic nephropathy in normotensive type 1 diabetic patients. Kidney Int 2001; 60:228

[73] Prevention of stroke by antihypertensive drug treatment in older persons with isolated systolic hypertension. Final results of Systolic Hypertension in the Elderly Program (SHEP). SHEP Cooperative Research Group. JAMA 1991;265:3255

8

Cardiac Biomarkers in End-Stage Renal Disease

Leo Jacobs, Alma Mingels and Marja van Dieijen-Visser
Department of Clinical Chemistry, Maastricht University Medical Centre (MUMC)
The Netherlands

1. Introduction

Patients with end-stage renal disease (ESRD) often suffer from cardiovascular complications and comorbidities. For example, 55% of ESRD patients suffer from congestive heart failure (CHF) and cardiovascular diseases account for the majority of deaths among ESRD patients (Herzog, Ma, & Collins, 1998; National Institutes of Health; National Institute of Diabetes and Digestive and Kidney Diseases; Bethesda, 2007). It is, therefore, of great importance to diagnose the underlying cardiac pathologies and to provide accurate risk stratification in ESRD patients.

Over the years, a number of accurate and sensitive biochemical markers have been introduced that have greatly advanced the diagnosis and risk stratification of cardiovascular diseases. The most prominent of these biochemical markers are the cardiac troponins (cTn, either T or I) and the brain natriuretic peptides (BNPs) and their use has revolutionized the diagnosis and risk stratification of acute coronary syndromes (ACS) and CHF respectively (A. S. Maisel et al., 2002; Thygesen, Alpert, & White, 2007). However, in the setting of ESRD, cardiac troponin concentrations can be elevated in the absence of apparent cardiac damage or clinical symptoms (Apple, Murakami, Pearce, & Herzog, 2004; Aviles et al., 2002; C. deFilippi et al., 2003; Havekes et al., 2006; Sommerer, Beimler, et al., 2007). Similarly, BNP and N-terminal proBNP (NT-proBNP) concentrations are virtually always increased in ESRD patients (Apple et al., 2004; Madsen et al., 2007). The presence of such continuously elevated cardiac troponin, BNP and NT-proBNP concentrations can interfere with their diagnostic and prognostic potential in ESRD patients (David et al., 2008; Pimenta et al., 2009; Wu et al., 2007).

In this chapter, we will elaborate on the frequency of these cardiac biomarker elevations and discuss the underlying mechanisms behind them. In addition, we discuss the diagnostic and prognostic impact of these elevations and present approaches to improve the usefulness of cTn, BNP and NT-proBNP measurements.

2. The cardiac troponins

The troponin complex consists of three proteins, troponin C (TnC), troponin I (TnI) and troponin T (TnT) that together with tropomyosin regulate the affinity of actin towards myosin during muscle contraction (Kobayashi, Jin, & de Tombe, 2008), as illustrated in Figure 1. The troponin complex is present in all striated muscles, but different isoforms of troponin I and T exist in skeletal and cardiac tissue. This tissue specific expression of **cardiac** troponin I (cTnI) and **cardiac** troponin T (cTnT) isoforms within the heart has enabled the development of immunoassays that can specifically detect troponin originating from the heart (Cummins, Auckland, & Cummins, 1987; Katus et al., 1989). Nowadays, the cTns have become the biomarker of choice for the detection of myocardial injury and play an integral part in the diagnosis of ACS. According to current guidelines, (Morrow et al., 2007; Thygesen, Alpert, & White, 2007) an AMI is diagnosed when an increase or decrease in cardiac biomarker concentrations (preferably cTn), above the 99th percentile of the upper reference limit (URL) is detected, in combination with evidence of myocardial ischemia, as detected, either by clinical symptoms, electrocardiographic changes or imaging evidence. Additionally, the guidelines state that the cTn-assays should be able to measure the 99th percentile concentrations with a coefficient of variation (CV) smaller than 10%(Thygesen, Alpert, & White, 2007). Ideally, blood samples for the measurements of cTn should be drawn on first assessment (after the onset of clinical symptoms) and 6-9 hours later in order to detect a rising or falling pattern, as can be interpreted from Figure 2. However, cTn levels can remain elevated for some time and the diagnostic window for diagnosing AMI can remain open for several days after the onset of symptoms (e.g. when a patients presents > 24 hours after onset of symptoms).

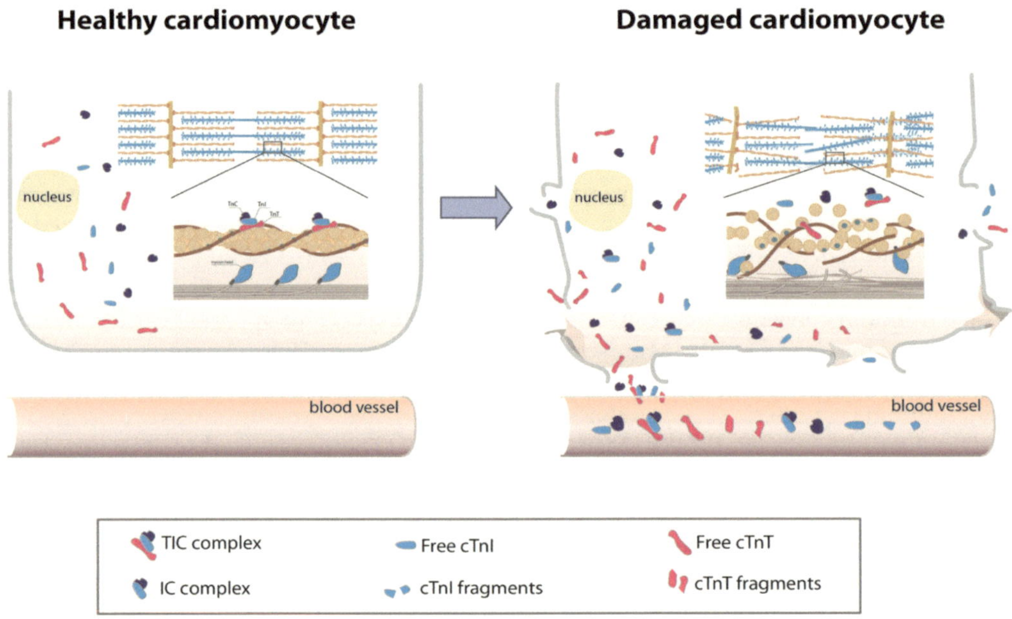

Fig. 1. The release of cTn from damaged cardiomyocytes.

Most of the studies investigating cTnT and cTnI elevations outside of AMI have been performed using immunoassays that lack sufficient analytical performance to accurately detect cTn concentrations in healthy subjects. As illustrated in Figure 3, most of the current cTn assays have either the limit of detection (LOD) of the assay higher than the reference concentrations or the CV exceeds 10% at the 99th URL (Giannitsis & Katus, 2004; Panteghini, 2006; Panteghini et al., 2004). Highly sensitive assays with the ability to accurately measure cTn values even in healthy subjects have been developed recently for cTnT (Giannitsis et al., 2010) and cTnI (F.S. Apple, 2009; Todd et al., 2007). The increased sensitivity may improve the prognostic power of cTn measurements and may enhance identification of subjects at

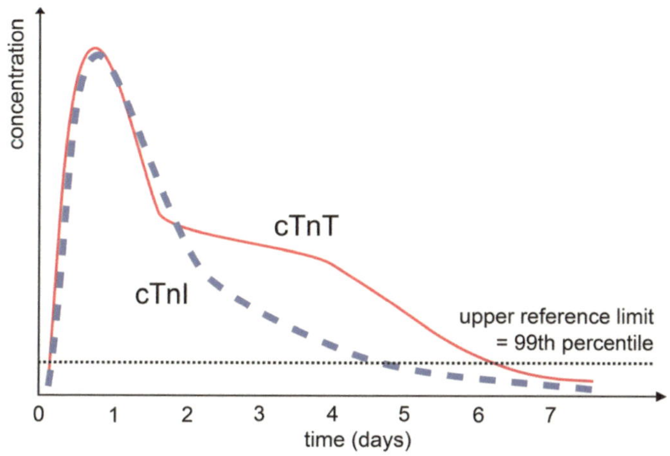

Fig. 2. The release kinetics of cTn after AMI.

risk. Indeed, two recent studies have shown the prognostic value of cTnT at previously undetectable levels in patients with stable coronary disease (Omland et al., 2009) and with stable chronic HF (Latini et al., 2007). Moreover, cTnT values measured by a high sensitive cTnT assay (hs-cTnT) that were undetectable with the conventional assay were found to be associated with the extent of coronary atherosclerosis (Laufer et al., 2010). Figure 1 visualizes the release of the cTns in response to cellular damage and figure 2 shows the typical release kinetics of the cTns seen after an acute myocardial infarction.

2.1 Cardiac troponin elevations in ESRD

In patients suffering from ESRD, cTn concentrations can be elevated in the absence of apparent cardiac damage or clinical symptoms (Apple et al., 2004; Aviles et al., 2002; C. deFilippi et al., 2003; Havekes et al., 2006; Sommerer, Beimler, et al., 2007). The exact frequency of these elevations varies somewhat between studies, depending on the patient inclusion criteria, the applied cut-off values and the troponin assay used. In general, cTnT has been found elevated more often than cTnI (roughly 53% for cTnT and 17% for cTnI as reviewed in (Kanderian & Francis, 2006)) although recent publications, using more sensitive assays suggest that the frequency of cTnT and cTnI elevations are similar (Hickman et al., 2007; Kumar, Michelis, Devita, Panagopoulos, & Rosenstock, 2010). It is important to note that the number of detected cTn elevations depends on the cut-offs that are used to define elevated values. As mentioned above, many cTn assays lack the sensitivity to accurately (<10% CV) measure the 99th percentile and the 10% CV is used as the diagnostic cut-off value. As a result the number of elevations will inevitably be lower when higher cut-off values are used. For example, in a study that we (Jacobs et al., 2009) performed in 32 ESRD patients we found that 38% of patients had cTnT elevations at baseline using the 10% CV cut-off, versus 63% using the 99th percentile cut-off with the contemporary 4th generation cTnT assay (Roche Diagnostics). Similarly cTnI concentrations where elevated above the 10% CV in 10% of the cases, compared to 50% elevations above the 99th percentile. Note that, the 10% CV is a property solely dependent on the sensitivity of the cTn assay and one should not compare cTn elevations above this level between assays. The introduction of guideline acceptable cTn assays that can accurate measure the 99th percentile will enable a better comparison of the frequencies of cTn elevations in ESRD patients.

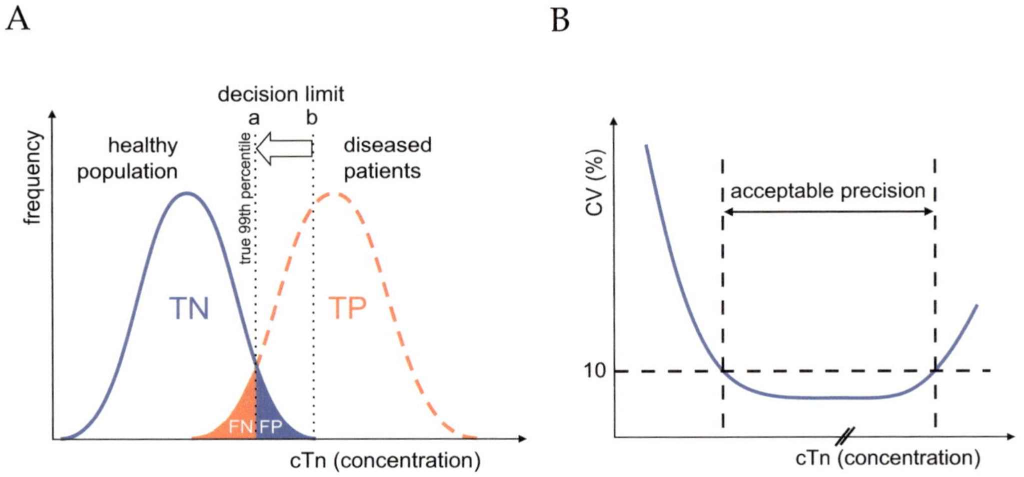

Fig. 3. (A) Biomarkers within the blood circulation follow a bell-shaped Gaussian distribution within a group of subjects. The diagnostic cut-off concentration for cTn is defined at the 99th percentile as measured in a healthy reference control group, so 1% of these subjects with the highest cTn concentrations are defined unhealthy (Apple et al., 2007; Morrow et al., 2007; Thygesen, Alpert, White, et al., 2007). At the time of definition, cTn concentrations were undetectable in all healthy individuals, as illustrated by decision limit 'b'. Improvements in the lower measuring range have lately resulted in cTn reference concentrations and thus also a true 99th percentile concentration. The lower decision limit is indicated by 'a'. However, this improvement in sensitivity = TP/(TP+FN) goes along with a worsening of the specificity = TN/(TN+FP). TP, number of subjects that were truly assigned positive; FN, number of subjects that were falsely assigned negative; TN, number of subjects that were truly assigned negative, FP, number of subjects that were falsely assigned positive; (B) A typical precision profile of an immunoassay. The diagnostic cutoff concentration should be measured with sufficient precision (coefficient of variation, CV = SD/mean <10%)(Panteghini et al., 2004).

In general, the use of more sensitive cTn assays will likely show that the presence of cTn elevations in ESRD patients might be even more frequent than previously thought. We found, that by using a more sensitive cTnT assay 94% of our patients had cTnT elevations above the 99th percentile with the hs-cTnT assay (Jacobs et al., 2009). Others have similarly found a larger amount of cTnI elevations in ESRD patients by using more sensitive cTnI assays (Hickman et al., 2007; Kumar et al., 2010).

With respect to the occurrence of cTn elevations in ESRD patients one should also take into account that the cTn concentrations in ESRD patients can vary over time, even in otherwise clinically stable patients. For example, by measuring cTn concentrations every two months, for a period of 6 months an additional number of patients with elevated cTn concentrations (at least once during the follow-up) could be identified (Jacobs et al., 2009). Similarly Roberts et al. have also shown longitudinal changes in the presence or absence of cTnT elevations in ESRD patients during a 1 year follow-up. In their study, cTnT values were measured 5 times and interestingly the patient survival decreased with increasing occurrence of cTnT elevations, i.e. the 1.7 year patients survival was 100%, 90% and 78% for patients with zero, one to four, or five out of five concentrations (Roberts et al., 2009). These findings are in line with above mentioned prognostic value of cTn elevations in ESRD patients. As such, assessing cTn concentrations at regular points in time would therefore appear as a sensible tool to increase clinical vigilance for the presence of myocardial damage and as a means for possible intervention. This is in agreement with previous studies which provided evidence for the increased ability of serial versus single cTn measurements to identify patients at risk for an event (Han, Lindsell, Ryan, & Gibler, 2005; Miller et al., 2007; Ooi, Zimmerman, Graham, & Wells, 2001; Roberts et al., 2004; Wayand, Baum, Schatzle, Scharf, & Neumeier, 2000).

2.1.1 Mechanisms underlying the cTn elevations

The underlying mechanisms behind these elevations have not been fully elucidated. The high incidence of coronary artery disease in ESRD patients (National Institutes of Health; National Institute of Diabetes and Digestive and Kidney Diseases; Bethesda, 2007) and the close relationship between cTn levels and the severity of coronary artery disease (C. deFilippi et al., 2003; Ooi, Isotalo, & Veinot, 2000) make the presence of subclinical ischemic cardiac damage a possible cause of cTn elevations. In this respect, it is also interesting to mention a study by DeFillipi et al. (C. R. deFilippi, Thorn, et al., 2007) who compared elevated cTnT values in 23 ESRD patients, with evidence of myocardial ischemia gathered by means of cardiovascular magnetic resonance (CMR) with late gadolinium enhancement (C. R. deFilippi, Thorn, et al., 2007). This study found that only a very small number of patients with elevated cTnT had CMR evidence of myocardial damage (0% of patients with cTnT <0.03 μg/L and 23% of patients with cTnT > 0.07 μg/L) (C. R. deFilippi, Thorn, et al., 2007). So, these patients, without known coronary artery disease and virtually no evidence of myocardial ischemia still had elevated cTnT values. These findings suggest there may be other than ischemia related reasons for the elevated levels of cTn. For example, the dialysis process itself can have a direct effect on cTn concentrations. There is some debate as to whether the dialysis process causes a decrease in cTn values (Montagnana et al., 2008) or an increase (Sommerer, Heckele, et al., 2007). In any case, different dialysis modalities like the use of high- or low- flux membranes and the method of vascular access can influence cTn concentrations (Lippi et al., 2008; Sommerer, Heckele, et al., 2007). For this reason, blood sampling times should be taken into account when measuring cTn concentrations and measurements are probably best performed pre-dialysis.

Another possible reason for the elevated cTn values in ESRD pertains to a decreased renal clearance of cTn. For example, the cTn half-life was shown to increase with the degree of renal impairment (Wiessner et al., 2007). Diris et al. (Diris et al., 2004) have shown the presence of immunoreactive cTnT fragments, which are small enough to be cleared by the kidneys and which might accumulate in ESRD patients. Others, however, have found only intact cTnT in patients with kidney failure, (Fahie-Wilson et al., 2006) and to date there is still a great deal of debate on the mechanisms underlying the cTn elevation in ESRD patients. Whatever the exact mechanism, the elevations should not be taken lightly as they are highly predictive for adverse cardiovascular events (Apple, Murakami, Pearce, & Herzog, 2002; Khan, Hemmelgarn, Tonelli, Thompson, & Levin, 2005; Sommerer, Beimler, et al., 2007).

2.2 Diagnosing AMI in ESRD

The presence of continuously elevated cTn concentrations can frustrate the diagnosis of AMI (eg. when ESRD patients are presenting with clinical symptoms). The National Academy of Clinical Biochemistry (NACB) has recognized this issue and has published guidelines that address this issue (Wu et al., 2007). These guidelines suggest that for patients with chronically elevated concentrations of cTn, changes in cTn (>20%) 6-9 hours after the onset of clinical symptoms are indicative of an AMI. To date, however, little is known about the analytical and biological variations of cTn in ESRD patients and >20% changes might also occur in the absence of clinical symptoms (Miller et al., 2007; Roberts et al., 2004). The lack of detailed knowledge of the biological variation in ESRD patients, in combination with the likely increase in the frequency of chronically elevated cTnT as a result of more sensitive measurements call for further refinement of the current guidelines. As the highly sensitive cTn assays will enable a more accurate assessment of the biological variation, the use of serial measurement in order to detect abnormal changes in cTn values will likely be incorporated into these refinements. A potential approach to incorporate the biological variation into the diagnosis of AMI could come from the use of reference change values (RCV) (Aakre & Sandberg, 2010). The RCV describes the change in a concentration between two time points, than can be perceived as significant, taking into account both the analytical and the individual (biological) variations and is calculated as follows:

$$RCV = z \times \sqrt{2} \times \sqrt{CV_A^2 + CV_I^2}$$

wherein z is the z score, which can be set at the desired level of statistical significance. The analytical variation is described by the CV_A and the individual (biological) variation by the CV_I (Omar, van der Watt, & Pillay, 2008). To date, there are only a few studies that investigated the RCV values for cTnT (Vasile, Saenger, Kroning, & Jaffe, 2010) and cTnI (Wu, Lu, Todd, Moecks, & Wians, 2009) in healthy subjects and more studies are needed to examine the strengths and weaknesses of using RCV values for the diagnosis of AMI. The CV_I for cTn can vary from population to population and can depend on the sampling time-intervals. For example, it has to be investigated if the variations in the cTn measurements seen in dialysis patients (i.e. (Hill, Cleve, Carlisle, Young, & McQueen, 2009; Jacobs et al., 2009)) are comparable to those in "healthy subjects" and if they are diagnostically relevant. So, in order to define the biological variations, clear rules need to be established with respect to the inclusion of subjects, sampling times, storage etc. Moreover, the variations in otherwise healthy subjects may vary from those in diseased populations.

3. The natriuretic peptides

The damage to the heart that is sustained during an AMI, but also other disorders that can impair left ventricular myocardial function, can lead to heart failure (HF). In HF there is a structural or functional cardiac disorder that impairs the ability of the ventricle to fill with or eject blood(Hunt, 2005). In effect, the pump-function of the heart is impaired, which may lead to symptoms of dyspnea, fatigue and fluid retention. In the population over the age of 65, the incidence of HF is about 1 per 100 and within this age group it is the leading cause of hospitalization (in the United States) (Lloyd-Jones et al., 2002). Considering the wide variety of causes underlying HF, the diagnosis and risk stratification in these patients is difficult. Over the years several advances have been made and the use of cardiac biomarkers, notably

Brain Natriuretic Peptide (BNP) and N-terminal proBNP (NT-proBNP) has greatly advanced the physicians ability to identify patients with HF(A. S. Maisel et al., 2002) and to provide accurate risk stratification in this population(Christ et al., 2007).
The natriuretic peptides encompass a number of hormones that are involved in the regulation of fluid homeostasis. These hormones include arterial natriuretic peptide (ANP), B-type natriuretic peptide (BNP) and C-type natriuretic peptide of which BNP is the most important marker for the diagnosis of congestive heart failure. Physiologically, BNP plays an important role in the regulation of blood pressure; it induces natriuresis and diuresis, acts as a vasodilator and inhibits the renin-angiotensin system (Levin, Gardner, & Samson, 1998). The synthesis of BNP begins in the ventricular myocytes with the production of a precursor protein (Pre-proBNP) that is intracellularly converted to the prohormone proBNP. This prohormone is released into the bloodstream in response to increased hemodynamic stress (i.e. mechanical stretch seen during volume overload). Upon release into the circulation, the proBNP is split into the biologically active BNP and the inactive NT-proBNP (figure 4), although recent data suggest that proBNP itself also remains present in the bloodstream (Lam, Burnett, Costello-Boerrigter, Rodeheffer, & Redfield, 2007).

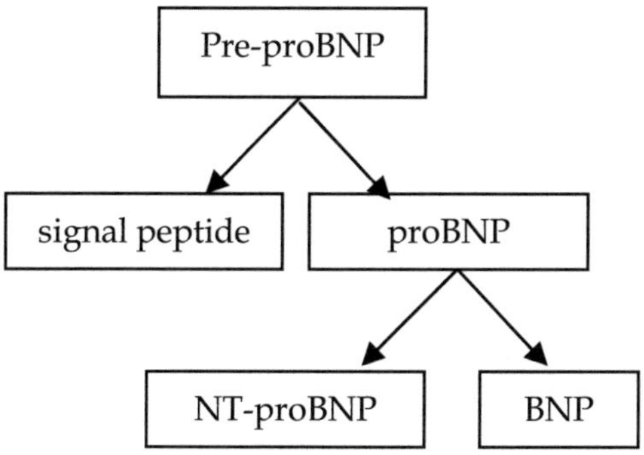

Fig. 4. The synthesis and release of BNP.

BNP and NT-proBNP concentrations correlate with the severity of left ventricular dysfunction (Wieczorek et al., 2002) and congestive heart failure (A. S. Maisel et al., 2002; Wieczorek et al., 2002) and are highly predictive of adverse events in patients who have suffered an AMI (Omland et al., 2002). Overall, BNP and NT-proBNP have equal diagnostic and prognostic value in chronic and acute heart failure (Clerico, Fontana, Zyw, Passino, & Emdin, 2007; Masson et al., 2006). However, NT-proBNP is more stable than BNP and can be collected in serum, heparin and EDTA plasma (Barnes, Collinson, Galasko, Lahiri, & Senior, 2004) , making NT-proBNP slightly more practical in use.
Clinically, the use of BNP and NT-proBNP has been particularly successful in the diagnosis of heart failure in patients with acute dyspnea and in ruling out heart failure (Hobbs et al., 2002) (Januzzi et al., 2005). There are, however, various factors that can influence the BNP and NT-proBNP concentrations which can interfere with their diagnostic and prognostic potential. For example, NT-proBNP is influenced by age, gender and obesity (A. Maisel, 2001; Mehra et al., 2004; Wang et al., 2002) and in particular by renal dysfunction (van Kimmenade et al., 2009; Vickery et al., 2005).

3.1 BNP and NT-proBNP elevations in ESRD

In patients with ESRD, the BNP and NT-proBNP concentrations are virtually always elevated above normal cut-off values (Apple et al., 2004; Madsen et al., 2007). There are several mechanisms that could explain the elevated BNP and NT-proBNP concentrations. In the first place there might be a lack of renal clearance as BNP and NT-proBNP have been shown to be inversely correlated to the glomerular filtration rate (reviewed in (C. DeFilippi, van Kimmenade, & Pinto, 2008). Interestingly, it is not clear if BNP and NT-proBNP are affected similarly by the reduction in renal clearance. Some reports mention that NT-proBNP is more strongly influenced by a decrease in renal function than BNP, (Vickery et al., 2005) whereas others state that they are equally dependent on the renal function for their clearance (van Kimmenade et al., 2009). It should be mentioned that the discrepancies between NT-proBNP and BNP increase with a decreasing glomerular filtration rate, as illustrated by the significantly higher NT-proBNP/BNP ratios in patients with a decreased renal function (Kemperman, van den Berg, Kirkels, & de Jonge, 2004; Srisawasdi, Vanavanan, Charoenpanichkit, & Kroll, 2010; van Kimmenade et al., 2009; Vickery et al., 2005). In particular in patients with a severely reduced renal function (eg. eGFR < 20) the NT-proBNP/BNP seems to increase exponentially (Srisawasdi et al., 2010; Vickery et al., 2005). Recent reports in ESRD patients suggest that the NT-proBNP/BNP ratio increases even further in patients receiving hemodialysis (Jacobs, Mingels, et al., 2010). This increase in the NT-proBNP ratio might not be the sole result of renal clearance and other mechanism such as the extra-renal clearance by circulating type-C natriuretic peptide receptor and by neural endopeptidases (Martinez-Rumayor, Richards, Burnett, & Januzzi, 2008) may play a role (van Kimmenade et al., 2009). Specifically in ESRD patients, there are several other factors that can influence BNP or NT-proBNP concentrations. For example, the dialysis process itself may influence BNP and NT-proBNP concentrations, like the type of dialysis membrane Interestingly, some find elevated levels of NT-proBNP after dialysis (Sommerer, Heckele, et al., 2007) whereas others find lower values (Madsen et al., 2007), and for BNP this might be different than for NT-proBNP (Wahl, Graf, Renz, & Fassbinder, 2004). Other parameters, related to the dialysis treatment, such as a patient's volume status could also affect NT-proBNP and BNP concentrations (Booth, Pinney, & Davenport, 2010; Jacobs, van de Kerkhof, et al., 2010) whereby, an increase in extracellular volume might induce left ventricular dilatation and subsequent increases in (NT-pro)BNP concentrations. More research is needed to understand the renal and extra-renal clearance of BNP and NT-proBNP and to identify ESRD related differences in the clearance or production of these peptides.

3.2 The clinical relevance of (NT-pro)BNP in ESRD

Regardless of the fact that virtually all ESRD patients have elevated (NT-pro)BNP values and that there is much uncertainty about the underlying reasons one should keep in mind that the (NT-pro)BNP concentrations still have a strong prognostic value in ESRD patients.
BNP and NT-proBNP are related to cardiovascular disease and all-cause mortality and thus their measurement remains of importance for diagnosis and risk stratification in ESRD patients (Apple et al., 2004; Madsen et al., 2007). Importantly the diagnostic and prognostic cut-off values for NT-proBNP in ESRD are significantly elevated compared to the cut-off values in patient with non or mildly impaired renal function. For example, in hemodialysis patients a NT-proBNP cut-off value ≥7200 ng/L could discriminate patients with LVD from

those without (David et al., 2008). More in general, DeFilippi et al found an upward shift in the optimal cut-off value for patients with a diminished renal function based on the estimated glomerular filtration rate (eGFR) (C. R. Defilippi, Seliger, Maynard, & Christenson, 2007). The optimal NT-proBNP cut-off for diagnosis of decompensated HF for patients (n=831) with eGFR <60 and ≥60 mL/min/1.73 m^2 was achieved at concentrations as high as 1200 ng/L and 900/450 ng/L (age ≥50/<50 years), respectively. For BNP, optimal cut-offs for patients with eGFR <30, 30-59, 60-90, >90 mL/min/1.73 m^2 were 225, 201, 104, and 71 ng/L, respectively. For optimal diagnostic performance of (NT-pro)BNP in ESRD patients, it is thus of great importance that appropriate cut-off concentrations will be developed.

4. Conclusion

While a reduced renal function and the dialysis treatment itself can have a significant influence on cardiac troponin and (NT-pro)BNP values they are strongly associated with adverse outcomes. Similarly, the cardiac troponins, which are often elevated above the diagnostic cut-off value for AMI provide valuable diagnostic and prognostic information in ESRD patients.

Considering the ESRD related processes that can influence the cardiac troponin and natriuretic peptide concentrations, more research is needed to define appropriate cut-off values for the diagnosis of AMI and CHF. As both cTn and (NT-pro)BNP concentrations are independently associated with cardiovascular mortality, their measurement is important for risk stratification and as a tool to increase clinical vigilance.

5. References

Aakre, K. M., & Sandberg, S. (2010). Can changes in troponin results be useful in diagnosing myocardial infarction? *Clin Chem, 56*(7), 1047-1049.

Apple, F. S., Jesse, R. L., Newby, L. K., Wu, A. H., Christenson, R. H., Cannon, C. P., et al. (2007). National Academy of Clinical Biochemistry and IFCC Committee for Standardization of Markers of Cardiac Damage Laboratory Medicine Practice Guidelines: analytical issues for biochemical markers of acute coronary syndromes. *Clin Chem, 53*(4), 547-551.

Apple, F. S., Murakami, M. M., Pearce, L. A., & Herzog, C. A. (2002). Predictive value of cardiac troponin I and T for subsequent death in end-stage renal disease. *Circulation, 106*(23), 2941-2945.

Apple, F. S., Murakami, M. M., Pearce, L. A., & Herzog, C. A. (2004). Multi-Biomarker Risk Stratification of N-Terminal Pro-B-Type Natriuretic Peptide, High-Sensitivity C-Reactive Protein, and Cardiac Troponin T and I in End-Stage Renal Disease for All-Cause Death. *Clin Chem, 50*, 2233-2235.

Aviles, R. J., Askari, A. T., Lindahl, B., Wallentin, L., Jia, G., Ohman, E. M., et al. (2002). Troponin T levels in patients with acute coronary syndromes, with or without renal dysfunction. *N Engl J Med, 346*(26), 2047-2052.

Barnes, S. C., Collinson, P. O., Galasko, G., Lahiri, A., & Senior, R. (2004). Evaluation of N-terminal pro-B type natriuretic peptide analysis on the Elecsys 1010 and 2010 analysers. *Ann Clin Biochem, 41*(Pt 6), 459-463.

Booth, J., Pinney, J., & Davenport, A. (2010). N-terminal proBNP--marker of cardiac dysfunction, fluid overload, or malnutrition in hemodialysis patients? *Clin J Am Soc Nephrol, 5*(6), 1036-1040.

Christ, M., Thuerlimann, A., Laule, K., Klima, T., Hochholzer, W., Perruchoud, A. P., et al. (2007). Long-term prognostic value of B-type natriuretic peptide in cardiac and non-cardiac causes of acute dyspnoea. *Eur J Clin Invest, 37*(11), 834-841.

Clerico, A., Fontana, M., Zyw, L., Passino, C., & Emdin, M. (2007). Comparison of the diagnostic accuracy of brain natriuretic peptide (BNP) and the N-terminal part of the propeptide of BNP immunoassays in chronic and acute heart failure: a systematic review. *Clinical chemistry, 53*(5), 813-822.

Cummins, B., Auckland, M. L., & Cummins, P. (1987). Cardiac-specific troponin-I radioimmunoassay in the diagnosis of acute myocardial infarction. *Am Heart J, 113*(6), 1333-1344.

David, S., Kumpers, P., Seidler, V., Biertz, F., Haller, H., & Fliser, D. (2008). Diagnostic value of N-terminal pro-B-type natriuretic peptide (NT-proBNP) for left ventricular dysfunction in patients with chronic kidney disease stage 5 on haemodialysis. *Nephrol Dial Transplant, 23*(4), 1370-1377.

DeFilippi, C., van Kimmenade, R. R., & Pinto, Y. M. (2008). Amino-terminal pro-B-type natriuretic peptide testing in renal disease. *Am J Cardiol, 101*(3A), 82-88.

deFilippi, C., Wasserman, S., Rosanio, S., Tiblier, E., Sperger, H., Tocchi, M., et al. (2003). Cardiac troponin T and C-reactive protein for predicting prognosis, coronary atherosclerosis, and cardiomyopathy in patients undergoing long-term hemodialysis. *Jama, 290*(3), 353-359.

Defilippi, C. R., Seliger, S. L., Maynard, S., & Christenson, R. H. (2007). Impact of renal disease on natriuretic Peptide testing for diagnosing decompensated heart failure and predicting mortality. *Clin Chem, 53*(8), 1511-1519.

deFilippi, C. R., Thorn, E. M., Aggarwal, M., Joy, A., Christenson, R. H., Duh, S. H., et al. (2007). Frequency and cause of cardiac troponin T elevation in chronic hemodialysis patients from study of cardiovascular magnetic resonance. *Am J Cardiol, 100*(5), 885-889.

Diris, J. H., Hackeng, C. M., Kooman, J. P., Pinto, Y. M., Hermens, W. T., & Van Dieijen-Visser, M. P. (2004). Impaired Renal Clearance Explains Elevated Troponin T Fragments in Hemodialysis Patients. *Circulation, 109*(1), 23-25.

F.S. Apple, M. M. M., D.P.Farris, S.A. Karimi, P.A. Simpson, L.T.Le. (2009). Serum 99th percentile reference value for the high sensitive Singulex cardiac troponin I assay. *Clinical Chemistry, 55*, A63.

Fahie-Wilson, M. N., Carmichael, D. J., Delaney, M. P., Stevens, P. E., Hall, E. M., & Lamb, E. J. (2006). Cardiac Troponin T Circulates in the Free, Intact Form in Patients with Kidney Failure. *Clin Chem, 52*(3), 414-420.

Giannitsis, E., & Katus, H. A. (2004). Comparison of cardiac troponin T and troponin I assays--implications of analytical and biochemical differences on clinical performance. *Clin Lab, 50*(9-10), 521-528.

Giannitsis, E., Kurz, K., Hallermayer, K., Jarausch, J., Jaffe, A. S., & Katus, H. A. (2010). Analytical validation of a high-sensitivity cardiac troponin T assay. *Clin Chem, 56*(2), 254-261.

Han, J. H., Lindsell, C. J., Ryan, R. J., & Gibler, W. B. (2005). Changes in cardiac troponin T measurements are associated with adverse cardiac events in patients with chronic kidney disease. *Am J Emerg Med, 23*(4), 468-473.

Havekes, B., van Manen, J. G., Krediet, R. T., Boeschoten, E. W., Vandenbroucke, J. P., & Dekker, F. W. (2006). Serum troponin T concentration as a predictor of mortality in hemodialysis and peritoneal dialysis patients. *Am J Kidney Dis, 47*(5), 823-829.

Herzog, C. A., Ma, J. Z., & Collins, A. J. (1998). Poor long-term survival after acute myocardial infarction among patients on long-term dialysis. *N Engl J Med, 339*(12), 799-805.

Hickman, P. E., Koerbin, G., Southcott, E., Tate, J., Dimeski, G., Carter, A., et al. (2007). Newer cardiac troponin I assays have similar performance to troponin T in patients with end-stage renal disease. *Ann Clin Biochem, 44*(Pt 3), 285-289.

Hill, S. A., Cleve, R., Carlisle, E., Young, E., & McQueen, M. J. (2009). Intra-individual variability in troponin T concentration in dialysis patients. *Clinical Biochemistry, 42*(10-11), 991-995.

Hobbs, F. D., Davis, R. C., Roalfe, A. K., Hare, R., Davies, M. K., & Kenkre, J. E. (2002). Reliability of N-terminal pro-brain natriuretic peptide assay in diagnosis of heart failure: cohort study in representative and high risk community populations. *Bmj, 324*(7352), 1498.

Hunt, S. A. (2005). ACC/AHA 2005 guideline update for the diagnosis and management of chronic heart failure in the adult: a report of the American College of Cardiology/American Heart Association Task Force on Practice Guidelines (Writing Committee to Update the 2001 Guidelines for the Evaluation and Management of Heart Failure). *J Am Coll Cardiol, 46*(6), e1-82.

Jacobs, L. H., Mingels, A. M., Wodzig, W. K., van Dieijen-Visser, M. P., Kooman, J. P., Srisawasdi, P., et al. (2010). Renal Dysfunction, Hemodialysis, and the NT-proBNP/BNP Ratio. *Am J Clin Pathol, 134*(3), 516-517.

Jacobs, L. H., van de Kerkhof, J., Mingels, A. M., Kleijnen, V. W., van der Sande, F. M., Wodzig, W. K., et al. (2009). Haemodialysis patients longitudinally assessed by highly sensitive cardiac troponin T and commercial cardiac troponin T and cardiac troponin I assays. *Ann Clin Biochem, 46*(Pt 4), 283-290.

Jacobs, L. H., van de Kerkhof, J. J., Mingels, A. M., Passos, V. L., Kleijnen, V. W., Mazairac, A. H., et al. (2010). Inflammation, overhydration and cardiac biomarkers in haemodialysis patients: a longitudinal study. *Nephrol Dial Transplant, 25*(1), 243-248.

Januzzi, J., James L., Camargo, C. A., Anwaruddin, S., Baggish, A. L., Chen, A. A., Krauser, D. G., et al. (2005). The N-terminal Pro-BNP Investigation of Dyspnea in the Emergency department (PRIDE) study. *The American Journal of Cardiology, 95*(8), 948-954.

Kanderian, A. S., & Francis, G. S. (2006). Cardiac troponins and chronic kidney disease. *Kidney Int, 69*(7), 1112-1114.

Katus, H. A., Remppis, A., Looser, S., Hallermeier, K., Scheffold, T., & Kubler, W. (1989). Enzyme linked immuno assay of cardiac troponin T for the detection of acute myocardial infarction in patients. *J Mol Cell Cardiol, 21*, 1349-1353.

Kemperman, H., van den Berg, M., Kirkels, H., & de Jonge, N. (2004). B-Type Natriuretic Peptide (BNP) and N-Terminal proBNP in Patients with End-Stage Heart Failure Supported by a Left Ventricular Assist Device. *Clin Chem, 50*(9), 1670-1672.

Khan, N. A., Hemmelgarn, B. R., Tonelli, M., Thompson, C. R., & Levin, A. (2005). Prognostic value of troponin T and I among asymptomatic patients with end-stage renal disease: a meta-analysis. *Circulation, 112*(20), 3088-3096.

Kobayashi, T., Jin, L., & de Tombe, P. P. (2008). Cardiac thin filament regulation. *Pflugers Arch, 457*(1), 37-46.

Kumar, N., Michelis, M. F., Devita, M. V., Panagopoulos, G., & Rosenstock, J. L. (2010). Troponin I levels in asymptomatic patients on haemodialysis using a high-sensitivity assay. *Nephrol Dial Transplant.*

Lam, C. S., Burnett, J. C., Jr., Costello-Boerrigter, L., Rodeheffer, R. J., & Redfield, M. M. (2007). Alternate circulating pro-B-type natriuretic peptide and B-type natriuretic peptide forms in the general population. *J Am Coll Cardiol, 49*(11), 1193-1202.

Latini, R., Masson, S., Anand, I. S., Missov, E., Carlson, M., Vago, T., et al. (2007). Prognostic value of very low plasma concentrations of troponin T in patients with stable chronic heart failure. *Circulation, 116*(11), 1242-1249.

Laufer, E. M., Mingels, A. M., Winkens, M. H., Joosen, I. A., Schellings, M. W., Leiner, T., et al. (2010). The extent of coronary atherosclerosis is associated with increasing circulating levels of high sensitive cardiac troponin T. *Arterioscler Thromb Vasc Biol, 30*(6), 1269-1275.

Levin, E. R., Gardner, D. G., & Samson, W. K. (1998). Natriuretic peptides. *N Engl J Med, 339*(5), 321-328.

Lippi, G., Tessitore, N., Montagnana, M., Salvagno, G. L., Lupo, A., & Guidi, G. C. (2008). Influence of sampling time and ultrafiltration coefficient of the dialysis membrane on cardiac troponin I and T. *Arch Pathol Lab Med, 132*(1), 72-76.

Lloyd-Jones, D. M., Larson, M. G., Leip, E. P., Beiser, A., D'Agostino, R. B., Kannel, W. B., et al. (2002). Lifetime risk for developing congestive heart failure: the Framingham Heart Study. *Circulation, 106*(24), 3068-3072.

Madsen, L. H., Ladefoged, S., Corell, P., Schou, M., Hildebrandt, P. R., & Atar, D. (2007). N-terminal pro brain natriuretic peptide predicts mortality in patients with end-stage renal disease in hemodialysis. *Kidney Int, 71*(6), 548-554.

Maisel, A. (2001). B-type natriuretic peptide levels: a potential novel "white count" for congestive heart failure. *J Card Fail, 7*(2), 183-193.

Maisel, A. S., Krishnaswamy, P., Nowak, R. M., McCord, J., Hollander, J. E., Duc, P., et al. (2002). Rapid measurement of B-type natriuretic peptide in the emergency diagnosis of heart failure. *N Engl J Med, 347*(3), 161-167.

Martinez-Rumayor, A., Richards, A. M., Burnett, J. C., & Januzzi, J. L., Jr. (2008). Biology of the natriuretic peptides. *Am J Cardiol, 101*(3A), 3-8.

Masson, S., Latini, R., Anand, I. S., Vago, T., Angelici, L., Barlera, S., et al. (2006). Direct Comparison of B-Type Natriuretic Peptide (BNP) and Amino-Terminal proBNP in a Large Population of Patients with Chronic and Symptomatic Heart Failure: The Valsartan Heart Failure (Val-HeFT) Data. *Clin Chem, 52*(8), 1528-1538.

Mehra, M. R., Uber, P. A., Park, M. H., Scott, R. L., Ventura, H. O., Harris, B. C., et al. (2004). Obesity and suppressed B-type natriuretic peptide levels in heart failure. *Journal of the American College of Cardiology, 43*(9), 1590-1595.

Miller, W. L., Hartman, K. A., Burritt, M. F., Grill, D. E., Rodeheffer, R. J., Burnett, J. C., Jr., et al. (2007). Serial biomarker measurements in ambulatory patients with chronic heart failure: the importance of change over time. *Circulation, 116*(3), 249-257.

Montagnana, M., Lippi, G., Tessitore, N., Salvagno, G. L., Targher, G., Gelati, M., et al. (2008). Effect of hemodialysis on traditional and innovative cardiac markers. *J Clin Lab Anal, 22*(1), 59-65.

Morrow, D. A., Cannon, C. P., Jesse, R. L., Newby, L. K., Ravkilde, J., Storrow, A. B., et al. (2007). National Academy of Clinical Biochemistry Laboratory Medicine Practice Guidelines: Clinical characteristics and utilization of biochemical markers in acute coronary syndromes. *Circulation, 115*(13), e356-375.

National Institutes of Health; National Institute of Diabetes and Digestive and Kidney Diseases; Bethesda, M. (2007). *U.S. Renal Data System, USRDS 2007 Annual Data Report: Atlas of Chronic Kidney Disease and End-Stage Renal Disease in the United States.*, 138-154.

Omar, F., van der Watt, G. F., & Pillay, T. S. (2008). Reference change values: how useful are they? *J Clin Pathol, 61*(4), 426-427.

Omland, T., de Lemos, J. A., Sabatine, M. S., Christophi, C. A., Rice, M. M., Jablonski, K. A., et al. (2009). A sensitive cardiac troponin T assay in stable coronary artery disease. *N Engl J Med, 361*(26), 2538-2547.

Omland, T., Persson, A., Ng, L., O'Brien, R., Karlsson, T., Herlitz, J., et al. (2002). N-terminal pro-B-type natriuretic peptide and long-term mortality in acute coronary syndromes. *Circulation, 106*(23), 2913-2918.

Ooi, D. S., Isotalo, P. A., & Veinot, J. P. (2000). Correlation of antemortem serum creatine kinase, creatine kinase-MB, troponin I, and troponin T with cardiac pathology. *Clin Chem, 46*(3), 338-344.

Ooi, D. S., Zimmerman, D., Graham, J., & Wells, G. A. (2001). Cardiac troponin T predicts long-term outcomes in hemodialysis patients. *Clin Chem, 47*(3), 412-417.

Panteghini, M. (2006). The new definition of myocardial infarction and the impact of troponin determination on clinical practice. *Int J Cardiol, 106*(3), 298-306.

Panteghini, M., Pagani, F., Yeo, K. T., Apple, F. S., Christenson, R. H., Dati, F., et al. (2004). Evaluation of imprecision for cardiac troponin assays at low-range concentrations. *Clin Chem, 50*(2), 327-332.

Pimenta, J., Sampaio, F., Martins, P., Carvalho, B., Rocha-Goncalves, F., Ferreira, A., et al. (2009). Aminoterminal B-type natriuretic peptide (NT-proBNP) in end-stage renal failure patients on regular hemodialysis: does it have diagnostic and prognostic implications? *Nephron Clin Pract, 111*(3), c182-188.

Roberts, M. A., Fernando, D., Macmillan, N., Proimos, G., Bach, L. A., Power, D. A., et al. (2004). Single and serial measurements of cardiac troponin I in asymptomatic patients on chronic hemodialysis. *Clin Nephrol, 61*(1), 40-46.

Roberts, M. A., Hare, D. L., Macmillan, N., Ratnaike, S., Sikaris, K., & Ierino, F. L. (2009). Serial increased cardiac troponin T predicts mortality in asymptomatic patients treated with chronic haemodialysis. *Ann Clin Biochem, 46*(Pt 4), 291-295.

Sommerer, C., Beimler, J., Schwenger, V., Heckele, N., Katus, H. A., Giannitsis, E., et al. (2007). Cardiac biomarkers and survival in haemodialysis patients. *Eur J Clin Invest, 37*(5), 350-356.

Sommerer, C., Heckele, S., Schwenger, V., Katus, H. A., Giannitsis, E., & Zeier, M. (2007). Cardiac biomarkers are influenced by dialysis characteristics. *Clin Nephrol, 68*, 392-400.

Srisawasdi, P., Vanavanan, S., Charoenpanichkit, C., & Kroll, M. H. (2010). The effect of renal dysfunction on BNP, NT-proBNP, and their ratio. *Am J Clin Pathol, 133*(1), 14-23.

Thygesen, K., Alpert, J. S., & White, H. D. (2007). Universal definition of myocardial infarction. *J Am Coll Cardiol, 50*(22), 2173-2195.

Thygesen, K., Alpert, J. S., White, H. D., Jaffe, A. S., Apple, F. S., Galvani, M., et al. (2007). Universal definition of myocardial infarction: Kristian Thygesen, Joseph S. Alpert and Harvey D. White on behalf of the Joint ESC/ACCF/AHA/WHF Task Force for the Redefinition of Myocardial Infarction. *Eur Heart J, 28*(20), 2525-2538.

Todd, J., Freese, B., Lu, A., Held, D., Morey, J., Livingston, R., et al. (2007). Ultrasensitive Flow-based Immunoassays using Single-Molecule Counting. *Clin Chem, 53*(11).

van Kimmenade, R. R., Januzzi, J. L., Jr., Bakker, J. A., Houben, A. J., Rennenberg, R., Kroon, A. A., et al. (2009). Renal clearance of B-type natriuretic peptide and amino terminal pro-B-type natriuretic peptide a mechanistic study in hypertensive subjects. *J Am Coll Cardiol, 53*(10), 884-890.

Vasile, V. C., Saenger, A. K., Kroning, J. M., & Jaffe, A. S. (2010). Biological and analytical variability of a novel high-sensitivity cardiac troponin T assay. *Clin Chem, 56*(7), 1086-1090.

Vickery, S., Price, C. P., John, R. I., Abbas, N. A., Webb, M. C., Kempson, M. E., et al. (2005). B-type natriuretic peptide (BNP) and amino-terminal proBNP in patients with CKD: relationship to renal function and left ventricular hypertrophy. *Am J Kidney Dis, 46*(4), 610-620.

Wahl, H. G., Graf, S., Renz, H., & Fassbinder, W. (2004). Elimination of the Cardiac Natriuretic Peptides B-Type Natriuretic Peptide (BNP) and N-Terminal proBNP by Hemodialysis. *Clin Chem, 50*(6), 1071-1074.

Wang, T. J., Larson, M. G., Levy, D., Leip, E. P., Benjamin, E. J., Wilson, P. W., et al. (2002). Impact of age and sex on plasma natriuretic peptide levels in healthy adults. *Am J Cardiol, 90*(3), 254-258.

Wayand, D., Baum, H., Schatzle, G., Scharf, J., & Neumeier, D. (2000). Cardiac troponin T and I in end-stage renal failure. *Clin Chem, 46*(9), 1345-1350.

Wieczorek, S. J., Wu, A. H., Christenson, R., Krishnaswamy, P., Gottlieb, S., Rosano, T., et al. (2002). A rapid B-type natriuretic peptide assay accurately diagnoses left ventricular dysfunction and heart failure: a multicenter evaluation. *Am Heart J, 144*(5), 834-839.

Wiessner, R., Hannemann-Pohl, K., Ziebig, R., Grubitzsch, H., Hocher, B., Vargas-Hein, O., et al. (2007). Impact of kidney function on plasma troponin concentrations after coronary artery bypass grafting. *Nephrol Dial Transplant.*

Wu, A. H., Jaffe, A. S., Apple, F. S., Jesse, R. L., Francis, G. L., Morrow, D. A., et al. (2007). National Academy of Clinical Biochemistry Laboratory Medicine Practice Guidelines: Use of Cardiac Troponin and B-Type Natriuretic Peptide or N-Terminal proB-Type Natriuretic Peptide for Etiologies Other than Acute Coronary Syndromes and Heart Failure. *Clin Chem, 53*(12), 2086-2096.

Wu, A. H., Lu, Q. A., Todd, J., Moecks, J., & Wians, F. (2009). Short- and long-term biological variation in cardiac troponin I measured with a high-sensitivity assay: implications for clinical practice. *Clin Chem, 55*(1), 52-58.

9

Cardiovascular Complications in Renal Diseases

Mohsen Kerkeni
Laboratory of Biochemistry
Human Nutrition and Metabolic Disorders
Faculty of Medicine
Monastir
Tunisia

1. Introduction

Patients with chronic renal disease (CRD) represent an important segment of Tunisian population, and mostly because of the high risk of cardiovascular disease (CVD) associated with renal insufficiency, detection and treatment of chronic renal disease is now a public health priority (Abderrahim E et al., 2001, Ben Maïz H et al., 2006, Counil E et al., 2008). The increased incidence of CVD is likely to be the result of a high prevalence of both traditional risk factors, such as diabetes mellitus, hypertension, dyslipidemia and smoking. Non traditional risk factors, such as hyperhomocysteinemia, oxidative stress and inflammation have been taken into account.

Homocysteine (Hcy) is an amino acid that circulates in the blood. An elevated serum concentration of homocysteine is a known risk factor for atherosclerosis and is associated with an increased risk of myocardial infraction and health. Accumulating evidence suggests that the Hcy thioester metabolite, hcy-thiolactone, has an important role in atherothrombosis. Hcy-thiolactone is a product of an error-editing reaction in protein biosynthesis, which forms when Hcy is mistakenly selected by methionyl-tRNA synthetase. The thioester chemistry of Hcy-thiolactone underlies its ability of form isopeptide bonds with protein lysines residues, which impairs or alters protein function. Protein targets for modification by Hcy-thiolactone include fibrogen, LDL, HDL, albumin, heamoglobin and ferritin. Pathophysiclogical consequences of protein N-homocyteinylation include protein and cell damage, activation of an adaptive immune response, synthesis of auto-antibodies against N-hcy-proteins, and enhanced thrombosis caused by N-hcy-fibrogen. The development of highly sensitive chemical and immunohistochemical assays has provided evidence for the contribution of the Hcy-thiolactone pathway to pathophysiology of the vascular system. In particular, conditions predisposing to atherosclerosis, such as genetic or dietary hyperhomocysteinemia, have been shown to lead to elevation of Hcy-thiolactone and N-hcy-protein.

Oxidative stress plays an important role in the pathogenesis of atherosclerosis and cardiovascular disease. Reactive oxygen species (ROS) production is toxic via their effects on cellular components such as denaturing proteins, membrane lipids and DNA. Oxidative

stress may be defined as an imbalance between the production and degradation of ROS such as superoxide anion, hydrogen peride, lipid peroxides and peroxynitrite. Enzymatic inactivation of ROS is achieved mainly by glutathione peroxydase (GPx), superoxidase dismutase (SOD) and catalase. GPx, the ubiquitous intracellular form and key antioxidant enzyme within most cells, including the endothelium, uses glutathione to reduce hydrogen peroxidase to water and lipid perides to their respective alcohols, and it also acts as a peroxynitrite reductase. In mice GPx deficiency results in abnormal vascular and cardiac function and structure. Similarly, SOD is represented by three different ubiquitously expressed enzymes that convert superoxide anion to hydrogen peroxide: cytosolic copper- and zinc-containing SOD, mitochondrial manganese-containing SOD and extracellular SOD. Extracellular SOD is most active in the vessel wall and has been shown to regulate the availability of nitric oxide by scavenging superoxide anion.
The presence of inflammation is an important element in the pathogenesis of atherosclerosis. Two pathaways are activated during the process: the protein kinase C and nuclear factor-kappa B (NF-kB) pathways. This lead to upregulation of genes that trigger the activation of angiotension converting enzyme, the local production of angiotensine II and the expression of adhesion molecules on the surface of endothelial cells. These events can result in endothelial dysfunction. The most extensively studied biomarker of inflammation in cardivasular disease is CRP. This is a circulating pentraxin that has a major role in human innate immune response and provides a stable plasma biomarker for low-grade systemic inflammation. It is predominantly produced in the liver. CRP has been implicated in multiple aspects of atherogenesis and plaque vulnerability, including expression of adhesion molecules, induction of NO, altered complement function and inhibition of intrinsic fibrinolysis. Procedures for its measurement are well standardized and automated and high-sensitivity assays (hs-CRP) are widely available. Increased CRP levels associated with increased prevalence of underlying atherosclerosis.
Studies of all Tunisian patients are nondialyzed chronic kidney disease, and with nondiabetic renal disease. Patients according to serum creatinine levels were sub-classified as follows: moderate renal failure, severe renal failure and end-stage renal disease. Etiologies of chronic renal disease in patients were chronic glomerular nephritis, chronic tubulointerstitial nephropathy, vascular nephropathy and unknown cause. Cardiovascular complications in all groups were diagnosed by echocardiography and electrocardiography. Patients with cardiovascular complications included cardiac insufficiency and left ventricular hypertrophy.

2. Homocysteine, paraoxonase activity and renal diseases

Homocysteine (Hcy) as a thiol-containing amino acid has gained great notoriety, since elevation of its plasma concentrations, a condition known as hyperhomocysteinemia, is correlated with many different diseases, in particular cardiovascular disease (Cavalca V et al., 2001, Kerkeni M et al., 2006), and end-stage renal disease (ESRD) (Ducloux D et al., 2000, Perna AF et al., 2004). Serum paraoxonase 1 (PON1) is an oxidant-sensitive enzyme that inhibits the atherogenic oxidation of low density lipoprotein (LDL). PON1 activity is also implicated in protection against cardiovascular disease (Mackness M et al., 2004). Some studies found that the paraoxonase protein (PON1), carried on high density lipoprotein (HDL), has homocysteine thiolactone (HcyT) hydrolase activity and protects against protein homocysteinylation in vitro (Jakubowski H et al., 2000, Jakubowski H, 2000). A possible molecular mechanism underlying hyperhomocysteinemia involves metabolic conversion of Hcy by methionyl-tRNA synthetase (MetRS) to HcyT, which then reacts with lysine residues in proteins, damaging their structure and impairing their physiological activities. HcyT is known to be cytotoxic in experimental animals and induces apoptotic death and proinflammation process in cultured human vascular endothelial and in primary human umbilical vein endothelial cells (HUVEC) (Kerkeni M et al., 2006). The extent of HcyT synthesis and protein homocysteinylation in human vascular endothelial cells depends on levels of Hcy, methionine, folate and HDL that are linked to vascular disease. In addition, hyperhomocysteinemia and paraoxonase activity are involved in the development of cardiovascular complications in patients with chronic renal disease and in patients undergoing hemodialysis.

We reported in previous studies that hyperhomocysteinemia, oxidative stress and paraoxonase activity are risk factors for cardiovascular disease and the severity of coronary artery disease in Tunisian population (Kerkeni M et al., 2008). The association between chronic renal disease, homocysteine and paraoxonase activity have been taken into account, and we reported that the development of cardiovascular complications related to end-stage renal disease (ESRD) (Kerkeni M et al., 2009). The coexistence of a high level of Hcy and a low PON1 concentration increases the severity of renal disease. In hyperhomocysteinemia condition, Hcy occurs in human blood in several forms. The most reactive is homocysteine thiolactone which it's detoxifies by Hcy-thiolactonase activity of PON1. We hypothesize that HcyT can also increase cellular toxicity in renal function via protein homocysteinylation participates in glomerular sclerosis and in the development of ESRD.

3. Endothelial NO synthase, methylenetetrahydrofolate reductase (MTHFR) gene polymorphisms and renal diseases

Epidemiologic studies have shown that dyslipidemia, diabetes mellitus, obesity, hypertension, and cigarette smoking are risk factors for cardiovascular complications. Assessment of these metabolic or lifestyle risk factors has, however, been ineffective in incompletely predicting the severity of renal disease and the development of CVD, suggesting that specific genetic predisposition should also be taken into account (Nordfors L et al., 2002).

The vascular endothelium modulates blood vessel wall homeostasis through the production of factors regulating vessel tone, coagulation state, cell growth, cell death, and leukocyte trafficking. One of the most important endothelial cell products is nitric oxide (NO), which is synthesized from L-arginine by enzyme endothelial nitric oxide synthase (eNOS). NO plays a key role in the relaxation of vascular smooth muscle, inhibits platelet and leukocyte adhesion to the endothelium, reduces vascular smooth muscle cell migration and proliferation, and limits oxidation of the atherogenic LDLs. NO may modulate homocysteine concentration directly by inhibiting methionine synthase, the enzyme that synthesizes methionine from homocysteine and 5-methyltetrahydrofolate. Alternatively, NO may modulate Hcy concentrations indirectly via folate catabolism by inhibiting the synthesis of ferritin, a protein that promotes the irreversible oxidative cleavage of folate. Although low folate concentrations are associated with hyperhomocysteinemia, which is a risk factor for atherosclerosis, the relative contributions of these potential mechanisms to Hcy modulation in vivo remain unclear.

Glomerular microcirculation is involved in the deterioration of renal function. Among several factors that regulate renal hemodynamics, NO (nitric oxide) has been reported to be critical. In the vascular endothelium, NO is produced by endothelial NO synthase (eNOS). NO production can be influenced by polymorphisms of the eNOS gene. Polymorphisms in exons may alter the three-dimensional structure of the enzyme, and those in introns may change the transcriptional activity (Tesauro M et al., 2000). These can lead to a decrease in NO production and, subsequently, an increase in arterial pressure or intraglomerular hypertension and produce renal damage. Previous studies have shown the polymorphisms of the eNOS gene are associated with the progression of nondiabetic end stage renal disease (ESRD). Several polymorphisms have been identified in the eNOS gene, among which is one located in exon 7 (G894T), which modifies its coding sequence ($Glu^{298}\rightarrow Asp$). The G894T polymorphism was reported to be associated with hypertension, diabetic nephropathy and ESRD (Shin Shin Y et al., 2004). Furthermore, in ESRD, mean total homocysteine levels are commonly elevated, and the methylenetetrahydrofolate reductase (MTHFR) gene polymorphisms may also be associated with renal disease. The eNOS and MTHFR gene polymorphisms have been shown to be associated with cardiovascular disease. We reported in previous studies that the eNOS and MTHFR gene polymorphisms were associated with the presence of cardiovascular disease (Kerkeni M et al., 2006a et b). However, the relationship between eNOS, MTHFR gene polymorphisms and cardiovascular disease in Tunisian patients with chronic renal disease has been examined. We investigated that (a) the relationship of these gene polymorphisms with the presence and the severity of renal disease, and (b) their relationships with CVD in these patients (Kerkeni M et al., 2009).

4. The mechanisms of homocysteine and paraoxonase activity to induce renal diseases

In our studies, prevalence of hyperhomocysteinemia was present in 94 % of Tunisian patients. We found that an increased Hcy levels in patients with moderate renal failure to ESRD. This observation was showed by numerous clinical studies, but the pathogenic role of increased Hcy Levels in the progression of ESRD remains controversial and the mechanisms how Hcy induced renal toxicity are still unknown. Recent studies showed the pathogenic action of Hcy in the glomeruli or in the kidney, such as local oxidative stress, endoplasmic reticulum stress, homocysteinylation, hypomethylation and glomerular mesangial cell apoptosis via activation of p38-mitogen-activated protein kinase (Yi F and Li PL, 2008). In hyperhomocysteinemia condition, Hcy occurs in human blood in several forms. The most reactive is homocysteine thiolactone (HcyT). It spontaneously homocysteinylates proteins impairing their structures and functions. An increase in HcyT can itself lead to inactivation of PON1 as it has been demonstrated by in vitro studies or negatively regulate PON1 gene expression. Furthermore, we showed in previous study that HcyT might possess stronger cytotoxicity and pro-inflammation properties in primary human umbilical vein endothelial cells. We hypothesize that HcyT can also increased cellular toxicity in renal function via protein homocysteinylation. There is considerable evidence that protein homocysteinylation participates in glomerular sclerosis and in the development of ESRD. In this regard, Perna et al. have reported that plasma homocysteinylation increased in ESRD patients subject to hemodialysis (Perna AF et al., 2006). It was demonstrated that in patients with terminal renal failure without dialysis protein homocysteinylation is significantly enhanced which may contribute to the atherogenesis and progression of ESRD in these patients. Another interesting mechanism that possible mediates glomerular injury or sclerosis induced by homocysteinylation is the irreversible homocysteinylation of long-lived proteins in connective tissue protein are especially susceptible to Hcy and HcyT attacks.

Hyperhomocysteinemia and a low PON1 activity were associated in patients with each etiology except the unknown cause. We showed an increased Hcy levels in patients with chronic tubulointerstitial nephropathy than patients with glomerular nephropathy. Hyperhomocysteinemia is able to promote glomerular damage and generate tubulointerstitial lesions. O'Riodan et al. showed that chronic endothelial nitric oxide synthase (eNOS) inhibition actuates endothethelial mesenchymal transformation in chronic kidney disease (O'Riordan E et al., 2007). Several studies have demonstrated that the bioavailability of NO is decreased in hyperhomocysteinemia. In addition, we found that patients with vascular nephropathies showed an increased hyperhomocysteinemia than patients with glomerular nephropathy. Hyperhomocysteinemia and a low PON1 activity were markedly associated in CRD patient with cardiovascular complications including cardiac insufficiency and left ventricular hypertrophy. Some studies have shown that hyperhomocysteinemia induced hypertension and ventricular hypertrophy. Given the similarity of pathological changes between glomerular injury and Hcy induced arterial damages, such as endothelial injury, cell proliferation or growth, increased matrix formation, and aggregated proteoglycan, it is assumed that an increase in plasma Hcy levels may also directly act on glomerular and tubulointerstitial cells, resulting in glomerular damage and tubulointerstitial lesions. Moreover, an impaired renal function will lead to a further increase in plasma Hcy levels which in turn exaggerates the progression of glomerular injury, resulting in a vicious cycle and consequent glomerulosclerosis and ESRD. In addition, Hcy may also produce detrimental actions or increase the risk of cardiovascular disease by decreasing plasma or tissue adenosine levels. It is well known that adenosine evokes several biological actions in the cardiovascular system and participates in the regulation of the renal function, including renal glomerular perfusion. It was demonstrated that chronic elevations of the plasma Hcy concentration in rats resulted in aretiosclerotic changes and glomerular dysfunction and sclerosis accompanied by sustained low level of plasma adenosine. Decreased adenosine concentrations during hyperhomocysteinemia may be due to an enhanced activity of a bidirectional enzyme, S-adenosylhomocysteine hydrolase. Due to space limitations, some other interesting topics related to the possible mechanisms mediating Hcy-induced glomerular and tubulointerstitial toxicities are not included, such as activation of proinflammatory factors, increased homocysteine thiolactone levels, and Hcy induced abnormal mitochondrial biogenesis.

5. The mechanisms of the eNOS and MTHFR gene mutations to induce renal diseases

We reported an association between the common G894T polymorphism of the eNOS and the presence of renal disease. We found that the eNOS 894T allele was markedly associated with severity of renal disease in patients with nondiabetic renal disease. Furthermore, eNOS G894T mutation was increased in CRD patients with cardiovascular complications included cardiac insufficiency and left ventricular hypertrophy. In the vascular endothelium, NO is produced by eNOS and implicated in numerous aspects of renal vascular control and function. It is thought to exert a vasculoprotective effect by modulation of kidney blood flow through counterbalancing the effects of the renin-angiotensin system. A deficiency of the endogenous vasodilatator NO has been implicated as a potential cause of chronic renal diseases and in end-stage renal failure. NO production can be influenced by polymorphisms of the eNOS gene. These can lead to a decrease in NO production and, subsequently, an increase in arterial pressure or intraglomerular hypertension and renal damage. Polymorphisms in exons may alter the three-dimensional structure of the enzyme, and may change the transcriptional activity (Tesauro M et al. 2000). The eNOS G894T variant leads to an amino acid substitution of aspartate for glutamate at position 298 of the protein. Tesauro et al. showed that an in vitro study the eNOS protein with aspartate, but not glutamate, at position 298 is subject to cleavage by endogenous protease and produces 35-kDa amino-terminal and 100-kDa carboxyl-terminal fragments. Nevertheless, Tesauro et al. found that significant potential structure changes in the Chou-Fasman secondary structure and pointed out that the coding region polymorphism has functional consequences.

We therefore speculate that, in vivo, the eNOS 894GT and 894TT genotype leads to alter NO production, endothelial dysfunction, promotes renal hemodynamic dysfunction, and aggravate the extent of renal disease. With chronic eNOS enzyme dysfunction, decreased NO production may contribute to raise cardiovascular complications as well as micro and marcovascular damage. Previous studies were interested the effect of MTHFR genotypes on total homocysteine in patients with renal failure. However, plasma total homocysteine increases as renal function declines; it is elevated in the vast majority of patients with ESRD. The glomerular filtration rate is a strong determinant of plasma homocysteine concentration, even in individuals with very mild renal dysfunction. As reviewed by Brasttstron and Wilcken, almost every study in which renal diseases has shown a highly significant positive correlation between serum creatinine and Hcy concentrations. The total Hcy levels increase in patients with moderate renal failure and can be >100 μM in patients with ESRD. Nevertheless, several studies showed that MTHFR C677T polymorphism aggravates hyperhomocysteinemia in hemodialysis patients. However, the association between MTHFR polymorphisms and the risk of cardiovascular disease in patients with renal disease remains controversial.

In our studies, MTHFR polymorphisms were not associated with the presence and the severity of renal disease in CRD patients, and we found also a lack association with cardiovascular complications in CRD patient. On the other hand, hyperhomocysteinemia was founded in these patients, and Hcy levels increased not only in ESRD patients but increased markedly in patients with cardiovascular complications. We hypothesize that the synergic effects of the eNOS G984T variant and hyperhomocysteinemia induced less NO production and contribute to the extent of severity of renal disease and induced cardiovascular damage.

6. Conclusion

Hyperhomocysteinemia and low PON1 activity are associated with chronic renal disease and markedly associated in Tunisian patients with cardiovascular complications. We postulate that with chronic toxicity induced by hyperhomocysteinemia may contribute to the severity of renal disease and increase the incidence of cardiovascular disease in patients. Some key targets in these pathogenic pathways must be identified to direct toward prevention or treatment of ESRD associated with hyperhomocysteinemia which is particularly important since so far there are no efficient Hcy lowering and Hcy detoxifying strategies being used in CRD patients. The G894T polymorphism of the eNOS gene is associated with the presence and the severity of renal disease in Tunisian population. The eNOS G984T variant and hyperhomocysteinemia both increase the extent of renal disease, and the development and progression of cardiovascular complications.

7. Acknowledgments

Author expresses his sincere appreciation to Prof. A. Miled (Laboratory of Biochemistry, CHU. F. Hached, Sousse, Tunisia) and Prof F. Trivin (Laboratory of Biochemistry, Saint-Joseph Hospital, Paris, France) for their continued direction and encouragement throughout the study.

8. References

Abderrahim E, Zouaghi K, Hedri H, et al. (2001). Renal replacement therapy for diabetic end-stage renal disease. Experience of a Tunisian hospital centre. *Diabetes Metab;* 27:584-90.

Ben Maïz H, Abderrahim E, Ben Moussa F, Goucha R, Karoui C(2006). Epidemiology of glomerular diseases in Tunisian from 1975 to 2005. Influence of changes in healthcare and society. *Bull Acad Natl Med;*190:403-16.

Cavalca V, Cighetti G, Bamonti F, et al. (2001). Oxidative stress and homocysteine in coronary artery disease. *Clin Chem;*47:887-92.

Counil E, Cherni N, Hkarrat M, Achour A, Trimech H. (2008). Trends of incidence dialysis patients in Tunisia between 1992 and 2001. *Am J Kidney Dis;*51:463-70.

Ducloux D, Motte G, Challier B, Gibey R, Chalopin JM. (2000). Serum total homocysteine and cardiovascular disease occurrence in chronic, stable renal transplant recipients: a prospective study. *J Am Soc Nephrol;*11:134-137.

Jakubowski H, Zhang L, Bardeguez A, and Aviv A. (2000). Homocysteine thiolactone and protein homocysteinylation in human endothelial cells: Implications for atherosclerosis. *Circ Res;*87:45-51.

Jakubowski H. (2000). Calcium-dependent human serum homocysteine thiolactone hydrolyse: A protective mechanism against protein N- homocysteinylation. *J Biol Chem;*275:3957-62.

Kerkeni M, Addad F, Chauffert M, et al. (2006a). Hyperhomocysteinemia, endothelial nitric oxide synthase polymorphism, and risk of coronary artery disease. *Clinical Chemistry;* 52: 53-58.

Kerkeni M, Addad F, Chauffert M, et al. (2006b). Hyperhomocysteinemia, methylenetetrahydrofolate reductase polymorphism and risk of coronary artery disease. *Ann Clin Biochem;* 43: 1-7.

Kerkeni M, Addad F, Chauffert M, et al. (2006). Hyperhomocysteinemia, paraoxonase activity and risk of coronary artery disease. *Clin Biochem;*39:821-5.

Kerkeni M, Added F, Ben Farhat M, et al. (2008). Hyperhomocysteinemia and parameters of antioxidative defence in Tunisian patients with coronary heart disease. *Ann Clin Biochem;*45:193-98.

Kerkeni M, Letaief A, Achour A, Miled A, Trivin F and Maaroufi K. (2009). Endothelial nitric oxide synthase, Methylenetetrahydrofolate reductase polymorphisms, and cardiovascular complication in Tunisian patients with nondiabetic renal disease. *Clinical Biochemistry* ;42:958-64.

Kerkeni M, Letaief A, Achour A, Miled A, Trivin F, and Maaroufi K. (2009). Hyperhomocysteinemia, paraoxonase concentration and cardiovascular complication in Tunisian patients with nondiabetic renal disease. *Clinical Biochemistry*;42:777-82.

Kerkeni M, Tnani M, Chuniaud L, et al. (2006). Comparative study on in vitro effects of homocysteine thiolactone and homocysteine on HUVEC cells: evidence for a stronger proapoptotic and proinflammation homocysteine thiolactone. *Mol Cell Biochem*;291:119-26.

Mackness M, Durrington P, Mackness B. (2004). Paraoxonase 1 activity, concentration and genotype in cardiovascular disease. *Curr Opin Lipidol*;15:399-404.

Nordfors L, Stenvinkel P, Marchlewska A, et al. (2002) Molecular genetics in renal medicine: what can we hope to achieve? *Nephrol Dial Transplant*;17:5-11.

O'Riordan E, Mendelev N, Patschan S, et al. (2007). Chronic NOS inhibition actuates endothelial mesenchymal transformation. *Am J Physiol Heart Circ Physiol*;292 :285-94.

Perna AF, Ingrosso D, Satta E, Lombardi C, Acanfora F, De Santo NG. (2004). Homocysteine metabolism in renal failure. *Curr Opin Clin Nutr Metab Care*;7:53-57.

Perna AF, Satta E, Acanfora F, Lombardi C, Ingrosso D, De Santo NG. (2006). Increased plasma protein homocysteinylation in hemodialysis patients. *Kidney Int*;69 :869-76.

Shin Shin Y, Hong Baek S, Yuk Chang K, et al. (2004). Relation between eNOS Glu298Asp polymorphism and progression of diabetic nephropathy. *Diabetes Research and Clinical Practice*;65:257-65.

Tesauro M, Thompson WC, Rogliani P, Qi L, Chaudhary PP, Moss J. (2000). Intracellular processing of endothelial nitric oxide synthase isoforms associated with differences in severity of cardiopulmonary diseases: cleavage of proteins with aspartate vs. glutamate at position 298. *Proc Natl Acad Sci USA*;97:2832-5.

Tesauro M, Thompson WC, Rogliani P, Qi L, Chaudhary PP, Moss J. (2000). Intracellular processing of endothelial nitric oxide synthase isoforms associated with differences in severity of cardiopulmonary diseases: cleavage of proteins with aspartate vs. glutamate at position 298. *Proc Natl Acad Sci USA*;97:2832-5.

Yi F, Li PL.(2008). Mechanisms of homocysteine induced glomerular injury and sclerosis. *Am J Nephrol*;28:524-264.

Part 2

Transplantation

10

Laparoscopic Transperitoneal and Retroperitoneal Nephrectomies in Children: A Change of Practice

Julio J. Báez[1], Gaston F. Mesples[2] and Alfredo E. Benito[3]
[1]Department of Pediatric Surgery and Pediatric Urology
Municipal Children's Hospital of Cordoba, National University of Cordoba, Cordoba
[2]Department of Pediatric Surgery and Pediatric Urology
Childrens Hospital Dr Lucio Molas, La Pampa
[3]Editor, Scientific Photography Specialist
Editorial Director of Recfot, Recursos Fotográficos - Córdoba
Argentina

1. Introduction

Over the past decade, nothing has changed the practice of pediatric urology as much as the expansion in the minimally invasive techniques for routine operations. The breadth of urologic pathology, which can be managed via the laparoscopic approach, continues to expand as technologies and surgical experience mature.

Mounting evidence has demonstrated that for many urologic procedures, pathology can be managed efficiently and effectively while significantly decreasing the pain and convalescence, traditionally associated with ablative and reconstructive open urologic procedures. The blossoming of laparoscopic surgery within urology has resulted in some challenges as the most common procedure, laparoscopic nephrectomy, remains technically demanding. The total nephrectomy with or without ureterectomy, might be indicated for multicystic dysplastic kidney, for destructed kidney by obstructive uropathy and for small kidney with hypertension. We discuss after the usefulness to remove or not multicystic dysplastic kidneys but this congenital malformation represents an excellent indication to begin our experience with laparoscopic surgery because the dissection is easy and hemostasis problems are quite nil.

Laparoscopic nephrectomy offers distinct benefits over standard open nephrectomy for nonmalignant disease in terms of cosmesis, reduced postoperative stay and less need for analgesia, and has become an increasingly popular method since its first report by Clayman et al in 1991 (Clayman et al., 1991) in adults and by Figenshau and associates in 1994 in children (Figenshau et al., 1994).

With the evolution of the endoscopic and minimally invasive techniques these conventional incisions have either been abandoned or significantly modified to reduce the morbidity to the child.

Renal dysplasia is a common kidney disorder, frequently associated with congenital uropathy that leads to renal failure in children with an incidence estimated in 1:3000 to

1:4300; they may arise de novo (primary) or be found in association with congenital obstruction of the urinary tract or vesico-ureteric reflux (VUR) (secondary).
The histologic term defining a malformed part or the whole kidney and the presence of primitive ducts lined with undifferentiated columnar epithelium and surrounded by undifferentiated fibromuscular collar with sometimes metaplastic elements such as cartilage. (Figure 1)

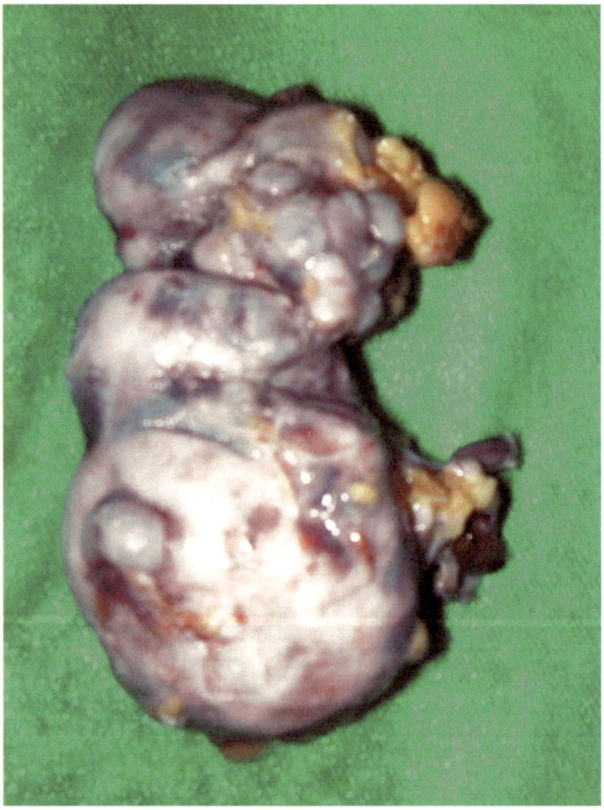

Fig. 1. Renal dysplasia is a kidney disorder defined as a malformed part or the whole kidney and the presence of primitive ducts lined with undifferentiated columnar epithelium and surrounded by undifferentiated fibromuscular collar with sometimes metaplastic elements such as cartilage.

In 1936, Schwartz (Schwartz, 1936) was the first to describe a "unilateral multicystic kidney in a specimen removed from a 7 month old boy suspected to have Wilms tumor or massive hydronephrosis.
In 1964 Pathak and Williams (Pathak & Williams, 1964) added the descriptive term dysplastic to these lesions citing the presence of embryonic mesenchyme and primitive renal components (cartilage and muscle).
Despite the frequent occurrence of renal dysplasia in association with obstructive urophaty, its pathogenesis remains unknown.
Abnormal metanephric differentiation in cases of renal dysplasia results in abnormal renal organization and poor development of renal elements.

Felson and Cussen (Felson & Cussen, 1975) in 1975 viewed the multicystic kidney as an extreme form of hydronephrosis that occurs secondary to atresia of the ureter or renal pelvis.

Cystic dysplasia of an entire upper pole can be seen in kidneys with duplicated collecting systems, especially associated with ureteroceles and bilateral cystic dysplasia also may be seen secondary to posterior urethral valves.

Shibata and Nagata (Shibata et al., 2001) report that nephron induction with filtrating function occurs before the development of cysts; early fetal urinary tract obstruction causes cystic formation in the developing nephrons, which subsequently disrupts nephron induction and tubular development and also cited the importance of abnormalities in the activity of transcription factor PAX2 and antiapoptosis protein bcl2 in the pathogenesis of renal dysplasia.

Matsell and colleagues (Matsell et al., 1996) propose that it may be abnormalities in branching of the ureteral bud that are responsible for progressive local hisptopathologic changes, supported by previous findings of abnormal metanephric development with ectopic ureteral orifices reported by Mackie and Stephens (Mackie & Stephens, 1975).

More recently, Spencer and Maizel (Spencer & Maizel, 1987) discovered that alterations in ureteral epithelial and mesenchymal cells by inhibition of glycosylation of the extracellular matrix could induced dysplasia without obstruction, that support the theory that dysplasia is the result of disruption in normal epithelial-mesenchymal interaction during the induction of renal tubules.

Recent studies have focused on finding the genes involved with renal development whose abnormal expressions are responsible for renal dysplasia.

Classically, kidney malformations including dysplasia are classified based on histology.

Recent advances in molecular biology and genetics have led Woolf and Winyard (Wolf & Winyard, 1998) to suggest a more straightforward classification to describe kidney malformations. The abnormalities can be divided into groups, based on the underlying cell biology, such as aberrant early development or defect in terminal maturation (Winyard & Chitty, 2001). The aberrant early development group, include dysplastic kidneys, whether large multicystic dysplastic kidneys or small organs with combination of hypoplasia-dysplasia and some obstructed kidneys.

Defects in terminal maturation are observed in polycystic kidney disease.

This category of renal disease is usually not associated with an obstructive uropathy and is mainly managed by nephrologists for the development of renal failure and hypertension.

Dysplastic kidneys can be any size, ranging between massive kidney with multiple large cyst up to 9 cm, to normal or small kidneys with or without cyst. (figure 2)

Dysplasia can be unilateral, bilateral, or segmental affecting only part of the kidney.

2. Diagnosis

The current classic presentation is the prenatal sonographic diagnosis, that could be made at 15 weeks of gestation, with typical appearance of multilocualted abdominal mass consisting of multiple thin walled cysts, which do not appear to connect, or circumferential cysts in kidneys of more normal size, associated with lower urinary tract obstruction, particularly in bilateral cases.

The amniotic fluid volume is usually normal in unilateral cases and with oligo or anhydramnios in bilateral cases. Small kidneys are difficult to detect prenatally and are commonly missdiagnosed as renal agenesis. Even with evident prenatal diagnosis, a post natal follow up is needed to confirm the diagnosis and search for associated anomalies (heart, spine, extremities, face, and umbilical cord, as up to 35% may have extrarrenal anomalies and these are more frequent in bilateral disease).

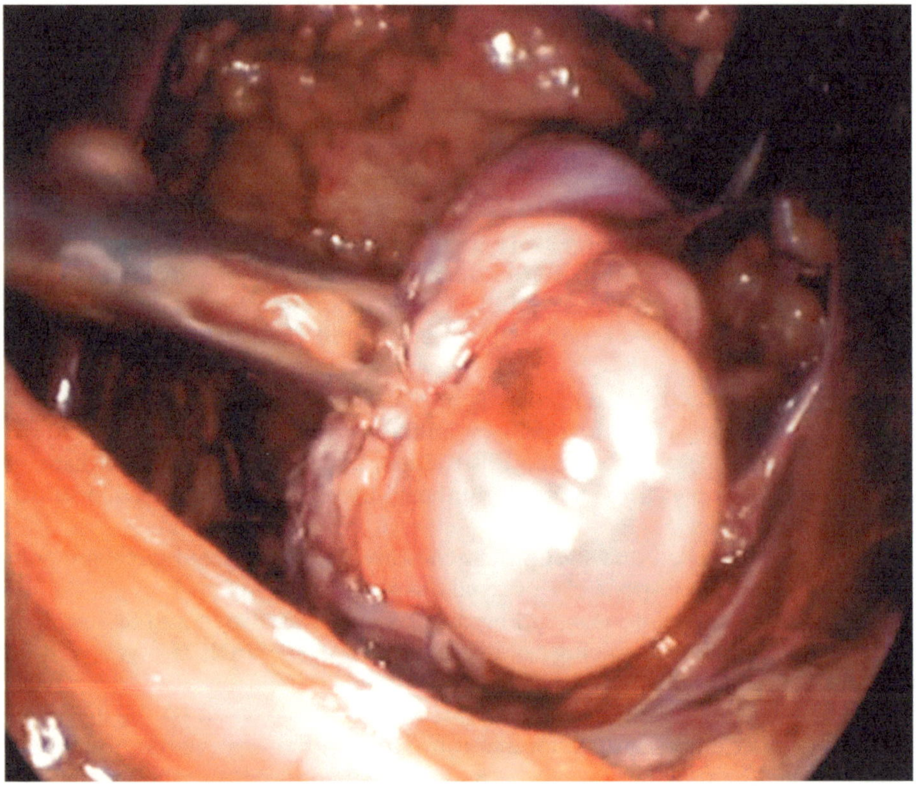

Fig. 2. Dysplastic kidneys can be any size, ranging between massive kidney with multiple large cyst up to 9 cm, to normal or small kidneys with or without cyst (typical multicystic dysplastic kidney appearing as a "bunch of grapes").

Previously before the routine antenatal ultrasound, the diagnosis was most often made in infancy in the presence of a palpable abdominal mass, which is found in 22% to 37% of the cases(12-13), flank pain, urinary tract infection or hypertension.

Ultrasound in combination with renal scintigraphy yields an accurate diagnosis of MCDK disease in 93% of suspected cases (Stuck et al., 1982).

Stuck et al have characterized ultrasound features of dysplastic kidney: presence of sharp interfaces between multiple, randomly arranged, and variable size cysts, the largest with nonmedial location; a lack of an identifiable renal sinus; and an absence of renal parenchyma (Strife et al., 1993). (figure 3)

Parenchymal imaging with Tc99m DMSA provide an excellent picture of functional parenchyma or defects indicating nonfunctioning parenchyma, but it has the inability to assess the excretory phase of renal function that makes it impossible to distinguish MCDK from hydronephrosis caused by UPJ obstruction. (Koff et al., 1980; Tyrrell et al., 1994) (figure 4)

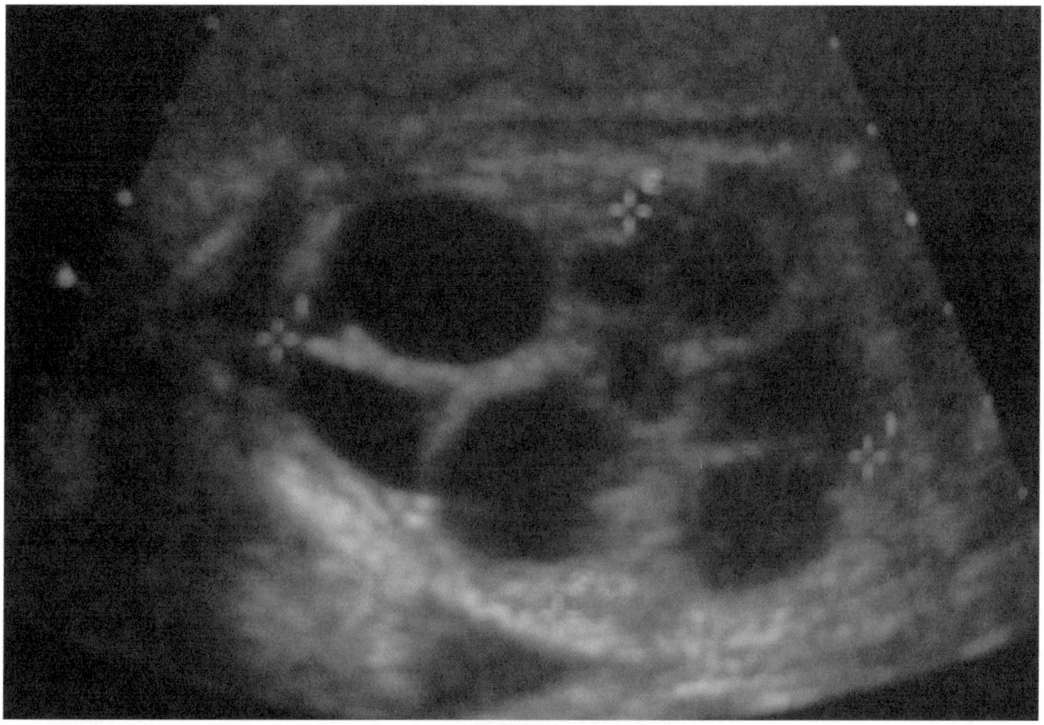

Fig. 3. Prenatal sonographic diagnosis of M.C.D.K. (presence of sharp interfaces between multiple, randomly arranged, and variable size cysts, the largest with nonmedial location; a lack of an identifiable renal sinus; and an absence of renal parenchyma).

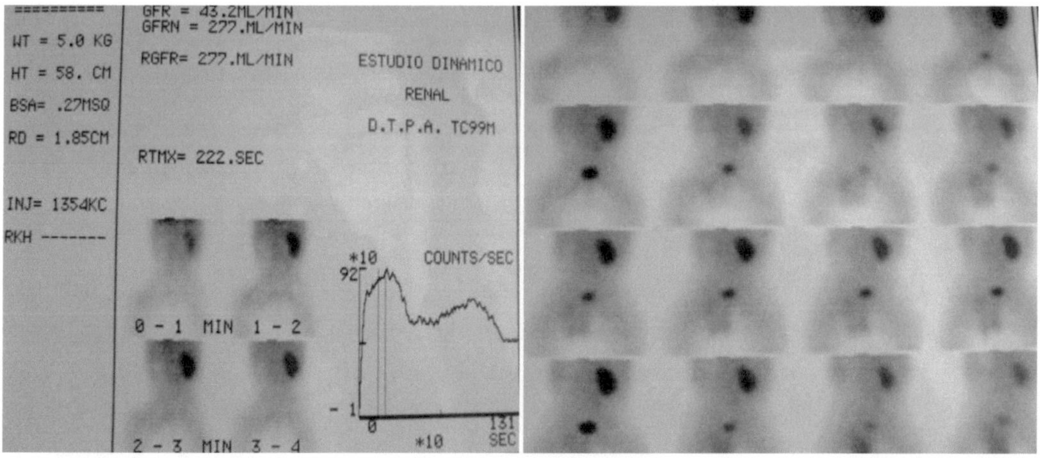

Fig. 4. Renal scintigraphy.All the kidneys removed showed renal function lower than 10% in D.T.P.A. (Parenchymal imaging with Tc 99mDMSA provide and excellent picture of functional parenchyma or defects indicating nonfunctioning parenchyma, but it has the inability to assess the excretory phase of renal function that makes impossible distinguish MCDK from hydronephrosis caused by UPJ obstruction).

If the diagnosis is unclear, a Nephro TAC or Uro MRI to differentiate MCDK from obstructive uropathy or duplex system is performed. (figure 5) (figure 6)

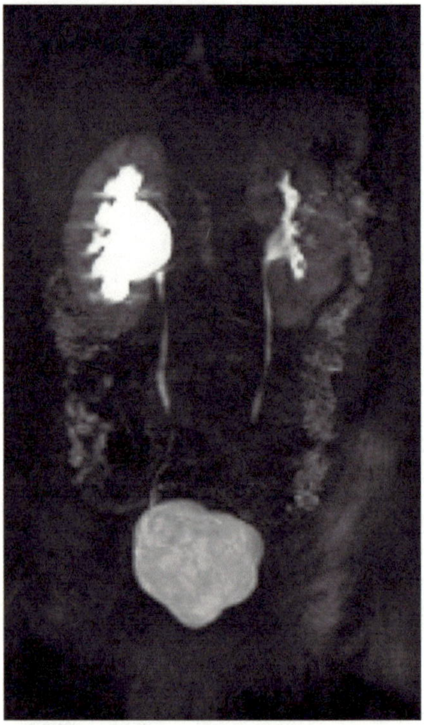

Fig. 5. Hydronephrosis in the right kidney with ureteropelvic junction obstruction by Uro MRI.

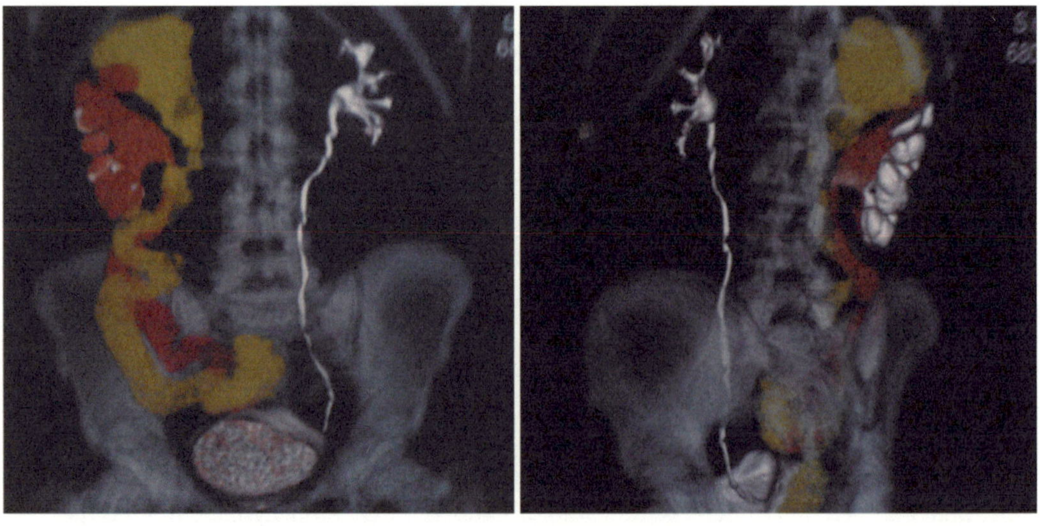

Fig. 6. Nephro TAC with 3 D reconstruction to differentiate MCDK from obstructive uropathy or duplex system.

Complete evaluation include VCUG; contralateral v.u.r has been reported to be associated in 15% to 28% of cases in literature.(Al-Khaldi et al., 1994; Aslam & Watson, 2006; Atiyeh et al., 1992; Karmazyn & Zerin, 1997) (figure 7)

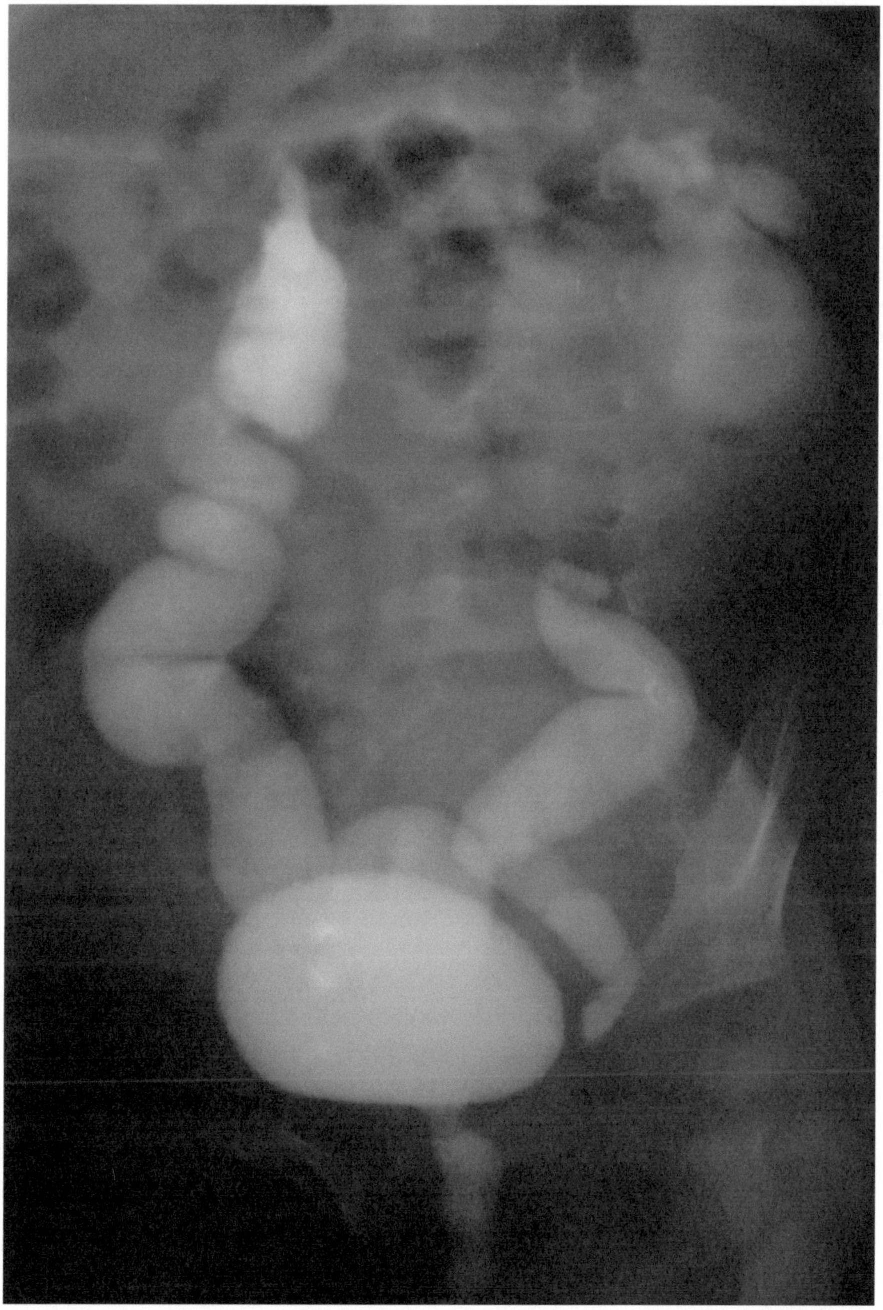

Fig. 7. Contralateral V.U.R has been reported to be associated in 15% to 28% of cases of M.C.D.K. in literature.

The improvement in our understanding of the natural history of some congenital renal anomalies, such as multicystic dysplastic kidney (MCDK), has caused some changes in management approach.
The treatment of MCDK has passed through different phases. It was originally suggested that dysplastic kidneys must be removed to avoid rare complications such as hypertension, infection or possible malignant transformation until the mid-1980s.
In the last decade, there has been a shift in the management of dysplastic kidneys from surgical removal to a conservative approach using serial US examination (Wacksman & Phipps, 1993; Gordon et al., 1988). This change in treatment is due to the perception that malignant transformation is a rare occurrence, and sequential US imaging of a large number of infants diagnosed with this problem has revealed that most of these structures involute over time without causing any problems.
In 2001 Oliveira et al found partial involution in 68%, complete involution in 21% and increase in unit size in 11%.The mean age at complete or partial involution of the lesion was 18 months.
In unilateral cases, there is often a compensatory hypertrophy of the contralateral kidney. (Oliveira et al., 2001)
In recent years, the argument has emerged again with regard to the management of dysplastic kidneys; several studies have recommended surgical removal because the natural history of the condition in the long term is still uncertain, and nephrectomy is more cost effective than conservative management, however an elective nephrectomy is no longer routinely performed in most of centers.
Patients with bilateral disease or associated genitourinary anomalies had a higher incidence of urinary tract infection and progression to renal failure (22% with obstruction and 14% with contralateral reflux).Rare complications as pain was reported as the only symptom in older patient with resolution after nephrectomy. (Ambrose et al., 1982)
Holloway et al report a huge cyst, that need percutaneous decompression to relieve the respiratory distress in infant. (Holloway & Weinstein, 1990)
In the registry of the American Academy of Pediatrics for dysplatic kidney 2.6% were associated with infection, hypertension was found in less than 1% (olders reports have demonstrated its resolution after nephrectomy).
Seeman et al (Seeman et al., 2001), monitored blood pressure in children and found anomalies only in those who had ultrasonographic, and or laboratory signs of contralateral kidney abnormalities.
In children neoplasia represents 25% of indications. This is to be expected in view of the higher incidence of malignancy in older patients and the higher proportion of children who present with congenital malformations. In a review of the literature, Perez (Perez et al., 1998) found multiple reports of malignancy arising in MCDK, including renal cell carcinoma (5 cases), malignant mesothelioma (1 case) and Wilms tumor (11 cases).
Narchi (Narchi, 2005) performed a systematic review of the literature managed conservatively; no children developed a Wilms tumor. But there is another argument favouring the association between Wilms tumor and MCDK; the finding of nephrogenic rest, recognized as precursors to nephroblastoma, which may remain quiescent or become hyperplastic, forming a nodule (adenomatous focus or nodular renal blastema) is possibly an early stage in tumor formation. (Beckwith et al., 1990)
Even though this association or the malignant degeneration is exceptional, a careful initial ultrasound examination is mandatory and any equivocal diagnosis with suspicious nature of the cyst should lead to surgical removal of the kidney.

Conservative follow up includes renal ultrasound every 3 to 4 months to age 3 years, every 6 months to age 5 years, and then every year to age 8 years. (Onal & Kogan, 2006)

The regimen would be costly when considered on a level compared with early nephrectomy. In some cases close long term follow up, with ultrasound and physical examination may be easier said than done, and rigid compliance may be unrealistic. In these cases, early surgical excision may be the best treatment.

We thought it pertinent to assess the effects of the last changes on the indications for nephrectomy in the paediatric age group.

A literature review revealed a limited number of publications on the indications for nephrectomy in children.

A few reports reviewed the indications in various age groups without any special mention of paediatric patients (Scott (Jr) & Selzman, 1966; Beisland et al., 2000).

Others reported on a small number of nephrectomies in children (Schmidt et al., 1992; Pearlman & Kobashigawa, 1968).

Laparoscopic nephrectomy offers advantages similar to the retroperitoneal approach for open surgery; Hamilton et al (Hamilton et al., 2000) found comparable results on transperitoneal laparoscopic nephrectomy with significant decrease in hospital stay after laparoscopic compared with open nephrectomy (22.5 vs 42.3 hours) with longer operative time in laparoscopic group (175.6 vs 120.2 min).

In laparoscopy the peritoneal cavity and its contents are avoided, minimizing risk of injury that may occur when mobilizing bowel, and avoiding potential future complications associated with intraperitoneal adhesions.

Here, we report our initial series of laparoscopic nephrectomies in paediatric patients, their indications, and the clinical presentation of this particular group of patients with various renal abnormalities that required nephrectomy.

In our experience, most MCDK's have ultimately been removed, reflux nephropathy was the second major indication for nephrectomy; whether VUR is associated with congenital dysplasia/hypoplasia that is not amenable to any form of postnatal therapy, or whether this form of treatment is unsuccessful in preventing' further renal damage; has yet to be clarified.

The decrease in the proportion of nephrectomies performed for PUJ (third main indication) obstruction is probably due to the vigorous use of antenatal scan to detect these cases as early as possible thus allowing proper follow up and intervention when required.

This is in agreement with the findings of Capolicchio and colleagues who demonstrated that early diagnosis of hydronephrosis provided by prenatal Ultrasonography is associated with less obstructive nephropathy (Capolicchio et al., 1999).

Laparoscopy is considered to be the standard technique in performing nephrectomies in children with renal benign disorders.

Many studies have shown the advantage of this, against open technique.

Nowadays, a laparoscopic nephrectomy can be performed in two ways, transperitoneal or retroperitoneal. (Collar R et al., 2001; Baez et al., 2003)

The first laparoscopic nephrectomy was performed by Clayman in 1991 using the transperitoneal technique on an 85 years old female patient.

The first to perform a retroperitoneoscopy with insufflation were Roberts (Roberts, 1976) in 1978 and Wickham (Wickham & Miller, 1979) in 1979.

Gaur and Kerbl in 1992 published the first cases of retroperitoneal laparoscopic nephrectomies in adults (Gaur et al., 1993; Kerbl et al., 1993), whereas Chandoke, Rassweiller and Valla did the same with children in 1993, 1994 and 1996 respectively. (Chandhoke et al., 1993; Rasweiller et al., 1994; Valla et al., 1996)

Since then a large amount of result have been published using both laparoscopic nephrectomy techniques.

The renal benign disorder continues to be the main indication for nephrectomy in children for non-functioning kidneys secondary to obstructive uropathy or reflux. Although laparoscopy nephrectomy is an easy and safe procedure, the indications for nephrectomy are still debatable. The acceptable indications for these cases are the increase in size of cysts or the rare complications of hypertension and infection.

Malignant renal tumors in children are not considered for laparoscopy (the most common is nephroblastoma that is large in size, frequently extending outside the kidney and with high risk of rupture during dissection), although recently cases of extractions of kidneys tumors have been published using both techniques. (Duarte et al., 2004; Etcheverry et al., 2002) In spite of this we have not included in our statistics oncologist indications, and in not one of the extracted materials malignant signs of tumors were found.

3. Technique

For the transperitoneal approach ,with patient in dorsal decubitus three ports were placed, one in the navel (10 mm optic device)the second and third ports(5 mm working ports) on the half clavicular line below the rib cage ,and one the same side, 2 cms above the level of the superior iliac spine; respectively; has shown the advantage of working in a wide space and with easier identifiable anatomic repairs and a more direct view of intraabdominal organs to avoid, and the umbilical port is well concealed, particularly for specimen removal. Nevertheless the access to the renal hilar region requires a considerable mobilization and retraction of the bowel.

Like other adult and paediatric surgeons (Lorenzo Gomez & Gonzales, 2003) used to working laparoscopically in the abdominal cavity, we opted for the transperitoneal approach to start our experience, which could affect the final results because these were the first patients in our learning curve.

Retroperitoneoscopic nephrectomy in children has several advantages over transperitoneal approaches .There is less risk of injury to adjacent organs such as the bowel, liver or spleen, with little risk of formation of intraperitoneal adhesions; and the retropeitoneum can be drained more effectively than the peritoneum.

Guilloneau and col demonstrated a lesser average time in performing nephrectomies by lumboscopy and comparing them with the laparoscopic approach (Guilloneau et al., 1996) this probably due to a direct entry via retroperitoneal in the renal cell without the necessity of abdominal dissection.

Lorenzo Gomez and R Gonzales, carried out an investigation comparing more than 330 procedures performed using both methods, were, the operating time for the retroperitoneal approach was also less. (Lorenzo Gomez & Gonzales, 2003)

The retroperitoneal approach needs a good anatomical knowledge that has been viewed by Himpens (Himpens, 1996). It has the disadvantage of smaller active space with an absence of intraabdominal structures easy to recognize like the liver or spleen. At the same time provides a direct and faster to the renal hillius avoiding bowel manipulation that could produce ileus and delay the recovery of the patient.

By this direct access to the kidney in an anatomic orientation with gravity facilitating exposure of the renal hilum, the artery lies posterior so it can be controlled without manipulating the vein, and this allows control of arteries prior to veins, according to the accepted practice, to prevent engorgement of the kidney and easier control of veins with less blood in them. The renal pelvis is posterior as well facilitating mobilization and exposure as needed. If open access to the kidney becomes urgent, it can be performed through a lumbotomy incision.
With the patient in the lateral decubitus and hyper extension of the problem side getting a better active place, on the lower end of the 12th rib a 10 mm port were placed for optic device, and the two working 5 mm ports, one above the of the iliac crests upper line and the other resting the external side of the lumbar complex muscle equidistant to the others. (figure 8)

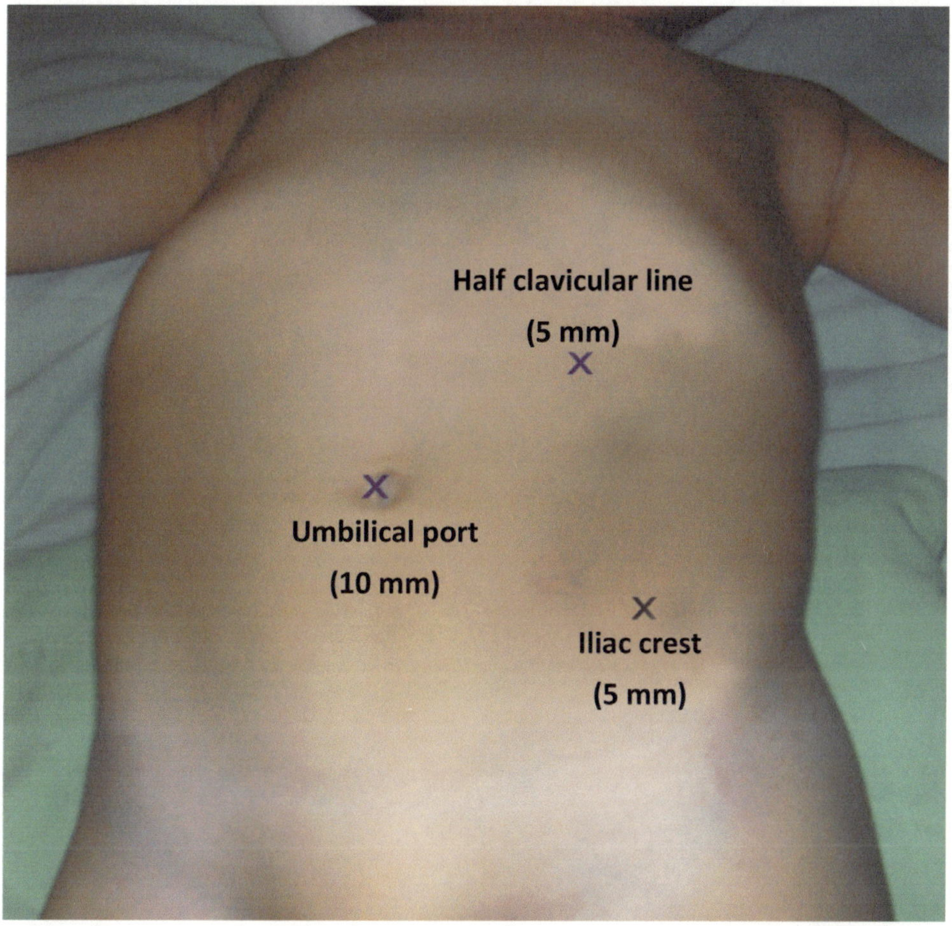

Fig. 8. Patient positioning for transperitoneal approach with the surgeon standing in the front of the abdomen, the child is positioned with the flank of the involved side elevated at 30 degree angle to facilitate the exposure after reflecting the colon. Three ports were placed, one in the navel (10 mm optic device) the second and third ports (5 mm working ports) on the half clavicular line below the rib cage ,and one the same side, 2 cms above the level of the superior iliac spine; respectively. A fourth trocar could be placed in the midaxillary line for exposure to retract the liver or spleen if needed.

After the introduction of the 10 mm port, the two mains landmarks- anterior part of the psoas muscle and the lower pole of the kidney, mobile with respiration-are recognized. (figure 9)

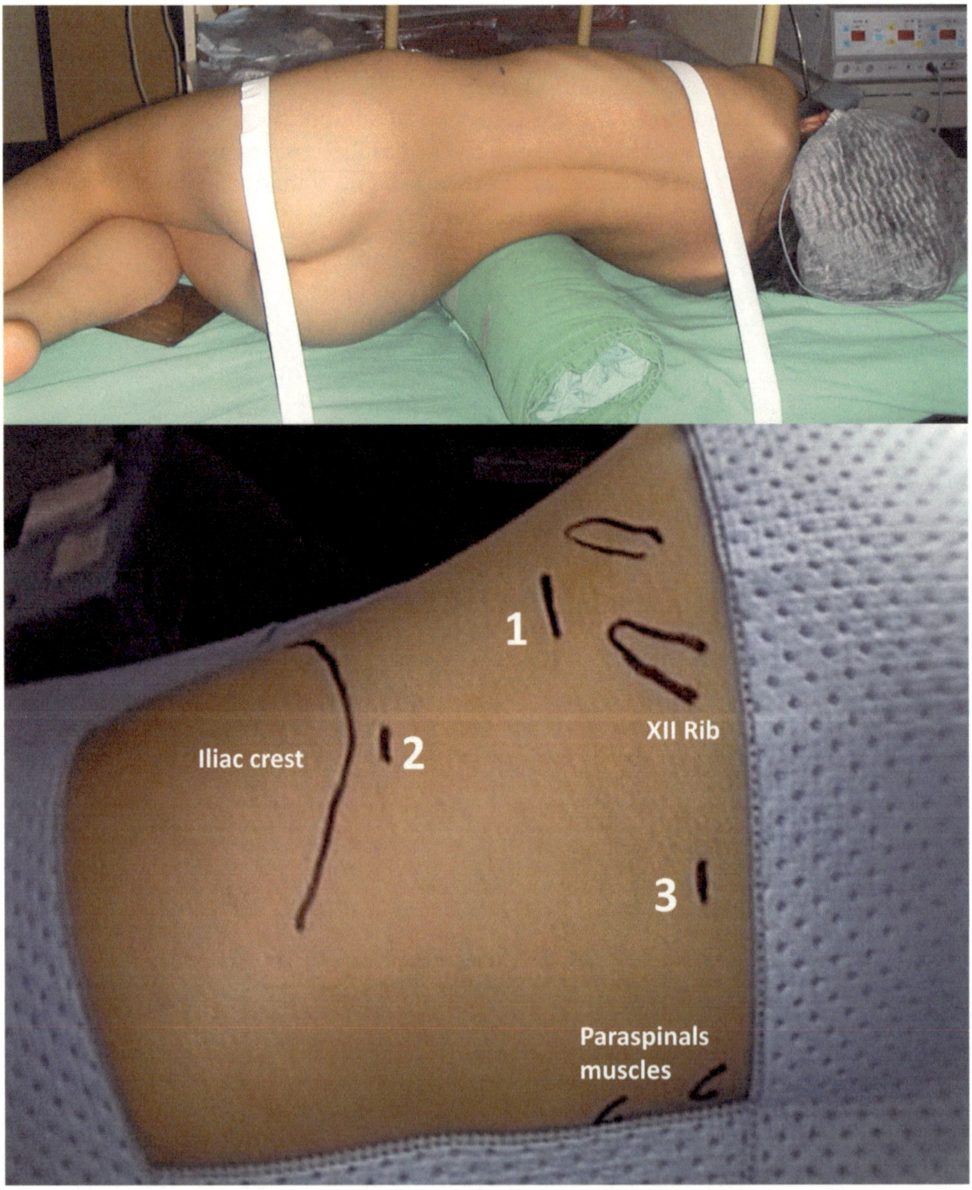

Fig. 9. Position for retroperitoneal approach. The patient is placed in the lateral decubitus position, exposing the involved side as in position for an open simple nephrectomy, with sufficient flexion of the operating table so as to expose the area of trocars placement: on the lower end of the 12th rib a 10 mm port were placed for optic device, and the two working 5 mm ports, one above the iliac crests upper line and the other resting on the external side of the lumbar complex muscle equidistant to the others.

The working space is progressively created by moving the tip of the telescope to free retroperitoneal fibrous tissues, taking care not to injury the peritoneum.
After the two faces and the two poles are completely freed, the kidney is mobilized to the top, and the renal vessel dissected via posterior approach, in the inferior part of the field where there are only one artery and one vein and not too close to the kidney were the vessels are divided in several branches. (figure 10)

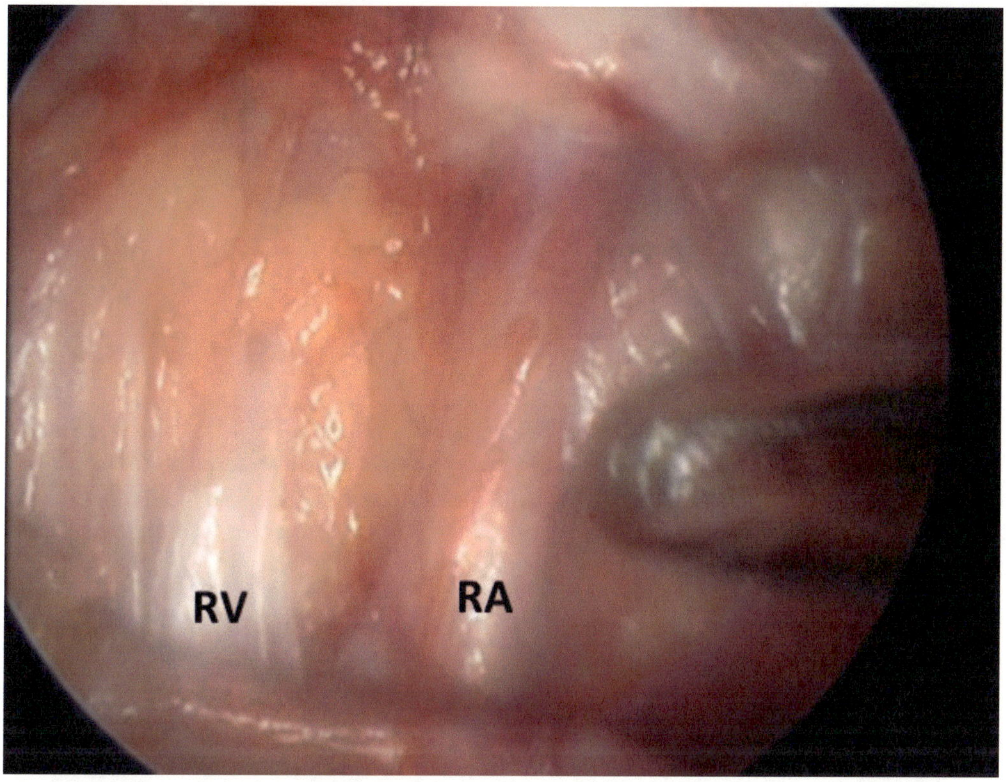

Fig. 10. Exposure and ligature of the renal pedicle which is identified and approached posteriorly. The kidney drops under gravity keeping the vessels under stretch. This allows careful two-instrument dissection of the vascular pedicle. At the left side the artery is dissected close the junction with the aorta and vena cava, and at the right side the renal vein is also exposed of it full length.

If the ilium dissection is difficult the ureter may serve as main reference it's easy to recognize in the retroperitoneal space and its dissection up to the kidney leads to the renal vessels.
After dissection of the renal pedicle, the vessels are clipped, ligated or coagulated, depending of the vessel diameter and the surgeon experience. (figure 11)
The ureterectomy could be limited to the lumbar portion in non-refluxing ureter; in presence of reflux or dilated ureter the dissection is distally followed and the ureter is ligated s close as possible to the ureterovesical junction.
For the material extraction in all cases the renal tissue was sufficiently thin enough to allow the extraction through the incision of the initial port without morcellation. (figure 12)

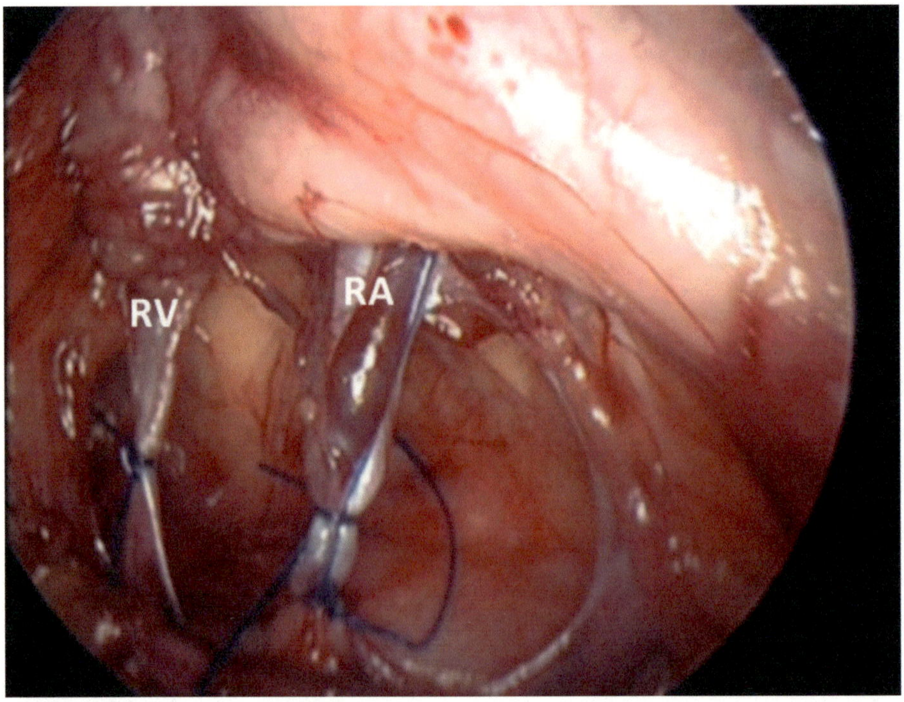

Fig. 11. After dissection of the renal pedicle, the vessels could be clipped, ligated or coagulated depending of the vessel diameter and the surgeon experience (in this case ligature of the renal pedicle with extracorporeal knots).

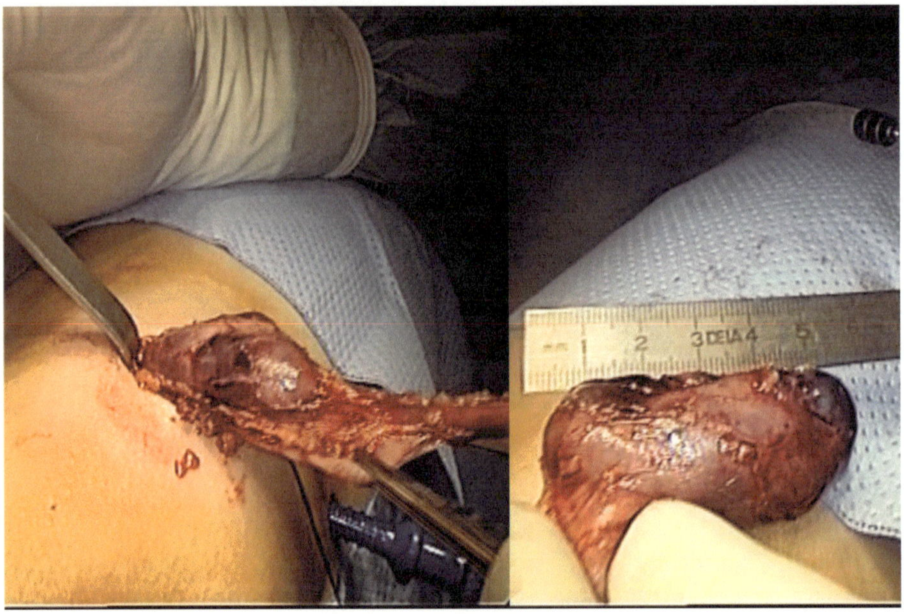

Fig. 12. For the material extraction in all cases the renal tissue was sufficiently thin enough to allow the extraction through the incision of the initial port without morcellation.

In our initial experience thirty two laparoscopic total nephrectomies were performed. On the beginning of our learning curve the first ten (10) patients were treated using the transperitoneal technique (group 1) whereas the rest using retroperitoneal technique(group 2).The indications for both groups were similar: V.U.R. 4 patients for group 1 and 6 for 2, hydronephrosis 3 patients for T.P. and 6 for R.P. and M.C.D.K. 3 patients for group 1 and 8 patients for group 2. (figure 13)

	Indications	
	Group 1	Group 2
V.U.R	4 patients	6 patients
Hydronephrosis	3 patients	6 patients
M.C.D.K.	3 patients	8 patients

Fig. 13. Main surgical indications for laparoscopic nephrectomy by both procedures (V.U.R.: vesicoureteral reflux, M.C.D.K.: Multi Cystic Dysplasic Kidney).

Two patients underwent upper pole laparoscopic heminephrectomies using the retroperitoneal approach have not been included in the final results.
1 case of retroperitoneal had to be converted due to massive hydronephrosis with perirrenal fibrosis.
Rasweiller et al. report a longer operating time in similar cases with a high probability of conversion for severe adhesions and fibrosis (Rasweiller et al., 1998), but Hemal et al. demonstrated that is feasible to perform retroperitoneal nephrectomies with massive hydronephrosis (more than 1000 mL of liquid in system). (Hemal et al., 1999)
But nevertheless like Valla et al. don't recommend the initial retroperitoneal practice on these types of patients. (Valla et al., 1996)
In the other case a transperitoneal nephrectomy changed into an open technique due to a problem with the equipment that occurred during surgery.
In the rest 28 laparoscopic operations performed there were no complications during surgery. During 2 retroperitoneal operations we had peritoneal perforations that did not cause any consequences, emphysema or pneumothorax. Hemodynamic changes and CO_2 diffusion were equal with the two laparoscopic techniques, in our results.
Postoperative management after transperitoneal or retroperitoneal nephrectomy does not require specific cares.
Both approaches were statistically similar with respect to complications during and after surgery, hospitalization and analgesic requirements.
All the patients could eat again within the first 24 hours .However those operated on using the retroperitoneal method were able to eat earlier than those the transabdominal way. It is important to clarify that in the first cases for all laparoscopic surgeries with intraabdominal technique, the post-surgery tolerance could have been delayed because of more conservative approach. Nevertheless 2 patients of the group 1 (T.P.) vomited at 10 and 12 hours after

surgery delaying the return to oral feeding. It is interesting to note, in many publications (Poddoubny et al., 2003; Ehrlich et al., 1994) in nephrectomies performed intraabdominally there are no details of events like nausea or vomiting early on after surgery, despite the fact that all achieve tolerance within the first 12-24 hrs.

A prospective and comparative study by Desai et al (Desai et al., 2005) using both techniques, in 5 out of 50 patients resulted in ileus that lasted longer than 48 hs in transabdominal nephrectomies.

However they could not associate this approach with a large incidence of ileus.

It is for this reason that today in our institution the laparoscopic retroperitoneal approach is the preferred method to perform nephrectomies. Despite this preference we have achieved our learning curve with transperitoneal approach and now we are quite willing to recommend it to those starting urologic laparoscopy.

The main advantage of a retroperitoneal approach is more direct and faster exposure (Doublet et al., 1996) without peritoneal transgression and without dissection and handling of intraperitoneal structures; avoid the risk of shoulder pain, omental evisceration or intestinal adhesions (Moore et al., 1995) and can be easily performed even after previous abdominal surgery.

The retroperitoneal approach had the disadvantage in the lack of natural cavity; the working space should be created with the risk of accidental peritoneal tear (Morgan (Jr) & Rader, 1992; Kumar et al., 2001) that induces pneumoperitoneum and reduces the working space and visibility. This incident could be avoided by careful preparation of the retroperitoneal space for insertion of anterior working ports. If that occurs at the beginning of the procedure, it is useful to close with purse string suture of the perforation or if it not possible, by inserting a Verress needle in the peritoneal cavity to desufflate the pneumoperitoneum continuously during the surgery.

The second disadvantage is that ergonomics of work is less, with reduced surgical field and it requires a greater learning curve and better surgical skills to perform. This problem was exposed by Erlich et al. (Ehrlich et al., 1994) who in the first retroperitoneal surgery stated that the limited working space precluded introduction of other retroperitoneal instrument.

Finally this initial study shows that there is comparable security and efficacy in both approaches but probably there exist specific situations in which a particular method is more suitable.

We believe that the option of the laparoscopic approach for the nephrectomy must depend on the preference and the individual training of each surgeon, and the choice of approach must be in accordance with each clinical situation emphasizing and recommending retroperitoneal procedures while the surgical skills of the surgeon can.

There has been an improvement in our understanding of the natural history of some congenital renal anomalies, such as multicystic dysplastic kidney (M.C.D.K.), which has caused some changes in management approach.

Minimally invasive procedures emphasize our goals of improving patient comfort and safety while adapting the laparoscopic procedures as closely as possible to the conventional surgical techniques. (El-Gonehimi et al., 2002)

Actually laparoscopic is considered to be the standard technique in performing nephrectomies in children with renal benign disorders.

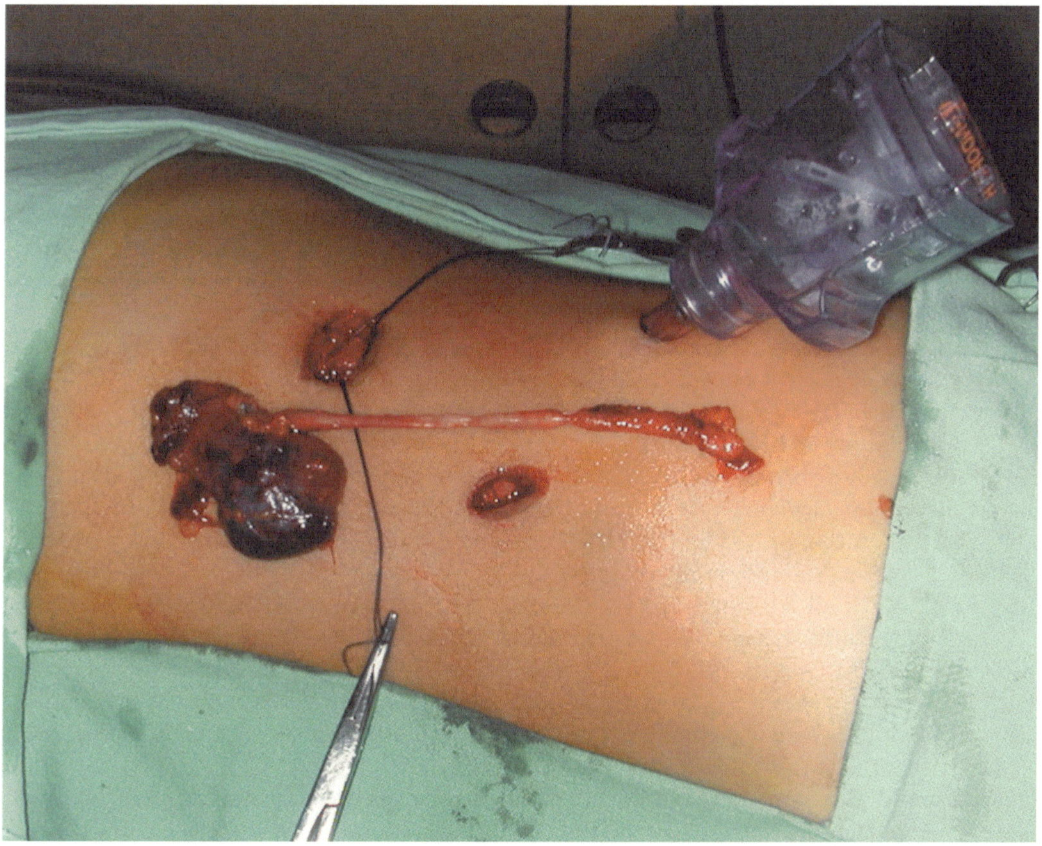

Fig. 14. In our institution the laparoscopic retroperitoneal approach is the preferred method to perform nephrectomies, but there is comparable security and efficacy in both approaches.

Conflict of interest
The authors have nothing to disclose.

Ethical approval
Ethical approval was not required.

4. References

[1] Clayman RV, Kavoussi LR, Soper NJ, et al (1991). *Laparoscopy nephrectomy.* N Engl J Med; 324:1370.
[2] Figenshau RS, Clayman RV, Kerbl D, et al (1994). *Laparoscopic nephrectomy in the child: initial report.* J Urol; 151:740-741.
[3] Schwartz J (1936). *An unusual unilateral multicystic kidney in an infant.* J Urol; 35:259.
[4] Pathak IG, Williams DI (1964). *Multicystic and cystic dysplastic kidneys.* Br J Urol; 36:318.
[5] Felson B, Cussen LJ (1975). *The hydronephrotic type of congenital multicystic disease of the kidney.* Semin Roentgenol; 10:113.
[6] Shibata S, Shigeta M, Shu U, et al (2001). *Initial pathological events in renal dysplasia with urinary tract obstruction in utero.* Virchows Arch; 439:560.

[7] Matsell DG, Bennett T, Goodyer P, et al (1996). *The pathogenesis of multicystic dysplastic kidney disease: insights from the study of fetal kidneys.* Lab Invest; 74:883.
[8] Mackie CG, Stephens SD (1975). *Duplex kidneys: a correlation of renal dysplasia with position of the ureteral orifice.* J Urol; 114:274
[9] Spencer JR, Maizel M (1987). *Inhibition of protein glycosylation causes renal dysplasia in the chick embryo.* J Urol; 138:94.
[10] Wolf AS, Winyard PJD (1998). *Advances in the cell biology and genetics of human kidney malformations.* J Am Soc Nephrol; 9:114-1125.
[11] Winyard P, Chitty L (2001). *Dysplastic and polycystic kidneys: diagnosis, associations and managements.* Prenat Diagn; 21.924-935.
[12] Gordon AC, Thomas DFM, Arthur RJ, et al (1988). *Multicystic dysplastic kidney: is nephrectomy still appropriate?* J Urol; 140:1231.
[13] Kessler OJ, Ziv N, Livne PM, et al (1998). *Involution rate of multicystic renal dysplasia.* Pediatrics; 102:1472.
[14] Stuck KJ, Koff SA, Silver TM (1982). *Ultrasonic features of multicystic dysplastic kidney: expanded diagnostic criteria.* Radiology; 143:217.
[15] Strife JL, Souza AS, Kirks DR, et al (1993). *Multicystic dysplastic kidney in children: US follow-up.* Radiology; 186:785.
[16] Koff SA, Thrall JH, Keyes (Jr) JW (1980). *Assessment of hydroureteronephrosis in children using diuretic radionuclide urography.* J Urol; 123:531.
[17] Tyrrell PNM, Boivin CM, Burrell DN, et al (1994). *Multicystic dysplastic kidney: another application of 99mTc MAG3.* Clin Radiol; 49:400.
[18] Al-Khaldi N, Watson AR, Zuccollo J, et al (1994). *Outcome of antenatally detected cystic dysplastic kidney disease.* Arch Dis Child; 70:520.
[19] Aslam M, Watson AR (2006). *Unilateral multicystic dysplastic kidney: long term outcomes.* Arch Dis Child; 91:820
[20] Atiyeh B, Husmann D, Baum M (1992). *Contralateral renal abnormalities in multicystic-dysplastic kidney disease.* J Pediatr; 121:65.
[21] Karmazyn B, Zerin JM (1997). *Lower urinary tract abnormalities in children with multicystic dysplastic kidney.* Radiology; 203:223
[22] Wacksman J, Phipps L (1993). *Report of the Multicystic Kidney Registry preliminary findings.* J Urol; 150:1870e2.
[23] Gordon AC, Thomas DF, Arthur RJ, Irving HC (1988). *Multicystic dysplastic kidney: is nephrectomy still appropriate?* J Urol; 140(5 Pt 2):1231e4.
[24] Oliveira EA, Diniz JS, Vilasboas AS, et al (2001). *Multicystic dysplastic kidney detected by fetal sonography:conservative management and follow up.* Pediatr Surg Int; 17:54-7.
[25] Ambrose SS, GouldRA, Trulock TS, Parrot TS (1982). *Unilateral multicystic renal disease in adults.* J Urol; 128:366-369
[26] Holloway WR, Weinstein SH (1990). *Percutaneous descompression :treatment for respiratory distress secondary to* multicystic dysplastic kidney. J Urol; 144:113-115.
[27] Seeman T, John U, BlahovaK et al (2001). *Ambulatory blood pressure monitoring in children with unilateral multicystic dysplastic kidney.* Eur J Pediatr; 160:78-83.
[28] Perez LM, Naidu SI, Joseph DB (1998). *Outcome and cost analysis of operative versus nonoperative management of neonatal multicystic dysplastic kidneys.* J Urol; 160:1207.
[29] Narchi H (2005). *Risk of Wilms' tumour with multicystic kidney disease: a systematic review.* Arch Dis Child; 90:147.

[30] Beckwith JB, Kiviat NB, Bonadio JF (1990). *Nephrogenic rests, nephroblastomatosis, and the pathogenesis of Wilms' tumor*. Pediatr Pathol; 10:1.

[31] Onal B, Kogan B (2006). *Natural history of patients with multicystic dysplastic kidney – what follow-up is needed?*. J Urol; 176:1607.

[32] Scott (Jr) RF, Selzman HM (1966). *Complications of nephrectomy: review of 450 patients and a description of a modification of the transperitoneal approach*. J Urol; 95:307e12.

[33] Beisland C, Medby PC, Sander S, Beisland HO (2000). *Nephrectomy e indications, complications and postoperative mortality in 646 consecutive patients*. Eur Urol; 37: 58e64.

[34] Schmidt A, Dietz HG, Schneider K (1992). *Long-term results after partial and unilateral nephrectomy in childhood*. Eur J Pediatr Surg; 2:269e73.

[35] Pearlman CK, Kobashigawa L. Nephrectomy: review of 200 cases. Am Surg 1968; 34:438e41.

[36] Hamilton BD, Gatti JM, Cartwright PC, Snow BW (2000). *Comparison of laparoscopic versus open nephrectomy in the pediatric population*. J Urol; 163:937-939.

[37] Capolicchio G, Leonard MP, Wong C, et al (1999). *Prenatal diagnosis of hydronephrosis: impact on renal function and its recovery after pyeloplasty*. J Urol; 162:1029e32.

[38] Collar R, Etcheverry R, Urrutia A, et al (2001). *Nefrectomía laparoscópica retroperitoeal en pediatría*. Rev de Cir Inf; 12(2):169-171.

[39] Baez JJN, Betolli M, Sentagne A, et al (2003). *Nefrectomía vía laparoscópica transperitoneal*. Rev Cir Inf; 13(3 y 4): 152-154.

[40] Roberts JA (1976). *Retroperitoneal endoscopy*. J Med Primatol; 5:124-127.

[41] Wickham JEA, Miller RA. Urinary calculus disease. The surgical treatment of urolithiasis 1979: 145-198.

[42] Gaur DD, Agarwal DR, Purhoit KC (1993). *Retroperitoneal laparoscopic nephrectomy: Initial case report*. J Urol; 149: 103-105.

[43] Kerbl K, Figenshau RS, Clayman RV, et al (1993). *Retroperitoneal laparoscopic nephrectomy: Laboratory and clinical experience*. J Endourol; 7:23-26.

[44] Chandhoke RS, Glansky S, Koyle M, Kaula NF (1993). *Pediatric retroperitoneal laparoscopic nephrectomy*. J Endourol; 138(suppl 7): 12.

[45] Rasweiller JJ, Henkel TO, Stoch D, et al (1994). *Retroperitoneal laparoscopic nephrectomy and other procedures in the upper retroperitoneum using a ballon disection technique*. Eur Urol; 25:229-236.

[46] Valla JS, Guilloneau B, Montupet Ph, et al (1996). *Retroperitoneal laparoscopic nephrectomy in children: preliminary report of 18 cases*. It J Ped Surg Sci; 10(1-2):35-37.

[47] Duarte JD, Denes F, Cristofani LM, et al (2004). *Laparoscopic nephrectomy for Wilms tumor after chemotherapy. Initial experience*. J Urol; 172:1438-1440.

[48] Etcheverry R, Collar R, Tobia Gonzales S, et al (2002). *Nefroma quístico en pediatría. Manejo quirúrgico con técnica videolaparoscópica retroperitoneal*. Rev de Cir Inf; 12(2):117-119.

[49] Lorenzo Gomez MF, Gonzales R (2003). *Laparoscopic nephrectomy in children: the transperitoneal vs the retroperitoneal approach*. Arch Esp urol; 56(4):401-413.

[50] Guilloneau B, Ballanger P, Lugagne PM, Valla JS, Vallancien G (1996). *Laparoscopic vs lumboscopic nephrectomy*. Eur Urol; 29(3):288-291.

[51] Himpens H (1996). *Technique, equipement and exposure for endoscopic retroperitoneal surgery*. Seminars in Laparosic surgery; 3-2-; 109-116.

[52] Rasweiller J, Fornara P, Weber M, et al (1998). *Laparoscopic nephrectomy: the experience of the laparoscopy working group of the German Urologic Association.* J Urol; 160(1):28.
[53] Hemal AK, Wadhwa SN, Kumar M, Gupta NP (1999). *Transperitoneal and retroperitoneal laparoscopic nephrectomy for giant hydronephrosis.* J Urol; 162:35-35.
[54] Valla JS, Guilloneau B, Montupet Ph, et al (1996). *Retroperitoneal laparoscopic nephrectomy in children: preliminary report of 18 cases.* It J Ped Surg Sci; 0(1-2):35-37.
[55] Poddoubny IV, Dronov AF, Kovarsky SL, et al (2003). *Laparoscopic nephrectomy and nephroureterectomy in 90 pediatric patients.* Ped Endosurg Inn Tech; 7(2):135-140.
[56] Ehrlich RM, Gershman A, Fuchs G (1994). *Laparoscopic renal surgery in children.* J Urol; 151:735-739.
[57] Desai MM, Strzempkowski B, Matin SF, et al (2005). *Prospective randomized comparison of transperitoneal versus retroperitoneal laparoscopic radical nephrectomy.* J Urol; 173(1):38-41.
[58] Doublet JD, Barretto HS, Degremont AC, Gattegno B, Thibault P (1996). *Retroperitoneal nephrectomy: comparison of laparoscopy with open surgery.* World J Surg; 713-716.
[59] Moore RG, Kavoussi LS, Bloom DA, et al (1995). *Postoperative adhesion formation after urological laparoscopy in the pediatric population.* J Urol; 153:792-795.
[60] Morgan C (Jr), Rader D (1992). *Laparoscopic unroofing of a renal cyst.* J Urol; 148:1835-1836.
[61] Kumar M, Kumar R, Hemal AK, Gupta NP (2001). *Complications of retroperitoneoscopic surgery at one centre.* BJU Int; 87:607-612.
[62] Ehrlich RM, Gershman A, Fuchs G (1994). *Laparoscopic renal surgery in children.* J Urol; 151:735-739.
[63] El-Gonehimi A, Farhat W, Bagli D, et al (2002). *Mentored retroperitoneal laparoscopic renal surgery in children: a safe approach to learning.* BJU Int; 89(s2):78.

11

Mechanisms of Calcineurin Inhibitor Nephrotoxicity in Chronic Allograft Injury

Craig Slattery[1], Hilary Cassidy[1], Olwyn Johnston[2], Michael P. Ryan[1] and Tara McMorrow[1]

[1]*Renal Disease Research Group, UCD School of Biomolecular and Biomedical Science UCD Conway Institute University College Dublin*

[2]*Division of Nephrology, University of British Columbia, Vancouver*

[1]*Ireland*

[2]*Canada*

1. Introduction

The first successful transplantation of a human kidney was performed more than 50 years ago by Murray and colleagues in 1954 between identical twins. The success of this transplantation was due to the fact that no significant rejection occurs between genetically identical twins and therefore immunosuppression was not necessary in this particular case (Merrill *et al.*, 1956). However, solid-organ transplantation could not be considered truly successful until the 1970's after significant technical and pharmacological advances. In particular, the discovery and development of the calcineurin inhibitors (CNIs) has made allograft transplantation routinely successful with greatly reduced risk of acute rejection. In the absence of pharmacological agents to address the primary pathological mechanisms involved, renal transplantation has now been the standard management of end stage renal failure for the past four decades (Wolfe *et al.*, 1999). Short-term renal allograft and allograft recipient survival rates have increased significantly during the last decade largely due to improved patient monitoring. However, allograft half-life beyond 1 year post-transplant remains largely unchanged. While rates of early allograft failure have significantly reduced, late renal allograft dysfunction remains a significant problem in the transplant population (de Fijter). Chronic allograft injury (CAI) is the most prevalent cause of allograft dysfunction in the first decade after transplantation. The term CAI is used to describe deterioration of renal allograft function and structure due to immunological processes (i.e. chronic rejection) and/or a range of simultaneous non-immunological factors such as CNI-induced nephrotoxicity, hypertension and infection. This chapter will outline the pathophysiology and etiology of CAI and the role that CNI nephrotoxicity plays in this disease process. It will also review experimental studies that have identified important molecular mechanisms involved and discuss strategies utilised to minimise the development and progression of CAI.

2. Chronic allograft injury

2.1 Definition and terminology

In 2006, a study analysed the US Transplantation Data United Network for Organ Sharing (UCLA and UNOS) Renal Transplant Registry database which contained more than 138,000 cases. The analysis showed that despite remarkable improvements in short-term graft outcomes, the allograft loss rate after the first year post-transplant had not significantly changed over the previous 10 years (Kaneku and Terasaki, 2006). Therefore, prolonging the survival of kidney allografts in the long term is the major focus of modern transplant medicine. The majority of renal allografts fail after a period of progressive functional decline which is associated with glomerulosclerosis, tubular atrophy, interstitial fibrosis, and arteriosclerosis. This process is referred to as chronic allograft injury (CAI). The terminology associated with CAI has been revised significantly during the last decade and so, for clarity, some time will be devoted to clearly defining the current nomenclature and its evolution. In the late 1990's, allograft failure more than 3 months after transplantation came to be designated as chronic allograft nephropathy. This term came into existence through use of the Banff classification scheme of kidney-transplant diseases which organised biopsy specimens into those with acute injuries versus those with chronic injuries (Racusen *et al.*, 1999). Chronic allograft nephropathy included at least four distinct entities that could not always be differentiated on biopsy (chronic rejection, chronic toxic effects of calcineurin inhibitors (CNIs); hypertensive vascular disease; and chronic infection, reflux, or both). The rationale for the term was that chronic allograft nephropathy was preferable to "chronic rejection," since this would imply that immunological mechanisms of injury were the primary pathological mechanism. Therefore, chronic allograft nephropathy was utilised as a cover-all term for cases where fibrosis was detected in the interstitium and where tubular atrophy was evident. However, CAI is a multifactorial process in which both immunological (e.g. antibody-mediated rejection) and non-immunological factors (e.g. ischemia–reperfusion injury, hypertension and CNI nephrotoxicity) play a role. These factors are not mutually exclusive and CAI most likely results from the combination of these multiple factors. Over time, all of these factors became synonymous with 'chronic allograft nephropathy' and disease entities with different etiologies were classified together leading to loss of important stratifying elements which would allow physicians to determine more specific diagnosis and treatments. Therefore, the terminology of 'chronic allograft nephropathy' was discouraged in the 8th Banff Conference in 2005 because it was felt that the term encouraged the misconception that chronic allograft injury is one specific disease rather than a collective term for non-specific scarring from all potential causes of chronic allograft dysfunction with fibrosis (Racusen and Regele, 2010). The new classification system replaced the term 'chronic allograft nephropathy' with *'interstitial fibrosis and tubular atrophy'* (IF/TA) with no evidence of any more specific etiology, and requires the recognition and recording of other specific morphological features such as polyomavirus nephropathy (immunostaining for SV40 antigen) or CNI nephrotoxicity (arteriolar hyalinosis with peripheral hyaline nodules in the absence of hypertension or diabetes). However, this new classification also has limitations and the usage of 'chronic allograft nephropathy' has persisted in leading academic journals and conference proceedings. For the purposes of this chapter, the most recent terminology conventions will be utilised.

2.2 Aetiology and pathophysiology of chronic allograft injury

CAI leads to chronic allograft dysfunction manifesting clinically as a decline in renal function and the development of hypertension and proteinuria (Sijpkens *et al.*, 2003). The half-life of cadaveric renal transplants is 12–14 years, with longer survival in living-donor grafts. Progressive deterioration of function with fibrotic changes accounts for about 35–40%

of all late allograft loss (Sijpkens *et al.*, 2003). The functional and structural changes observed during CAI share striking similarities with those observed in other forms of chronic progressive kidney disease. Histologically, CAI is characterised by atherosclerosis, glomerulosclerosis, interstitial fibrosis, and tubular atrophy (Paul, 1995; Paul, 1995). Ultimately, progressive decrease in the functional nephron mass is the major pathophysiological process. While multiple mechanisms contribute to the reduction in functional nephron mass, renal tubulointerstitial fibrosis (TIF) is considered the final common mechanism leading to end-stage renal disease regardless of the initiating insult (Iwano and Neilson, 2004; Guarino *et al.*, 2009; Liu, 2009). It has been demonstrated in both experimental and clinical studies that TIF correlates more consistently with renal functional impairment than glomerular damage (Nath, 1998). TIF is characterised by the gradual loss of the tubular epithelium, progressive accumulation of fibroblasts and alpha smooth muscle actin (α-SMA)-positive myofibroblasts and accumulation of extracellular matrix (ECM) components in the tubular interstitium (Masszi *et al.*, 2004). This accumulation occurs because of a pathological imbalance in the production and degradation of ECM. The exact mechanism by which tubulointerstitial fibrosis results in renal functional decline is not fully clear, however a number of factors are thought to contribute including obliteration of postglomerular capillaries (Kang *et al.*, 2002), formation of atubular glomeruli (Marcussen, 1995) and tubular atrophy (Strutz *et al.*, 2002). Concomitant with the development of interstitial fibrosis is the fate of cells of the tubulointerstitium. As fibrosis progresses, tubular cells and peritubular capillaries decrease in number and ultimately disappear. Interstitial fibroblasts become activated and increase in number, and there is notable infiltration of inflammatory cells into the interstitial compartment (Eddy, 1996; Eddy, 2005).

3. Calcineurin inhibitors – Immunosuppressive agents

Prior to the discovery of calcineurin inhibitors (CNIs) in the 1970s, attempts at solid organ transplantation had consistently failed due to rejection of the allograft by the recipient's immune system. Over the past 40 years, immunosuppressive agents have revolutionised solid organ transplantation. In their absence, progressive immune-mediated injury occurs in transplanted organs. The general mechanisms of action of all current and established immunosuppressive therapies operate based on their primary site of action. The immunosuppressants agents can be classified as inhibitors of transcription (cyclosporine, tacrolimus), inhibitors of nucleotide synthesis (azothioprine, mycophenolate mofetil, leflunomide) and inhibitors of growth factor signal transduction (sirolimus, leflunomide (Suthanthiran and Strom, 1994; Suthanthiran *et al.*, 1996). The initial and maintenance therapy of such immunosuppressive agents prevents allograft rejection.

In the United States, there was a marked improvement in both short and long-term kidney graft survival from cadaveric and living donors between 1988 and 1996 (Hariharan *et al.*, 2000). During this period also the use of tacrolimus steadily increased as cyclosporine use decreased. In 1993, 95% of patients undergoing kidney transplant were using cyclosporine while only 2% used tacrolimus. This was followed by a gradual decline in the use of cyclosporine, down to 30% in 2002 in the United States according to the US Department of Health Organ Procurement and Transplantation Network 2003. The reasons for this conversion are most likely related to multi-centre trial data which has suggested lower acute rejection rates with tacrolimus (Pirsch *et al.*, 1997). Today, both CNIs are pivotal in the prevention of allograft rejection and are part of more than 90% of immunosuppressive protocols used in organ transplantation.

3.1 Cyclosporine A

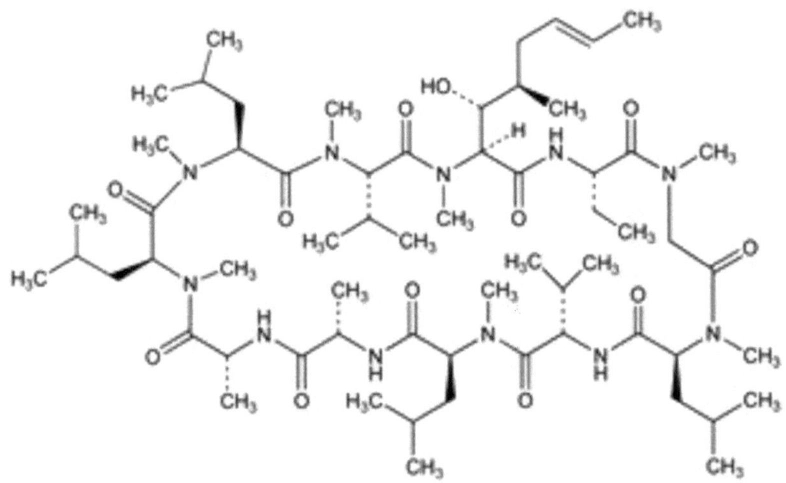

Fig. 1. Chemical Structures of CsA (Adapted from www.medicinescomplete.com)

3.1.1 Discovery

Members of the cyclosporine family were first isolated in 1970 from mycelia of two strains of the soil fungus, Fungi Imperfecti of the species *Tolypocladium infatum* (Ruegger *et al.*, 1976). Cyclosporine A (CsA) was first identified by a group in Sandoz Ltd., Basel, Switzerland, who were conducting routine screening for novel agents with fungal antibiotic activity. On investigation, it was observed that while CsA completely blocked T-cell activation, the same concentrations of CsA were not cytotoxic to cells and did not block the proliferation of other cell types suggesting that CsA could make a useful immunosuppressive agent (Borel, 1976; Borel *et al.*, 1976; Borel *et al.*, 1977). Further work by Borel *et al.* lead to the purification of CsA and the initiation of *in vitro* and *in vivo* testing of the immunosuppressive and toxic effects of CsA. The first clinical uses of CsA took place in 1978 following a kidney transplantation (Calne *et al.*, 1978), and bone marrow transplantation (Powles *et al.*, 1978). In 1983, CsA was registered for organ transplantation in Switzerland, under the registered trademark of Sandimmune. Later that same year, the drug was registered in the United States. By 1985, the first clinical trials of CsA in the treatment of autoimmune diseases had begun (Borel, 1986; Borel and Gunn, 1986). Since its clinical introduction in 1983, CsA revolutionised the field of organ transplantation (Calne, 1986).

3.1.2 Pharmacokinetics

CsA is a neutral, lipophilic cyclic endecapeptide consisting of 11 amino acids, with a molecular weight of 1203 daltons. The peptide is essentially insoluble in water and contains four amide groups, all of which are intra-molecularly hydrogen bonded in both the tetragonal and orthorhombic crystal structures (Stevenson *et al.*, 2003). CsA is soluble in organic solvents and stable in solution at temperatures below 30°C. It is however sensitive to light, cold, and oxidation (IARC International Agency for Research on Cancer 1990). CsA is not compatible with alkali metals, aluminium and heat. Carbon monoxide, carbon dioxide, nitrogen oxides, hydrogen chloride gas and phasogene constitute the hazardous combustion or decomposition products associated with CsA (Sigma Chemical Co. 2002).CsA is readily absorbed because it is a highly lipophilic molecule, despite being a peptide. While oral administration is the preferred route of CsA prophylaxis, its absorption may be incomplete, slow and erratic thus suggesting a major drawback of oral formulation. The bioavailability of oral CsA averages about 30% (Holt *et al.*, 1994) and large inter- and intrapatient variations in CsA absorption have been observed partly due to the unpredictable bioavailability of CsA following oral administration. These variations most likely reflect differences in the seperation of CsA from its vehicle in the intestine. Genetic variations in cytochrome P450 and P-glycoprotein may also be involved (Rivory *et al.*, 2000). Many factors can affect CsA absorption, however the presence of normal serum low-density lipoprotein levels, co-administration of CsA with food and prolonged therapy have been shown to improve the drugs absorption (Bennett *et al.*, 1996). Obesity may also be an influential factor due to CsA being a hydrophobic compound with preferential distribution to adipose tissue and lipoproteins (Cather *et al.*, 2001).

CsA is significantly metabolised in the liver by the cytochrome P450 (CYP) 3A4 system, largely by hydroxylation and N-demethylation (Whalen *et al.*, 1999). It is extensively biotransformed to approximately 15 metabolites, which are almost completely eliminated via the biliary system. Less than 3% of the parent compound is excreted in urine and thus higher blood levels of CsA do not occur in patients with renal dysfunction (Lim *et al.*, 1996). CsA plasma levels peak in 2 to 4 hours and the serum half life ranges from 6.3 hours to 20.4 hours. The therapeutic concentration in whole blood is between 40 and 200 ng/mL.

3.1.3 Clinical use and mechanism of action

CsA is primarily renowned as a powerful immunosuppressant for use in organ transplantation to prevent graft rejection in kidney, liver, heart, lung and combined heart-lung transplants (Li *et al.*, 2003). In addition, it is used to prevent rejection following bone marrow transplantation and in the prophylaxis of host-versus-graft disease. It is also used in the treatment of psoriasis, atopic dermatitis, encephalomyelitis, rheumatoid arthritis, nephrotic syndrome, and uveoretinitis (Cather *et al.*, 2001; Gordon and Ruderman, 2006).

CsA is a potent inhibitor of cell-mediated immunity, and a less potent inhibitor of humoral immunity. While the precise molecular mechanism of CsA action is incompletely understood, the major pathway involves inhibition of calcineurin and subsequent inhibition of the expression of the interleukin-2 (IL-2) gene in activated T-cells (Kronke *et al.*, 1984). CsA binds to cyclophilin, a cytoplasmic propyl peptidyl isomerase and undergoes conformational changes converting CsA to an active formulation. The CsA-cyclophilin complex then binds with high affinity to calcineurin, a Ca^{2+}-dependent serine-threonine phosphatase (Liu, 1993). In T-lymphocytes, calcineurin is activated by a rise in cytoplasmic Ca^{2+} which occurs after T-cell receptor activation by antigen recognition. Calcineurin then dephosphorylates the cytoplasmic form of the transcription factor NFAT (nuclear factor of activated T-cells), allowing NFAT to translocate to the nucleus where, in combination with its nuclear form, fos or jun, it initiates transcription of the T-cell growth factor IL-2 (Jain *et al.*, 1993; Jain *et al.*, 1993; Wesselborg *et al.*, 1996). The CsA-cyclophilin complex binds to and inhibits calcineurin, thereby blocking NFAT dephosphorylation, IL-2 transcription and T-cell growth resulting in immunosuppression (Fruman *et al.*, 1992). In addition, CsA has recently been found to inhibit the JNK and p38 signalling pathway activity triggered by antigen recognition in T-cells (Matsuda and Koyasu, 2000). The presence of all three target pathways for CsA in T-cells may explain the high specificity of its immunosuppressive effects. The mechanism of action of CsA is summarised in Figure 2.

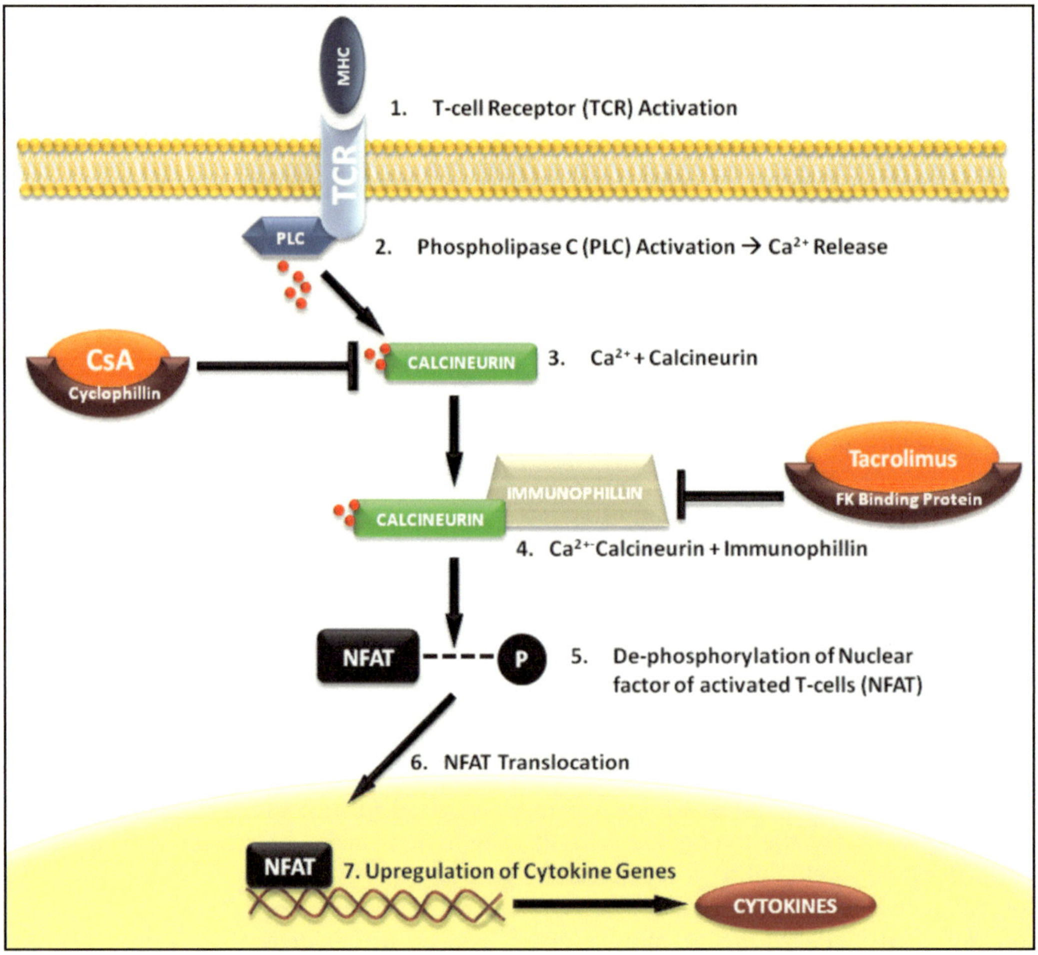

Fig. 2. Mechanism of Action of Calcineurin Inhibitors CsA and Tacrolimus

3.2 Tacrolimus (FK506)

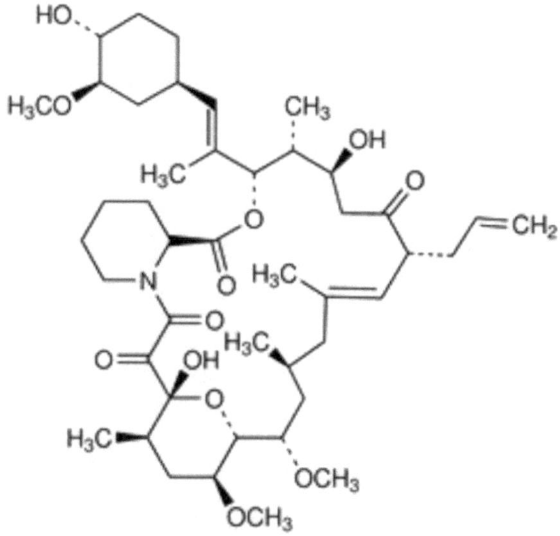

(Adapted from www.medicinescomplete.com)

Fig. 3. Chemical Structure of tacrolimus (FK506)

3.2.1 Discovery

Tacrolimus, also known as FK506 or Prograf®, is a macrolide compound that was isolated by Fujisawa researchers from the culture broth of a soil microorganism *Streptomyces tsukubaensis* near Mount Tsukuba, Japan in 1984 (Kino and Goto, 1993). By 1987, the marked immunosuppressive properties of tacrolimus were confirmed following extensive *in vitro* and *in vivo* testing (Kino and Goto, 1993), thereby identifying what would become a cornerstone of immunosuppressive prophylaxis after solid organ transplantation. Tacrolimus was first launched in Japan in 1993, for prevention of allograft rejection in liver or kidney transplant patients. In the US, tacrolimus (Prograf®) was approved for prevention of rejection in liver transplant recipients in 1994, and in kidney transplant recipients in 1997. In 2003, tacrolimus was used as initial immunosuppression in 67% of kidney recipients and 89% of liver recipients (UNOS United Network for Organ Sharing 2004). It wasn't until the mid-1990s that tacrolimus became available in Europe (Pratschke *et al.*, 1998).

Tacrolimus is a potent immunosuppressive agent that is effective in allograft prophylaxis after organ transplantation. While it has been shown to be 10 to 100 times more potent than CsA (Goto *et al.*, 1991), tacrolimus has significantly reduced the incidence and severity of acute rejection rates in organ transplantation (Kaplan *et al.*, 2003; Toz *et al.*, 2004). In addition, patients receiving tacrolimus therapy require less concomitant corticosteroid therapy thus reducing the risk of adverse corticosteroid-associated side effects (Busuttil and Holt, 1997).

3.2.2 Pharmacokinetics

Tacrolimus is a 23-membered macrolide structure ($C_{44}H_{69}NO_{12}$) with a molecular weight of 822 Da (Christians *et al.*, 1992). As a result of cis-trans isomerism of the C-N amide bonds, tacrolimus forms two rotamers in a ratio 2:1. It is soluble in alcohols, halogenated hydrocarbons, and ether but just minimally soluble in aliphatic hydrocarbons and water (Christians *et al.*, 1992).

Tacrolimus is available for use in liquid, oral or topical formulations. Following intravenous administration, tacrolimus undergoes extensive tissue distribution and binds tightly to erythrocytes (Yura *et al.*, 1999). It is metabolised by the intestinal and hepatic cytochrome P450 system to at least nine metabolites (Christians *et al.*, 1992). A review by Kelly and Kahan reported that CYP3A4 is primarily responsible for the metabolism of tacrolimus (Kelly and Kahan, 2002). The demethylated metabolites exhibit an immunosuppressive activity up to 70% of that of the parent compound (Iwasaki *et al.*, 1993). Excretion of tacrolimus is mainly via the biliary system in the form of several metabolites.

The oral formulation is composed of capsules of a solid dispersion of tacrolimus in hydroxypropyl methylcellulose (Lake *et al.*, 1995). Following oral administration of this highly lipophilic drug, absorption is not complete, with its bioavailability ranging from 10-60%. It reaches maximum blood levels after 1-2 hours after dosing and its half-life ranges from 8-24 hours. It has been postulated that interactions with the proximal small intestinal CYP enzymes may affect pharmacokinetics and absorption of the drug, thus attributable for the low and highly variable oral bioavailability (Lampen *et al.*, 1995). Drug level monitoring is critical as tacrolimus has a high inter-individual variability and a narrow therapeutic index (Jusko, 1995).

3.2.3 Clinical use and mechanism of action

Tacrolimus is a potent immunosuppressive agent that is effective in allograft prophylaxis after organ transplantation, for therapy of acute rejection and in treatment of different immune diseases (Lampen *et al.*, 1995). In addition to its powerful immunosuppressive properties, tacrolimus ointment (tacrolimus ointment) has been utilised in the treatment of moderate to severe atopic eczema (atopic dermatitis) which is unresponsive to conventional therapy. During atopic eczema, the skin's immune system is, to some degree, overactive in its protection. Tacrolimus works by suppressing such over-activity i.e., its therapeutic efficacy is attributed to its immunomodulatory effects on different immune cell types (Lan *et al.*, 2004).

The mechanism of action of tacrolimus is similar to that of CsA but involves binding of tacrolimus to the cytoplasmic immunophilin, FK binding protein 12 (FKBP12). The tacrolimus-FKBP complex then mediates inhibition of calcineurin's phosphatase activity and the subsequent, NFAT-dependent production of IL-2 and other cytokines. While tacrolimus is extremely effective in allograft prophylaxis after organ transplantation, the onset of nephrotoxicity is a major drawback that limits its use clinically (Katari *et al.*, 1997). A significant number of additional toxicities have been reported following administration of tacrolimus. Such toxicities include neurotoxicity (Veroux *et al.*, 2002), which has been suggested to be linked to the inhibition of calcineurin phosphatase, cardiomyopathy (Seino *et al.*, 2003), anaemia, chronic diarrhoea (Webster *et al.*, 2005), post-transplant diabetes mellitus (Araki *et al.*, 2006), and lymphoproliferative disease (Caillard *et al.*, 2006) and infections (Griffith *et al.*, 1994). The mechanism of action of tacrolimus is summarised in Figure 2.

3.3 Calcineurin inhibitor toxicity

While CsA and tacrolimus differ in their molecular structure and intracellular binding characteristics, both compounds ultimately inhibit calcineurin. Inhibition of the calcineurin-

NFAT pathway by CNIs is not specific to immune cells and it can lead to toxic changes in addition to immunosuppressive effects. Furthermore, there is evidence to suggest that the molecular effects of CNIs are not limited to NFAT dependent mechanisms.

Several adverse effects have been reported following CNI administration. These include acute and chronic renal dysfunction, haemolytic-uraemic syndrome, electrolyte disturbances (hyperkalaemia, hypomagnesaemia, and hypocalcaemia), tubular acidosis, defects in urinary concentrating ability, hepatotoxicity, neurotoxicity, dyslipidaemia, gingival hyperplasia, hypertrichosis, malignancies, and increased risk of cardiovascular events (Burdmann *et al.*, 1995; Li *et al.*, 2004). Hypertension is another common adverse reaction to CNIs and is thought to be associated with the decrease in renal function (Ponticelli, 2005). CNI-induced hypertension is however reversible upon decrease or cessation of dose. Female transplant recipients taking CsA during pregnancy tend to have an increased number of premature deliveries in addition to low birth weight offspring, thus suggesting that CsA crosses the placental barrier (Cather *et al.*, 2001).

The most significant toxic side effect of CNI administration is nephrotoxicity (Burdmann *et al.*, 1995; Li *et al.*, 2004; Ponticelli, 2005). This includes both acute and chronic nephrotoxic effects. Acute CNI nephrotoxicity is largely characterised by hemodynamically induced renal dysfunction which is generally fully reversible by cessation or decrease of the drug (Cattaneo *et al.*, 2004). While the majority of available data on acute toxicity relates to CsA, tacrolimus effects are believed to be similar (Lloberas *et al.*, 2008). Evidence suggests that the hemodynamic disruption observed in acute CNI nephrotoxicity is mediated by inappropriate activation of the renin-angiotensin system (RAS). RAS activation stimulates production of potent vasoconstricting factors such as angiotensin II, endothelin and thromboxane, while also suppressing the synthesis of vasodilating prostacyclins, prostaglandin E2, and nitric oxide (NO) (Wissmann *et al.*, 1996; Lamas, 2005). RAS appears to be activated by the direct action of CsA on juxtaglomerular cells and by indirectly by induced renal arteriolar vasoconstriction (Kurtz *et al.*, 1988). A relatively rare complication related to acute CNI nephrotoxicity is hemolytic uremic syndrome (HUS). Since 1980, the number of case reports describing transplant patients who developed acute arteriolopathy and severe renal impairment consistent with HUS while on CsA or tacrolimus, has steadily increased (Cattaneo *et al.*, 2004). The primary pathology is an extensive thrombotic process in the renal microcirculation with several glomerular capillaries occluded by thrombi extending from the afferent arterioles and containing platelet aggregates (Medina *et al.*, 2001). The mechanism by which CNIs induce this acute obliterating arteriolopathy remains ill-defined. However, the renal vascular endothelium is likely the primary target. Endothelial cell injury disrupts the synthesis of vasodilatory and antithrombotic substances, while promoting the generation of vasoconstrictive and aggregating mediators promoting the development of HUS and renal failure (Cattaneo *et al.*, 2004).

While the basis of acute CNI nephrotoxicity is primarily hemodynamic, features of tubular damage are also often observed. Acute CNI nephrotoxicity is often accompanied by significant vacuolisation of tubular epithelial cells likely induced by enlargement of the endoplasmic reticulum and increased lysosomal volume (Morozumi *et al.*, 1986; Morozumi *et al.*, 2004). These effects may be the result of localised ischemia downstream of CNI-induced intrarenal vasoconstriction, however evidence suggests that CNIs, and CsA in particular has direct cytotoxic effects on tubular epithelial cells. CsA induces endoplasmic reticulum stress and cell death by induction of pro-apoptotic proteins (Healy *et al.*, 1998;

Pallet *et al.*, 2008; Pallet *et al.*, 2008). Similar effects on tubular cells were observed with tacrolimus (Du *et al.*, 2009; Du *et al.*, 2009).

While acute CNI nephrotoxicity is generally reversible, long-term exposure to CNIs can lead to irreversible damage to renal structure and function. Chronic CNI nephrotoxicity is characterised by histological lesions that are associated with irreversible and progressive interstitial renal fibrosis which correlates with diminishing renal function (Cattaneo *et al.*, 2004). Typical histopathological changes include arteriolar hyalinosis, tubular atrophy, interstitial fibrosis, thickening and fibrosis of the Bowman's capsule, and focal, segmental or global glomerular sclerosis (Williams and Haragsim, 2006). The development of these chronic alterations most likely involves a combination of CNI-induced hemodynamic changes and direct toxic effect of CNIs on tubular epithelial cells. Arteriolar hyalinosis (hyaline deposits around afferent arterioles) is a characteristic sign of chronic CNI toxicity. Hyaline deposits progressively replace necrotic vascular smooth muscle cells. The cause of smooth muscle cell necrosis is unclear but may be a consequence of calcineurin-NFAT inhibition (Nieves-Cintron *et al.*, 2007). If the hyaline deposits are large they can cause significant narrowing of vascular lumen and may promote the progression of chronic CNI injury (Mihatsch *et al.*, 1998).

Arteriolopathy and narrowing of the renal vasculature lumen can be considered major contributors to the development of chronic CNI nephrotoxicity but it is increasingly evident that the direct effects of CNIs on the tubular epithelial cells of the nephron play a major role in the progression and development of interstitial fibrosis during CAI. Free radicals and reactive oxygen species are produced in response to local ischemia and cell death in the tubulointerstitium. Another significant factor involved in the progression of chronic interstitial changes is the profibrotic cytokine transforming growth factor beta 1 (TGF-β1). TGF-β1 promotes the development of interstitial fibrosis by inhibiting ECM degradation, stimulating production of ECM proteins by modulating the normal function of tubular epithelial cells and resident interstitial fibroblasts (McMorrow *et al.*, 2005; Slattery *et al.*, 2005; Feldman *et al.*, 2007; Hertig *et al.*, 2008). These mechanisms will be disussed in detail below. However, the events that likely contribute to fibrosis in CAI are summarised in Figure 4.

They can be arbitrarily divided into three phases (Mannon, 2006; Mannon and Kirk, 2006). In the initiation phase, there is tissue injury, which may occur by either antigen dependent or independent insults. Regardless of the aetiology of the initiating event, the result is the fibrogenesis phase, consisting of inflammatory and proliferative responses, regulated by cytokines, chemokines and growth factors. This cascade of events results in the matrix accumulation phase. This is due to either increased production and/or reduced degradation of matrix, ultimately resulting in fibrosis.

4. Molecular mechanisms of CNI-induced chronic allograft injury

As described earlier, during CAI the decline in renal function correlates most closely with the degree of TIF. Therefore the molecular mechanisms contributing to the development of TIF have been a major research focus. Over the last decade, the molecular mechanisms underlying CNI nephrotoxicity have been extensively studied in our laboratory and others utilising a variety of *in vitro* and *in vivo* model systems, and clinical cohort studies. Particular focus has been on the direct effects of CsA and tacrolimus on the tubular interstitium and the principal cells that reside there; the tubular epithelial cells and interstitial fibroblasts.

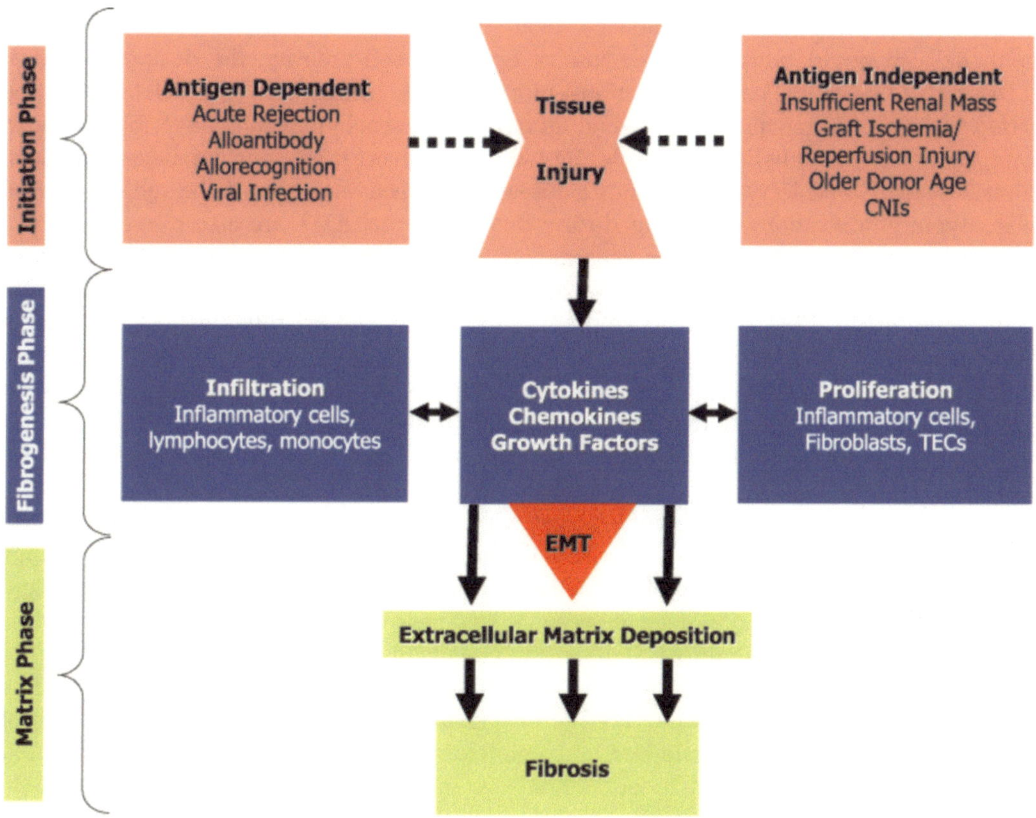

Fig. 4. Schema of the development of fibrosis in chronic allograft nephropathy (Adapted from Mannon, 2006)

4.1 *In vitro* data

Work from our laboratory has demonstrated that both CsA and tacrolimus have direct effects on proximal and distal tubular epithelial cells ranging from cell death and disruption of normal barrier function, to pro-fibrotic and phenotype altering effects. For the purposes of this discussion, the focus will be on effects relating to fibrosis and TIF in CNI nephrotoxicity. The majority of this work has focused on the effects of CsA on proximal tubular epithelial cells (PTECs).

The primary pathological features observed in the tubulointerstitium during TIF are interstitial ECM accumulation, decreased numbers of functioning tubular epithelial cells and increased numbers of activated fibroblasts (termed myofibroblasts). Accumulated evidence suggests that these events do not occur in isolation but are functionally linked. It is accepted that the main source of the ECM that accumulates during TIF is the myofibroblasts. However, the source of these myofibroblasts has been, and remains a point of debate. Previously, it was held that the increase in myofibroblasts was due to infiltrating circulatory fibroblasts which became active in the interstitium. However, significant in vitro evidence has demonstrated that a major source of myofibroblasts is the tubular epithelium itself through a process termed epithelial-mesenchymal transition (EMT). Under normal physiological conditions, epithelial to mesenchymal transitions are important events in embryonic morphogenesis (Hay and Zuk, 1995). Embryonic mesenchymal cells emerge from epithelial cell populations following loss of epithelial cell polarity, the disappearance of differentiated epithelial cell-cell junctions, reorganisation of the actin cytoskeleton, and the redistribution of organelles. Conversely, embryonic mesenchymal cells have the ability to completely regain epithelial phenotypes by the reverse process, mesenchymal-to-epithelium transition (MET) (Thiery, 2003). From a disease perspective, many of the molecular and phenotypic modifications occurring during developmental EMT are also observed in the most aggressive metastatic cancer cells and in fibrotic diseases (Thiery, 2003). Therefore EMT has emerged as a potentially central element in the development of metastatic tumours and tissue fibrosis. EMT is a stepwise progression in which numerous phenotypic changes occur leading to the loss of epithelial markers and function and the acquisition of a more (myo)fibroblast-like phenotype. The myofibroblast is a morphological intermediate between fibroblasts and smooth muscle cells. Like fibroblasts, they have the ability to produce and secrete large quantities of ECM components such as collagen I and III and fibronectin, and like smooth muscle cells they express α-smooth muscle actin (α-SMA) conferring the ability to contract and equipping the myofibroblast with enhanced locomotive ability. Thus, EMT may contribute significantly to renal failure through the accumulation of ECM and perhaps more significantly, through loss of epithelial cells leading to reduced tubular integrity and function. The PTEC may no longer be regarded as passive victims in renal disease, but as active contributors to renal fibrosis (Becker and Hewitson, 2000).

Yang and Liu (Yang and Liu, 2001) proposed that at the cellular level, EMT involves a number of coordinated events that are both necessary and sufficient for the completion of the EMT process. Using an optimised, sub-cytotoxic dose of CsA (4.2μM) a number of cell characteristics were examined in our laboratory including morphology and cytoskeletal arrangement, epithelial junctional integrity, expression of epithelial markers (e.g. E-cadherin), expression of myofibroblast markers (e.g. α-smooth muscle actin) and cell motility (Selection depicted in Figure 5). Human proximal tubular epithelial cells exposed to CsA exhibited major morphological changes associated with mesenchymal phenotypes. CsA treatment also resulted in significant cytoskeletal rearrangement, stress fibre formation and the development of filopodea. A number of important phenotypic markers were affected by CsA treatment. ZO-1 and E-cadherin expression were downregulated, while expression of the myfibroblast marker α-SMA was strongly induced. Treatment with CsA significantly enhanced the migratory ability of tubular epithelial cells. This effect was of great importance in relation to renal fibrosis as the ability of the myofibroblast to migrate into the interstitium contributes significantly to disease progression. *In vivo,* CsA has been observed to have significant effects on renal tubular ultrastructure causing a characteristic, stripped fibrosis (Morales *et al.*, 2001). However, the link between these morphological changes and EMT had not been previously made. This model of CsA-induced EMT was the first published example of drug-induced EMT in the literature (McMorrow *et al.*, 2005; Slattery *et al.*, 2005).

Having established that CsA did induce EMT in proximal tubular epithelial cells, the mechanisms underlying the effects were examined. Using microarray generated gene expression profiles and specific inhibitors, the major mediators of CsA-EMT were elucidated. Unsurprisingly, TGF-β1 was found to figure prominantly in the inductionof EMT. However, it was the mechanism of TGF-β1 induction by CsA which proved most interesting.CsA-induced TGF-β1 production appeared to be dependent on protein kianse C beta (PKC-β) activity (Slattery *et al.*, 2008). This was of interest as PKC-β is currently under investigation as a significant contributor to the development of diabetic nephropathy. These results suggested that the mechanisms underlying the development of diabetic nephropathy and CsA nephropathy may be common and so similar therapeutic strategies could be employed in both disease situations. Further experimental work identified the E2A transcription factors (E12 and E47) as downstream mediators of the effects of CsA on E-cadherin expression (Slattery *et al.*, 2006; Slattery *et al.*, 2008).

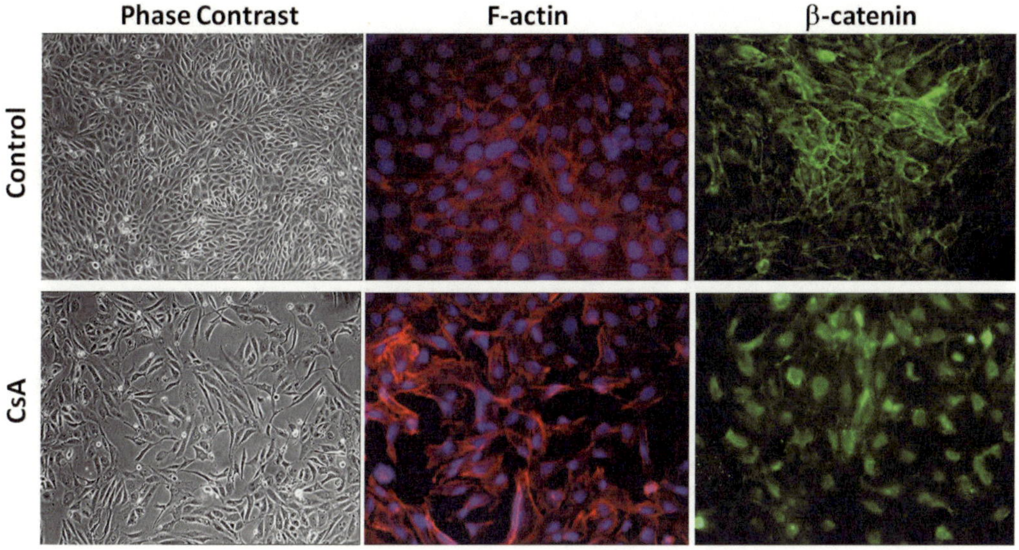

Fig. 5. Effects of CsA on normal PTEC morphology, F-actin distribution and β-catenin distribution in PTECs. (Adapted from Slattery et al. 2005)

4.2 *In vivo* data - Animal models and clinical studies

In parallel with *in vitro* studies, an *in vivo* rodent model of CsA-induced CAI was also established to investigate the mechanisms involved (O'Connell *et al.*). CsA nephrotoxicity was induced in CD-1 mice by daily CsA administration for 4 weeks. Mirroring *in vitro* findings, decreased E-cadherin and increased α-SMA expression was observed. In addition, TGF-β1 was significantly increased by CsA treatment in this *in vivo* model. In addition to investigating the molecular mechanism of CsA-induced nephrotoxicity, we have also focused on identifying novel diagnostic techniques to identify patients at risk of developing CAI in advance of currently used techniques such as proteinuria and creatinine monitoring. At present, a histological diagnosis with a renal transplant biopsy is the 'gold standard' for determining CAI. Therefore the development of novel, predictive indicators of CAI would be highly desirable. One strategy utilised to identify novel biomarkers has been urinary proteomic analysis in both the CsA mouse model (O'Connell *et al.* 2011) and in a clinical patient cohort (Johnston *et al.*, 2011) (Depicted in Figures 6 and 7 respectively). In the animal studies significant alterations in urinary podocin and uromodulin were observed which may be indicative of damage to the glomeruli and tubules after CsA treatment. Furthermore, E-cadherin, superoxide dismutase and vinculin levels in the urine may be early indicators of CsA nephrotoxicity.

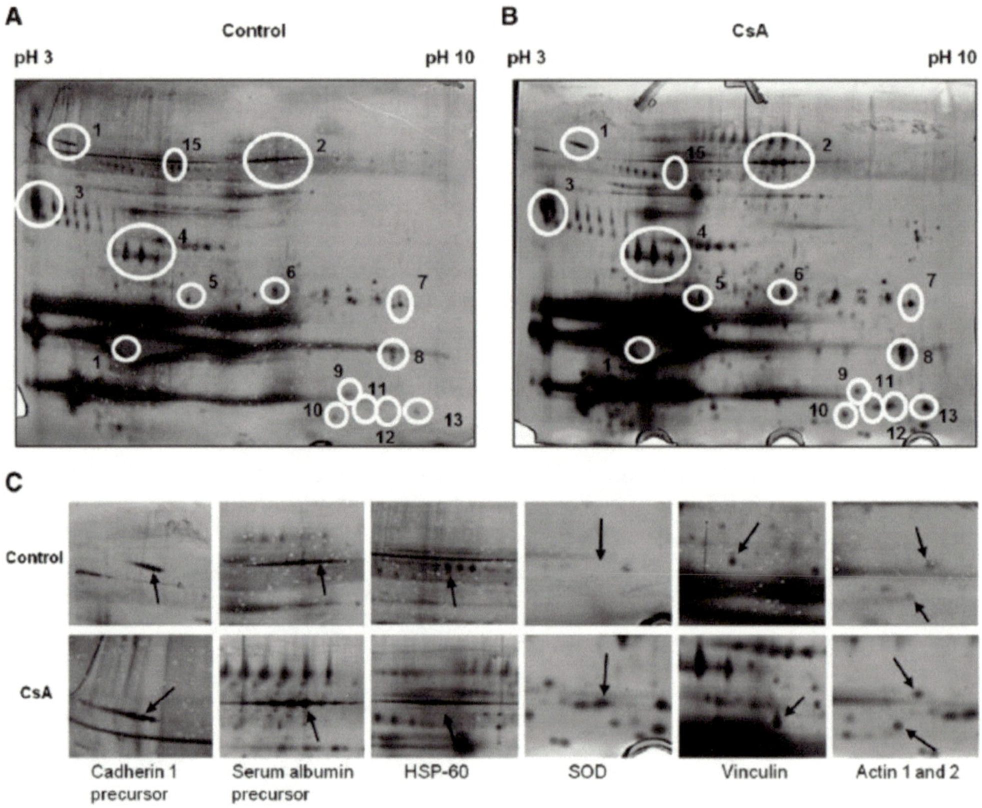

Fig. 6. Analysis of urinary proteins in a CsA-induced mouse model of CNI nephrotoxicity by 2D gel electrophosesis (Adapted from O'Connell *et al.* 2011).

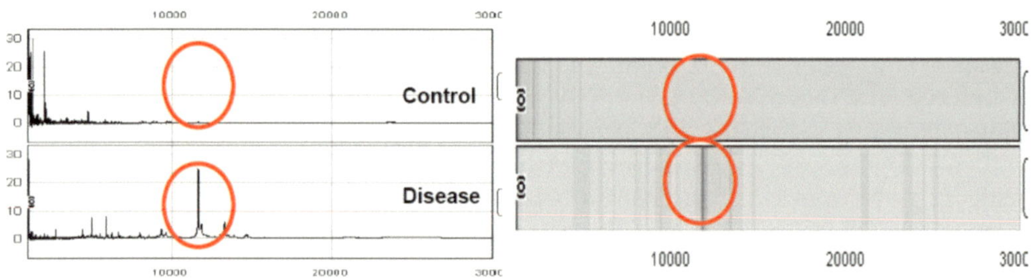

Fig. 7. Analysis of urinary proteins in clinical patient urine samples using ProteinChip and SELDI-TOF analysis (Adapted from Johnston *et al* 2011).

In the human clinical studies, 34 renal transplant recipients with histologically proven CAI and 36 patients with normal renal transplant function were compared. High-throughput urinary proteomic profiles were generated using ProteinChip arrays and surface-enhanced laser-desorption/ionisation time-of-flight mass spectrometry (SELDI-TOF-MS). Following SELDI, biomarker pattern software analysis was performed which led to the identification of a novel biomarker pattern that could distinguish patients with CAN from those with normal renal function. One of the identified proteins was β2 microglobulin which was a powerful distinguishing factor between CAI patients and control patients. Further validation is required to determine if this β2 microglobulin protein biomarker will allow for diagnosis of CAN by non-invasive methods in a clinical setting but this study clearly shows the potential of urinary proteomics to identify patients at risk of developing CAI.

5. Conclusion

In the continued absence of therapeutic strategies to prevent and/or reverse fibrosis which is the primary pathological driving force in chronic kidney disease, renal transplantation remains the primary treatment for end stage renal failure. It follows that calcineruin inhibitors will continue to be heavily utilised in anti-allograft rejection therapies. Therefore, furthering our understanding of the molecular basis of CNI nephrotoxicity must remain a major research topic with the goal of developing therapeutic strategies to reduce or eliminate the development of chronic allograft injury.

6. Acknowledgments

Work detailed in this chapter was supported by the UCD Conway Institute of Biomolecular and Biomedical Research under the Programme for Research in Third Level Institutions (PRTLI) administered by the Higher Education Authority (HEA). This work was also supported by Science Foundation Ireland, the Health Research Board of Ireland, Enterprise Ireland, the EU 7th Framework grant "SysKid", HEALTH-F2-2009-241544, and by a research bursary from the Irish Nephrological Society and Amgen Ltd. Craig Slattery is a Government of Ireland Research Fellow supported by the Irish Research Council for Science, Engineering and Technology.

7. References

Araki, M., S. M. Flechner, H. R. Ismail, L. M. Flechner, L. Zhou, I. H. Derweesh, D. Goldfarb, C. Modlin, A. C. Novick and C. Faiman (2006). Posttransplant diabetes mellitus in kidney transplant recipients receiving calcineurin or mTOR inhibitor drugs. *Transplantation* 81(3): 335-41.

Becker, G. J. and T. D. Hewitson (2000). The role of tubulointerstitial injury in chronic renal failure. *Curr Opin Nephrol Hypertens* 9(2): 133-8.

Bennett, W. M., A. DeMattos, D. J. Norman, M. M. Meyer and A. Olyaei (1996). Which cyclosporin formulation? *Lancet* 348(9021): 205.

Borel, J. F. (1976). Comparative study of in vitro and in vivo drug effects on cell-mediated cytotoxicity. *Immunology* 31(4): 631-41.

Borel, J. F. (1986). Immunological properties of ciclosporin (Sandimmune). *Contrib Nephrol* 51: 10-8.

Borel, J. F., C. Feurer, H. U. Gubler and H. Stahelin (1976). Biological effects of cyclosporin A: a new antilymphocytic agent. *Agents Actions* 6(4): 468-75.

Borel, J. F., C. Feurer, C. Magnee and H. Stahelin (1977). Effects of the new anti-lymphocytic peptide cyclosporin A in animals. *Immunology* 32(6): 1017-25.

Borel, J. F. and H. C. Gunn (1986). Cyclosporine as a new approach to therapy of autoimmune diseases. *Ann N Y Acad Sci* 475: 307-19.

Burdmann, E. A., T. F. Andoh, C. C. Nast, A. Evan, B. A. Connors, T. M. Coffman, J. Lindsley and W. M. Bennett (1995). Prevention of experimental cyclosporin-induced interstitial fibrosis by losartan and enalapril. *Am J Physiol* 269(4 Pt 2): F491-9.

Busuttil, R. W. and C. D. Holt (1997). Tacrolimus (FK506) is superior to cyclosporine in liver transplantation. *Transplant Proc* 29(1-2): 534-8.

Caillard, S., C. Lelong, F. Pessione and B. Moulin (2006). Post-transplant lymphoproliferative disorders occurring after renal transplantation in adults: report of 230 cases from the French Registry. *Am J Transplant* 6(11): 2735-42.

Calne, R. Y. (1986). The current state of renal transplantation. *Kidney Int Suppl* 19: S23-4.

Calne, R. Y., D. J. White, S. Thiru, D. B. Evans, P. McMaster, D. C. Dunn, G. N. Craddock, B. D. Pentlow and K. Rolles (1978). Cyclosporin A in patients receiving renal allografts from cadaver donors. *Lancet* 2(8104-5): 1323-7.

Cather, J. C., W. Abramovits and A. Menter (2001). Cyclosporine and tacrolimus in dermatology. *Dermatol Clin* 19(1): 119-37, ix.

Cattaneo, D., N. Perico, F. Gaspari and G. Remuzzi (2004). Nephrotoxic aspects of cyclosporine. *Transplant Proc* 36(2 Suppl): 234S-239S.

Christians, U., F. Braun, M. Schmidt, N. Kosian, H. M. Schiebel, L. Ernst, M. Winkler, C. Kruse, A. Linck and K. F. Sewing (1992). Specific and sensitive measurement of FK506 and its metabolites in blood and urine of liver-graft recipients. *Clin Chem* 38(10): 2025-32.

de Fijter, J. W. Rejection and function and chronic allograft dysfunction. *Kidney Int Suppl*(119): S38-41.

Du, J. F., S. Y. Li and B. Yu (2009). Rapamycin--rather than FK506--might promote allograft tolerance induced by CD4+CD25+ regulatory T cells. *Surgery* 146(3): 526-7; author reply 527-8.

Du, S., N. Hiramatsu, K. Hayakawa, A. Kasai, M. Okamura, T. Huang, J. Yao, M. Takeda, I. Araki, N. Sawada, A. W. Paton, J. C. Paton and M. Kitamura (2009). Suppression of NF-kappaB by cyclosporin a and tacrolimus (FK506) via induction of the C/EBP family: implication for unfolded protein response. *J Immunol* 182(11): 7201-11.

Eddy, A. A. (1996). Molecular insights into renal interstitial fibrosis. *J Am Soc Nephrol* 7(12): 2495-508.

Eddy, A. A. (2005). Progression in chronic kidney disease. *Adv Chronic Kidney Dis* 12(4): 353-65.

Feldman, G., B. Kiely, N. Martin, G. Ryan, T. McMorrow and M. P. Ryan (2007). Role for TGF-beta in cyclosporine-induced modulation of renal epithelial barrier function. *J Am Soc Nephrol* 18(6): 1662-71.

Fruman, D. A., C. B. Klee, B. E. Bierer and S. J. Burakoff (1992). Calcineurin phosphatase activity in T lymphocytes is inhibited by FK 506 and cyclosporin A. *Proc Natl Acad Sci U S A* 89(9): 3686-90.

Gordon, K. B. and E. M. Ruderman (2006). The treatment of psoriasis and psoriatic arthritis: an interdisciplinary approach. *J Am Acad Dermatol* 54(3 Suppl 2): S85-91.

Goto, S., S. M. Stepkowski and B. D. Kahan (1991). Effect of FK 506 and cyclosporine on heart allograft survival in rats. *Transplant Proc* 23(1 Pt 1): 529-30.

Griffith, B. P., K. Bando, R. L. Hardesty, J. M. Armitage, R. J. Keenan, S. M. Pham, I. L. Paradis, S. A. Yousem, K. Komatsu, H. Konishi and et al. (1994). A prospective randomized trial of FK506 versus cyclosporine after human pulmonary transplantation. *Transplantation* 57(6): 848-51.

Guarino, M., A. Tosoni and M. Nebuloni (2009). Direct contribution of epithelium to organ fibrosis: epithelial-mesenchymal transition. *Hum Pathol* 40(10): 1365-76.

Hariharan, S., C. P. Johnson, B. A. Bresnahan, S. E. Taranto, M. J. McIntosh and D. Stablein (2000). Improved graft survival after renal transplantation in the United States, 1988 to 1996. *N Engl J Med* 342(9): 605-12.

Hay, E. D. and A. Zuk (1995). Transformations between epithelium and mesenchyme: normal, pathological, and experimentally induced. *Am J Kidney Dis* 26(4): 678-90.

Healy, E., M. Dempsey, C. Lally and M. P. Ryan (1998). Apoptosis and necrosis: mechanisms of cell death induced by cyclosporine A in a renal proximal tubular cell line. *Kidney Int* 54(6): 1955-66.

Hertig, A., D. Anglicheau, J. Verine, N. Pallet, M. Touzot, P. Y. Ancel, L. Mesnard, N. Brousse, E. Baugey, D. Glotz, C. Legendre, E. Rondeau and Y. C. Xu-Dubois (2008). Early epithelial phenotypic changes predict graft fibrosis. *J Am Soc Nephrol* 19(8): 1584-91.

Holt, D. W., A. Johnston, N. B. Roberts, J. M. Tredger and A. K. Trull (1994). Methodological and clinical aspects of cyclosporin monitoring: report of the Association of Clinical Biochemists task force. *Ann Clin Biochem* 31 (Pt 5): 420-46.

Iwano, M. and E. G. Neilson (2004). Mechanisms of tubulointerstitial fibrosis. *Curr Opin Nephrol Hypertens* 13(3): 279-84.

Iwasaki, K., T. Shiraga, K. Nagase, Z. Tozuka, K. Noda, S. Sakuma, T. Fujitsu, K. Shimatani, A. Sato and M. Fujioka (1993). Isolation, identification, and biological activities of oxidative metabolites of FK506, a potent immunosuppressive macrolide lactone. *Drug Metab Dispos* 21(6): 971-7.

Jain, J., P. G. McCaffrey, Z. Miner, T. K. Kerppola, J. N. Lambert, G. L. Verdine, T. Curran and A. Rao (1993). The T-cell transcription factor NFATp is a substrate for calcineurin and interacts with Fos and Jun. *Nature* 365(6444): 352-5.

Jain, J., Z. Miner and A. Rao (1993). Analysis of the preexisting and nuclear forms of nuclear factor of activated T cells. *J Immunol* 151(2): 837-48.

Johnston, O., H. Cassidy, S. O'Connell, A. O'Riordan, W. Gallagher, P. B. Maguire, K. Wynne, G. Cagney, M. P. Ryan, P. J. Conlon and T. McMorrow (2011). Identification of β2-microglobulin as a urinary biomarker for chronic allograft nephropathy using proteomic methods. *Proteomics Clin Appl.* DOI: 10.1002/prca.201000160.

Jusko, W. J. (1995). Analysis of tacrolimus (FK 506) in relation to therapeutic drug monitoring. *Ther Drug Monit* 17(6): 596-601.

Kaneku, H. K. and P. I. Terasaki (2006). Thirty year trend in kidney transplants: UCLA and UNOS Renal Transplant Registry. *Clin Transpl*: 1-27.

Kang, D. H., J. Kanellis, C. Hugo, L. Truong, S. Anderson, D. Kerjaschki, G. F. Schreiner and R. J. Johnson (2002). Role of the microvascular endothelium in progressive renal disease. *J Am Soc Nephrol* 13(3): 806-16.

Kaplan, B., J. D. Schold and H. U. Meier-Kriesche (2003). Long-term graft survival with neoral and tacrolimus: a paired kidney analysis. *J Am Soc Nephrol* 14(11): 2980-4.

Katari, S. R., M. Magnone, R. Shapiro, M. Jordan, V. Scantlebury, C. Vivas, H. A. Gritsch, J. McCauley, T. Starzl, A. J. Demetris and P. S. Randhawa (1997). Tacrolimus nephrotoxicity after renal transplantation. *Transplant Proc* 29(1-2): 311.

Kelly, P. and B. D. Kahan (2002). Review: metabolism of immunosuppressant drugs. *Curr Drug Metab* 3(3): 275-87.

Kino, T. and T. Goto (1993). Discovery of FK-506 and update. *Ann N Y Acad Sci* 685: 13-21.

Kronke, M., W. J. Leonard, J. M. Depper, S. K. Arya, F. Wong-Staal, R. C. Gallo, T. A. Waldmann and W. C. Greene (1984). Cyclosporin A inhibits T-cell growth factor gene expression at the level of mRNA transcription. *Proc Natl Acad Sci U S A* 81(16): 5214-8.

Kurtz, A., R. Della Bruna and K. Kuhn (1988). Cyclosporine A enhances renin secretion and production in isolated juxtaglomerular cells. *Kidney Int* 33(5): 947-53.

Lake, J. R., K. J. Gorman, C. O. Esquivel, R. H. Wiesner, G. B. Klintmalm, C. M. Miller, B. W. Shaw and J. A. Gordon (1995). The impact of immunosuppressive regimens on the cost of liver transplantation--results from the U.S. FK506 multicenter trial. *Transplantation* 60(10): 1089-95.

Lamas, S. (2005). Cellular mechanisms of vascular injury mediated by calcineurin inhibitors. *Kidney Int* 68(2): 898-907.

Lampen, A., U. Christians, F. P. Guengerich, P. B. Watkins, J. C. Kolars, A. Bader, A. K. Gonschior, H. Dralle, I. Hackbarth and K. F. Sewing (1995). Metabolism of the immunosuppressant tacrolimus in the small intestine: cytochrome P450, drug interactions, and interindividual variability. *Drug Metab Dispos* 23(12): 1315-24.

Lan, C. C., Y. H. Kao, S. M. Huang, H. S. Yu and G. S. Chen (2004). FK506 independently upregulates transforming growth factor beta and downregulates inducible nitric oxide synthase in cultured human keratinocytes: possible mechanisms of how tacrolimus ointment interacts with atopic skin. *Br J Dermatol* 151(3): 679-84.

Li, C., S. W. Lim, B. K. Sun and C. W. Yang (2004). Chronic cyclosporine nephrotoxicity: new insights and preventive strategies. *Yonsei Med J* 45(6): 1004-16.

Li, C., C. W. Yang, W. Y. Kim, J. Y. Jung, J. H. Cha, Y. S. Kim, J. Kim, W. M. Bennett and B. K. Bang (2003). Reversibility of chronic cyclosporine nephropathy in rats after withdrawal of cyclosporine. *Am J Physiol Renal Physiol* 284(2): F389-98.

Lim, K. K., W. P. Su, A. L. Schroeter, C. J. Sabers, R. T. Abraham and M. R. Pittelkow (1996). Cyclosporine in the treatment of dermatologic disease: an update. *Mayo Clin Proc* 71(12): 1182-91.

Liu, J. (1993). FK506 and cyclosporin, molecular probes for studying intracellular signal transduction. *Immunol Today* 14(6): 290-5.

Liu, Y. (2009). New insights into epithelial-mesenchymal transition in kidney fibrosis. *J Am Soc Nephrol* 21(2): 212-22.

Lloberas, N., J. Torras, G. Alperovich, J. M. Cruzado, P. Gimenez-Bonafe, I. Herrero-Fresneda, M. Franquesa, I. Rama and J. M. Grinyo (2008). Different renal toxicity profiles in the association of cyclosporine and tacrolimus with sirolimus in rats. *Nephrol Dial Transplant* 23(10): 3111-9.

Mannon, R. B. (2006). Therapeutic targets in the treatment of allograft fibrosis. *Am J Transplant* 6(5 Pt 1): 867-75.

Mannon, R. B. and A. D. Kirk (2006). Beyond histology: novel tools to diagnose allograft dysfunction. *Clin J Am Soc Nephrol* 1(3): 358-66.

Marcussen, N. (1995). Atubular glomeruli in chronic renal disease. *Curr Top Pathol* 88: 145-74.

Masszi, A., L. Fan, L. Rosivall, C. A. McCulloch, O. D. Rotstein, I. Mucsi and A. Kapus (2004). Integrity of cell-cell contacts is a critical regulator of TGF-beta 1-induced epithelial-to-myofibroblast transition: role for beta-catenin. *Am J Pathol* 165(6): 1955-67.

Matsuda, S. and S. Koyasu (2000). Mechanisms of action of cyclosporine. *Immunopharmacology* 47(2-3): 119-25.

McMorrow, T., M. M. Gaffney, C. Slattery, E. Campbell and M. P. Ryan (2005). Cyclosporine A induced epithelial-mesenchymal transition in human renal proximal tubular epithelial cells. *Nephrol Dial Transplant* 20(10): 2215-25.

Medina, P. J., J. M. Sipols and J. N. George (2001). Drug-associated thrombotic thrombocytopenic purpura-hemolytic uremic syndrome. *Curr Opin Hematol* 8(5): 286-93.

Merrill, J. P., J. E. Murray, J. H. Harrison and W. R. Guild (1956). Successful homotransplantation of the human kidney between identical twins. *J Am Med Assoc* 160(4): 277-82.

Mihatsch, M. J., M. Kyo, K. Morozumi, Y. Yamaguchi, V. Nickeleit and B. Ryffel (1998). The side-effects of ciclosporine-A and tacrolimus. *Clin Nephrol* 49(6): 356-63.

Morales, J. M., A. Andres, M. Rengel and J. L. Rodicio (2001). Influence of cyclosporin, tacrolimus and rapamycin on renal function and arterial hypertension after renal transplantation. *Nephrol Dial Transplant* 16 Suppl 1: 121-4.

Morozumi, K., I. Shinmura, I. Gotoh, A. Yoshida, T. Fujinami, K. Uchida, N. Yamada, Y. Tominaga, Y. Nakanishi, T. Kanoh and et al. (1986). Studies on nephrotoxicity of cyclosporine in human renal allograft and rat. *Dev Toxicol Environ Sci* 14: 153-6.

Morozumi, K., A. Takeda, K. Uchida and M. J. Mihatsch (2004). Cyclosporine nephrotoxicity: how does it affect renal allograft function and transplant morphology? *Transplant Proc* 36(2 Suppl): 251S-256S.

Nath, K. A. (1998). The tubulointerstitium in progressive renal disease. *Kidney Int* 54(3): 992-4.

Nieves-Cintron, M., G. C. Amberg, C. B. Nichols, J. D. Molkentin and L. F. Santana (2007). Activation of NFATc3 down-regulates the beta1 subunit of large conductance, calcium-activated K+ channels in arterial smooth muscle and contributes to hypertension. *J Biol Chem* 282(5): 3231-40.

O'Connell, S., C. Slattery, M. P. Ryan and T. McMorrow Identification of novel indicators of cyclosporine A nephrotoxicity in a CD-1 mouse model. *Toxicol Appl Pharmacol* 252(2): 201-10.

Pallet, N., N. Bouvier, A. Bendjallabah, M. Rabant, J. P. Flinois, A. Hertig, C. Legendre, P. Beaune, E. Thervet and D. Anglicheau (2008). Cyclosporine-induced endoplasmic reticulum stress triggers tubular phenotypic changes and death. *Am J Transplant* 8(11): 2283-96.

Pallet, N., M. Rabant, Y. C. Xu-Dubois, D. Lecorre, M. H. Mucchielli, S. Imbeaud, N. Agier, A. Hertig, E. Thervet, C. Legendre, P. Beaune and D. Anglicheau (2008). Response of human renal tubular cells to cyclosporine and sirolimus: a toxicogenomic study. *Toxicol Appl Pharmacol* 229(2): 184-96.

Paul, L. C. (1995). Chronic renal transplant loss. *Kidney Int* 47(6): 1491-9.

Paul, L. C. (1995). Experimental models of chronic renal allograft rejection. *Transplant Proc* 27(3): 2126-8.

Pirsch, J. D., J. Miller, M. H. Deierhoi, F. Vincenti and R. S. Filo (1997). A comparison of tacrolimus (FK506) and cyclosporine for immunosuppression after cadaveric renal transplantation. FK506 Kidney Transplant Study Group. *Transplantation* 63(7): 977-83.

Ponticelli, C. (2005). Clinical experience with everolimus (Certican): a summary. *Transplantation* 79(9 Suppl): S93-4.

Powles, R. L., A. J. Barrett, H. Clink, H. E. Kay, J. Sloane and T. J. McElwain (1978). Cyclosporin A for the treatment of graft-versus-host disease in man. *Lancet* 2(8104-5): 1327-31.

Pratschke, J., T. Steinmuller, W. O. Bechstein, R. Neuhaus, S. G. Tullius, S. Jonas, G. Schumacher, W. Luck, M. Becker and P. Neuhaus (1998). Orthotopic liver transplantation for hepatic associated metabolic disorders. *Clin Transplant* 12(3): 228-32.

Racusen, L. C. and H. Regele The pathology of chronic allograft dysfunction. *Kidney Int Suppl*(119): S27-32.

Racusen, L. C., K. Solez, R. B. Colvin, S. M. Bonsib, M. C. Castro, T. Cavallo, B. P. Croker, A. J. Demetris, C. B. Drachenberg, A. B. Fogo, P. Furness, L. W. Gaber, I. W. Gibson, D. Glotz, J. C. Goldberg, J. Grande, P. F. Halloran, H. E. Hansen, B. Hartley, P. J. Hayry, C. M. Hill, E. O. Hoffman, L. G. Hunsicker, A. S. Lindblad, Y. Yamaguchi and et al. (1999). The Banff 97 working classification of renal allograft pathology. *Kidney Int* 55(2): 713-23.

Rivory, L. P., H. Qin, S. J. Clarke, J. Eris, G. Duggin, E. Ray, R. J. Trent and J. F. Bishop (2000). Frequency of cytochrome P450 3A4 variant genotype in transplant population and lack of association with cyclosporin clearance. *Eur J Clin Pharmacol* 56(5): 395-8.

Ruegger, A., M. Kuhn, H. Lichti, H. R. Loosli, R. Huguenin, C. Quiquerez and A. von Wartburg (1976). [Cyclosporin A, a Peptide Metabolite from Trichoderma polysporum (Link ex Pers.) Rifai, with a remarkable immunosuppressive activity]. *Helv Chim Acta* 59(4): 1075-92.

Seino, Y., M. Hori and T. Sonoda (2003). Multicenter prospective investigation on cardiovascular adverse effects of tacrolimus in kidney transplantations. *Cardiovasc Drugs Ther* 17(2): 141-9.

Sijpkens, Y. W., Doxiadis, II, M. J. Mallat, J. W. de Fijter, J. A. Bruijn, F. H. Claas and L. C. Paul (2003). Early versus late acute rejection episodes in renal transplantation. *Transplantation* 75(2): 204-8.

Slattery, C., E. Campbell, T. McMorrow and M. P. Ryan (2005). Cyclosporine A-induced renal fibrosis: a role for epithelial-mesenchymal transition. *Am J Pathol* 167(2): 395-407.

Slattery, C., T. McMorrow and M. P. Ryan (2006). Overexpression of E2A proteins induces epithelial-mesenchymal transition in human renal proximal tubular epithelial cells suggesting a potential role in renal fibrosis. *FEBS Lett* 580(17): 4021-30.

Slattery, C., M. P. Ryan and T. McMorrow (2008). E2A proteins: regulators of cell phenotype in normal physiology and disease. *Int J Biochem Cell Biol* 40(8): 1431-6.

Slattery, C., M. P. Ryan and T. McMorrow (2008). Protein kinase C beta overexpression induces fibrotic effects in human proximal tubular epithelial cells. *Int J Biochem Cell Biol* 40(10): 2218-29.

Stevenson, C. L., M. M. Tan and D. Lechuga-Ballesteros (2003). Secondary structure of cyclosporine in a spray-dried liquid crystal by FTIR. *J Pharm Sci* 92(9): 1832-43.

Strutz, F., M. Zeisberg, F. N. Ziyadeh, C. Q. Yang, R. Kalluri, G. A. Muller and E. G. Neilson (2002). Role of basic fibroblast growth factor-2 in epithelial-mesenchymal transformation. *Kidney Int* 61(5): 1714-28.

Suthanthiran, M., R. E. Morris and T. B. Strom (1996). Immunosuppressants: cellular and molecular mechanisms of action. *Am J Kidney Dis* 28(2): 159-72.

Suthanthiran, M. and T. B. Strom (1994). Renal transplantation. *N Engl J Med* 331(6): 365-76.

Thiery, J. P. (2003). Epithelial-mesenchymal transitions in development and pathologies. *Curr Opin Cell Biol* 15(6): 740-6.

Toz, H., S. Sen, M. Sezis, S. Duman, M. Ozkahya, S. Ozbek, C. Hoscoskun, G. Atabay and E. Ok (2004). Comparison of tacrolimus and cyclosporin in renal transplantation by the protocol biopsies. *Transplant Proc* 36(1): 134-6.

Veroux, P., M. Veroux, C. Puliatti, W. Morale, D. Cappello, M. Valvo and M. Macarone (2002). Tacrolimus-induced neurotoxicity in kidney transplant recipients. *Transplant Proc* 34(8): 3188-90.

Webster, A., R. C. Woodroffe, R. S. Taylor, J. R. Chapman and J. C. Craig (2005). Tacrolimus versus cyclosporin as primary immunosuppression for kidney transplant recipients. *Cochrane Database Syst Rev*(4): CD003961.

Wesselborg, S., D. A. Fruman, J. K. Sagoo, B. E. Bierer and S. J. Burakoff (1996). Identification of a physical interaction between calcineurin and nuclear factor of activated T cells (NFATp). *J Biol Chem* 271(3): 1274-7.

Whalen, R. D., P. N. Tata, G. J. Burckart and R. Venkataramanan (1999). Species differences in the hepatic and intestinal metabolism of cyclosporine. *Xenobiotica* 29(1): 3-9.

Williams, D. and L. Haragsim (2006). Calcineurin nephrotoxicity. *Adv Chronic Kidney Dis* 13(1): 47-55.

Wissmann, C., F. J. Frey, P. Ferrari and D. E. Uehlinger (1996). Acute cyclosporine-induced nephrotoxicity in renal transplant recipients: the role of the transplanted kidney. *J Am Soc Nephrol* 7(12): 2677-81.

Wolfe, R. A., V. B. Ashby, E. L. Milford, A. O. Ojo, R. E. Ettenger, L. Y. Agodoa, P. J. Held and F. K. Port (1999). Comparison of mortality in all patients on dialysis, patients on dialysis awaiting transplantation, and recipients of a first cadaveric transplant. *N Engl J Med* 341(23): 1725-30.

Yang, J. and Y. Liu (2001). Dissection of key events in tubular epithelial to myofibroblast transition and its implications in renal interstitial fibrosis. *Am J Pathol* 159(4): 1465-75.

Yura, H., N. Yoshimura, T. Hamashima, K. Akamatsu, M. Nishikawa, Y. Takakura and M. Hashida (1999). Synthesis and pharmacokinetics of a novel macromolecular prodrug of Tacrolimus (FK506), FK506-dextran conjugate. *J Control Release* 57(1): 87-99.

12

Malignancy Following Renal Transplantation

A. Vanacker and B. Maes
Heilig-Hartziekenhuis Roeselare-Menen
Belgium

1. Introduction

After transplantation, there is an increase in the incidence of a wide variety of malignancies compared to the general population, due to the chronic use of immunosuppressive agents. They appear to have a more aggressive behavior and a worse outcome. As a result, among recipients of renal transplantation, malignancy is the third most common cause of patient death with graft function, after cardiovascular diseases and infections. Since management and outcomes of the cardiovascular and infectious complications are improving, malignancy after transplantation will probably become more important (Briggs, 2001).
In this chapter, we will focus on the increased cancer incidence in solid organ transplant recipients, in order to emphasize the clinical importance of this topic in renal transplant patients. Since skin cancer and post-transplantation lymphoproliferative disorder PTLD are most strikingly increased after renal transplantation, we will study them in detail. There is some evidence that individual immunosuppressive agents have a different role in the development of post-transplantation malignancy. The available data on this will be discussed. Finally, based on the currently available international guidelines, we will propose an appropriate prevention and early detection program for patients undergoing renal transplantation.

2. Epidemiology and risk factors

Cancer risk is a major problem after renal transplantation. There is much data on the incidence of cancer after renal transplantation, mostly derived from large transplant registries. One of the largest is an American report (by the United States Renal Data System USRDS) on more than 35,000 patients who received a first renal transplantation (deceased or living donor). The incidence of malignancies during the first 3 years after transplantation was examined compared with the general US population. Three years after transplantation, a cumulative incidence of 7.5% for non-skin malignancy and 7.4% for skin cancer (excluding melanoma) was noted. Compared to the general population, there was especially an important increase in the incidence of Kaposi's sarcoma, non-Hodgkin's lymphoma and nonmelanoma skin cancers (more than 20-fold) and kidney cancer (approximately 15-fold). By contrast, the more common solid cancers in the general population (e. g. breast, lung, prostate, colorectal, uterine and ovarian cancer) were only slightly increased in incidence in transplant recipients (roughly twofold higher). Since cancer appears to be more common among haemodialysis patients (because of the correlation between uremia and abnormalities in the immune system), an additional comparison between the population of transplant recipients and haemodialysis patients on the waiting list was performed, in order to assess whether this increased incidence was attributed to the presence of end-stage renal disease (ESRD) or could really be related to the post-transplantation setting. For some malignancies, the risk was similar between both groups; however, several cancers (in particular for non-melanoma skin cancers, melanoma, Kaposi's sarcoma, non-Hodgkin's and Hodgkin's lymphoma, cancer of the mouth, cancer of the kidney, oesophageal cancers and leukaemia) are clearly more common after transplantation compared to patients on the waiting list (Kasiske et al., 2004).

A cohort study using data of 28,855 patients from an Australia and New Zealand Dialysis and Transplant Registry (ANZDATA) found similar results. When excluding non-melanoma skin cancer, they reported a slightly increased incidence of malignancy in patients with ESRD receiving dialysis compared to the general population (standardised incidence ratio SIR 1.35), which increased significantly after renal transplantation (SIR 3.27) (Vajdic CM et al., 2006). A Danish retrospective cohort study also showed that the major increase in incidence of malignancy occurs after transplantation and not during dialysis: SIR after transplantation 3.6 versus 1.4 during dialysis, both compared with the general population (Birkeland et al., 2000). In general, we can conclude that the risk of *de novo* malignancies is increased in transplant recipients, with a relative risk 3-5 times that of the general population. In table 1, we summarize the relative risk of certain malignancies compared to the general population and patients with ESRD on the waiting list.

The increased risk of developing malignancy after renal transplantation can in the first place be attributed to the use of immunosuppressive medication, which may damage DNA, lead to malignant transformation of cells and may interfere with normal immunosurveillance to neoplastic cells (allowing uncontrolled growth). It is clear that the intensity and duration of immunosuppressive therapy impacts cancer risk. Whether the type of immunosuppressive agent used also plays an important role in the development of secondary malignancy is a controversial issue. We will focus on this issue in more detail further in this chapter.

Moreover, some common viral infections after transplantation are linked to the development of certain malignancies: Kaposi's sarcoma (associated with human herpes virus 8, HHV8), non Hodgkin's lymphoma NHL and Hodgkin's lymphoma (Epstein-Barr virus, EBV), hepatocellular carcinoma (hepatitis B and C virus, HBV and HCV), cancer of cervix, vulva/vagina, penis, anus and oral cavity and pharynx (human papilloma virus, HPV). Some of those malignancies occur with the highest incidence in transplant recipients, compared to the general population. It is suggested that this could be explained by the impaired immune control of viral oncogenes.

Besides the etiological role of the intensity and duration of immunosuppression and infection by oncogenic viruses, also the genetic background of the host, chronic pretransplantation dialysis treatment, the patient's age at the time of transplantation, pre-transplant malignancy and established carcinogenic exposures (such as exposure to ultraviolet UV light, total sun burden, analgesic abuse and tobacco smoking) play an important role in the occurrence of malignancy after renal transplantation (Dantal & Pohanka, 2007; Morath et al., 2004).

The average time to presentation differs for other type of malignancies. Post-transplantation lymphoproliferative disorder PTLD can occur more early after transplantation, with 20% of PTLD occurring in the first year after renal transplantation. In contrast, skin cancer becomes more common with time.

	Vs. general population	Vs. patients on the waiting list
More common tumours:	2	Similar
Colon		"
Lung		"
Prostate		"
Stomach		"
Oesophagus		2.7
Pancreas		Similar
Ovary		"
Breast		"
Testicular cancer	3	Similar
Bladder cancer		
Melanoma	5	2.2
Leukemia		1.6
Hepatobiliary tumours		Similar
Cervical tumours		"
Vulvovaginal tumours		"
Renal cell cancer	15	1.4
Kaposi's sarcoma	> 20	9
Non-Hodgkin's lymphoma		3.3
Non-melanoma skin cancer		2.6

Table 1. Standardised incidence ratio (SIR) of cancer after transplantation, compared with the general US population and with patients with end-stage renal disease ESRD (adapted from Kasiske et al., 2004)

3. Skin cancer

Skin cancer is the most common cancer type following renal transplantation in Caucasian transplant recipients, occurring in more than 50% of patients in high incidence areas (such as Australia) after 20 years of renal transplantation. The incidence increases with the duration of immunosuppressive therapy. They occur at younger age (10 to 15 years younger than in the general population) and in multiple sites. Moreover, they are more aggressive and more likely to recur after resection. For that reason, they can cause serious morbidity and may have a life-threatening course.

As in the immunocompetent population, sun exposure (UV radiation, causing genetic mutations in epidermal keratinocytes that affect cell cycle regulation) is the major risk factor of developing skin cancer. In transplant patients, an additional important risk factor is the duration and intensity of immunosuppression. For that reason, skin cancer is 2 to 3 times more common after heart transplantation (requiring higher levels of immunosuppression), compared to kidney transplantation. It has been suggested that certain immunosuppressive medications (like azathioprine AZA and cyclosporine CsA) are associated with greater risk of skin cancer due to photosensitizing and mutagenic effects and that others (like mTOR inhibitors) may have antiproliferative effects (Kovach & Stasko, 2009). We will discuss this in detail in below (see '5. Immunosuppressive drugs and the risk of malignancy after transplantation').

3.1 Types of skin cancer

Skin cancer includes squamous cell carcinoma SCC, basal cell carcinoma BCC, malignant melanomas, Merkel cell carcinoma and Kaposi's sarcoma. In contrast to the general population, there is a predominance of SCC over BCC in renal transplant recipients, with a ratio of SCC to BCC of 4:1.

3.1.1 Squamous cell carcinoma SCC

Squamous cell carcinoma SCC arises from atypical keratinocytes of the epidermis. It occurs most commonly in sun exposed areas and is usually associated with precursor lesions like actinic keratoses, Bowen's disease (SCC in situ), viral warts and/or keratoacanthomas. The risk of SCC is 60 to 100 times greater than in the general population. The lesions appear as small red, keratotic, hard nodules that occasionally ulcerate. The pathogenesis is multifactorial, with cumulative sun exposure as most important factor. Also infection with human papillomavirus (HPV, particularly oncogenic HPV 5 and 8 strains) plays an important role in the development of SCC, with HPV being detected in 65 to 90% of SCC of transplant recipients. Other risk factors are fair skin, age, the level of immunosuppression, duration of pretransplantion dialysis, ionizing radiation, chronic inflamed skin (like scars or chronic ulcers) and possibly smoking. SCC is more aggressive in transplant recipients than in the general populations, resulting in higher risk of local recurrence (14% of patients), regional and distant metastasis (6-9% of patients) and mortality. In patients with metastases, disease-specific survival is approximately 50%. Treatment consists of complete local excision and lymphadenectomy if necessary. In immunocompromised patients with the initial presentation of aggressive SCCs, Mohs micrographic surgery should be administered in order to minimize the risk of recurrence and tissue loss. Mohs micrographic surgery includes removal of the tumour followed by immediate frozen section histopathologic examination of margins with subsequent re-excision of tumour-positive areas and final closure of the defect. When more than one lymph node is affected or when there is extracapsular spread, adjuvant radiotherapy should be considered. Systemic chemotherapy can be used for metastatic SCC (Kovach & Stasko, 2009).

3.1.2 Basal cell carcinoma BCC

Basal cell carcinoma BCC arises from the basal layer of the epidermis and its appendages. It occurs on sun-exposed skin, most commonly on the face or head (up to 70%). Common sites are eyelid margins, nose folds, lips and around and behind the ears. The incidence of BCC is increased by a factor 10 to 16 in transplant recipients, compared to the general population. Intense intermittent sun exposure is important in the pathogenesis of BCC, in contrast with SCC were the cumulative sun exposure plays an important role. Other risk factors for developing BCC are similar as for SCC. According to the clinical presentation, BCC can be divided in three sub-groups: nodular BCC (a pink or flesh-colored papule, often with a translucent, 'pearly' appearance and a teleangiectatic vessel, sometimes with central erosion), superficial BCC (a slightly scaly, light red papule or plaque) and morpheaform BCC (smooth, flesh-colored, or very lightly erythematous papules or plaques, frequently atrophic). As for SCC, treatment of BCC consists of local excision (Mohs surgery) with or without lymphadenectomy. Metastases of BCC are very rare even in immunosuppressed patients. However, BCC can cause serious local destruction, necessitating surgery and resulting in significant cosmetic deformity (Kovach & Stasko, 2009).

3.1.3 Malignant melanoma

Malignant melanomas arise from melanocytes. To detect a malignant melanoma, new or changing pigmented lesions should be examined with special attention for A, assymmetry; B, border irregularity; C, color variation/dark black color; D, diameter more than 6 mm; and E, evolution or change. Malignant melanomas can be classified into lentigo malignant melanomas (arising on sun-exposed skin of older individuals), superficial spreading malignant melanomas (most common, occurring in 70%, especially in Caucasian people), nodular malignant melanomas, acral lentiginous melanomas (arising on palms, soles and nail beds, commonly in more darkly pigmented persons), malignant melanomas on mucous membranes and miscellaneous forms. The risk of developing melanoma is 3.6 times greater in renal transplant recipients than in the general population. Risk factors for the development of post-transplant malignant melanomas are the presence of atypical nevi, history of blistering sunburns, immunosuppression, fair skin, a personal or family history of malignant melanomas, older age at the time of transplantation and the use of depleting anti-lymphocyte antibodies.

While SCC and BCC are rarely lethal, melanoma is a potentially fatal malignancy. The most prognostic factor is tumour thickness (Breslow depth). Patients diagnosed with malignant melanoma with a tumour thickness of less than 1 mm have an excellent outcome. However, if there is lymph node involvement or distant metastasis, survival rate is low with a 5-year survival of respectively 30% and less than 10% in immunocompetent persons. Outcome for posttransplant lesions with < 2 mm thickness is similar to the general population, while for lesions > 2 mm thickness prognosis is significantly worse (Matin et al., 2008). Treatment of melanoma consists of surgical excision, with reexcision of margins according to the thickness of the tumour. Sentinel node biopsy is recommended for patients with clinically negative nodes if Breslow depth is more than 1 mm. Reduction or change of the immunosuppressive regimen should be considered, balancing the prognosis of the tumour and the risk of graft rejection (Zwald FO et al., 2010).

3.1.4 Kaposi's sarcoma

Kaposi's sarcoma KS is a vascular neoplasm, characterized by reddish-brown or purple-blue plaques or nodules on cutaneous or mucosal surfaces, including the skin, lungs, gastrointestinal tract and lymphoid tissue. KS has been associated with the reactivation of latent human herpes virus 8 (HHV-8) infection or donor-to-recipient transfer of HHV-8-infected progenitor cells. The incidence of KS is 20 times increased in renal transplant recipients. It occurs frequently early after renal transplantation, with an average time to development after transplantation of 13 to 21 months. It is more common in male transplant recipients, with a male to female ratio ranging from 2:1 to 4:1. Most cases occurs in patients from Mediterranean, Jewish, Arabic, Caribbean or African ethnic groups. The treatment of Kaposi's sarcoma in renal transplant patients primarily consists of a reduction or discontinuation of the immunosuppressive medication, and possibly a conversion to alternative immunosuppressive agents like mTOR inhibitors (as will be discussed below) (Antman & Chuang, 2000; Campistol & Schena, 2007).

3.2 Prevention

As for immunocompetent individuals, prior exposure to solar ultraviolet radiation (UVR) is the predominant risk factor for development of cutaneous malignancies. In patients at high-risk, primary prevention including the avoidance of sun exposure (especially during peak hours of radiation), use of protective clothing and use of an effective sunscreen (protection factor >15) for unclothed body parts (head, neck, hands and arms) is very important. Early detection of skin cancer is essential to reduce disfiguring surgery and to prevent mortality from advanced or metastatic lesions. For this reason, patients should be aware of the increased risk of skin cancer and perform regular self-screening. Annual skin examination by a dermatologist is recommended, especially in high-risk patients (e.g. patients with a history of skin cancer, fair-skin, living in high sun-exposure climates, having occupations with sun exposure or having had significant sun exposure as a child). Treatment of premalignant lesions (actinic keratoses, viral warts) is advised in order to prevent progression to SCC. This can be done with liquid nitrogen cryosurgery, excision, and curettage or with topical therapies such as 5-fluorouracil (which interferes with DNA synthesis and cell proliferation) or imiquimod 5% cream (a topical imidazoquinolone immunomodulator stimulating local cell-mediated immune response directed against tumoral and viral antigens). When actinic keratoses or viral warts persist with these therapies, biopsy is required to rule out progression to SCC (Kovach & Stasko, 2009).

There are several studies suggesting that retinoids (vitamin A derivates, available in topical and oral preparations) may be beneficial to the treatment and/or prevention of non-melanoma skin tumours after solid organ transplantation. They are said to influence a broad spectrum of cellular functions through interactions with nuclear receptors. Topical retinoids are used to control actinic keratoses and to diminish SCC recurrence. Oral retinoids (most common acitretin) has been advised for patients with multiple and/or recurrent skin cancers. Chen et al. reviewed three small randomized controlled clinical trials on the use of oral retinoids as preventive agents in the development of skin cancer. The first trial was a cross-over trial with 23 high-risk patients. Compared to the acitretin period (25 mg daily), a 42% increase in the incidence of SCC was seen in the drug-free period. In the second trial, 44 high-risk patients were randomized to receive acitretin 30 mg daily or placebo. After 6 months of follow-up, 18 new skin cancers developed in the placebo group, whereas only 2 new skin cancers developed in the acitretin group. The last trial compared two different dose regimens (0.2 mg/kg/day versus 0.4 mg/kg/day) in 26 renal transplant recipients and did not find a significant difference in development of skin cancers between the two groups. While the first two trials included only high-risk patients, the last included any stable renal transplant recipient, which could explain the lack of benefit (Chen et al., 2005). After cessation of therapy, rebound phenomena with development of large numbers of cutaneous malignancies are reported. For that reason, oral retinoids should always be given as long-term maintenance therapy.

The major factor, however, limiting the use of oral retinoids in the prevention of skin cancer is the poor tolerance associated with it. Adverse effects include headaches, mucocutaneous side effects, musculoskeletal symptoms and hyperlipidaemia. Cheilitis has been reported in 70 to 100% of patients. In conclusion, in recipients with multiple and/or recurrent skin cancers, the use of systemic retinoids, such as low-dose acitretin (dose between 0.2 and 0.4 mg/kg/day), could be advised for months/years, if well tolerated. Gradual dose escalation to an effective dose in combination with monitoring of symptoms and laboratory findings and proactive management of adverse effects rather than discontinuation of therapy is recommended (Kovach et al, 2006; Otley et al., 2006).

4. Post-transplantation lymphoproliferative disorder PTLD

Post-transplantation lymphoproliferative disorder PTLD is a heterogeneous group of diseases characterized by abnormal lymphoid proliferation, that develop in a recipient of a solid-organ transplantation or bone marrow allograft. It is the second most frequent cancer after transplantation after skin cancer, with an overall incidence of 1 to 2% after kidney transplantation (30 to 50 times higher than in the general population). PTLD frequently arises from B lymphocytes, but can rarely also originate from T-cell proliferation. It is the most frequent malignancy during the first post-transplantation year, when the level of immunosuppression is the highest. There is a strong association with Epstein-Barr virus (EBV) infection, with 98% of cases associated with latent EBV infection. An increase in the EBV viral load in peripheral blood is often detected before development of PTLD. This EBV infection leads to B cell proliferation in the setting of decreased T-cell immune surveillance due to immunosuppressive treatment. Only 10 of almost 100 viral genes in the EBV DNA are expressed in latently infected B cells, including two oncogenes latent membrane protein type 1 LMP-1 and type 2 LMP-2. The number of expressed viral genes is reduced to diminish the recognition of cytotoxic T cells.

PTLD can be divided in three distinct morphologic groups, according to the World Health Organization classification, each containing some subtypes:

- Early disease (55% of cases), characterized by diffuse B cell hyperplasia of polyclonal nature, with no signs of malignant transformation. This has a good prognosis after reduction of immunosuppression.
- Polymorphic PTLD (30%), usually polyclonal B cell proliferation with evidence of early malignant transformation, such as clonal cytogenetic abnormalities and immunoglobulin gene rearrangements.
- Monomorphic PTLD (15%), characterized by monoclonal B cell proliferation with malignant cytogenetic abnormalities and immunoglobulin rearrangements. This includes high-grade invasive lymphoma of B or T lymphocyte centroblasts. It is associated with the worst outcome.

In table 2, the clinical and pathological features and the management of the different groups is summarized (Magee et al., 2008).

The clinical manifestations from PTLD are extremely variable and it often presents in a nonspecific way. Early PTLD (first year after transplantation) presents often with an infectious mononucleosis-like presentation, with prominent B-cell symptoms (fever, night sweats and weight loss) and rapid enlargement of the tonsils and cervical nodes. Late PTLD (more than 1 year after transplantation) has often a more gradual clinical course and fewer systemic symptoms. In half of the patients, extra-nodal disease is present, with involvement of gastrointestinal tract (stomach, intestine), lungs, skin, liver, central nervous system or frequently the allograft itself. It is of major importance to recognize early clinical signs and symptoms of PTLD. PTLD is often associated with elevated serum markers such as lactate dehydrogenase LDH. For an accurate diagnosis of PTLD, tissue biopsy is required. Fluorodeoxyglucose (FDG)-positron emission tomography (PET/CT) is an important tool in the diagnosis, staging and post-treatment evaluation.

Prognosis of PTLD varies according to clonality and extent of disease. However, in general, PTLD has a poor prognosis with a 1-year mortality of approximately 40%. The most important risk factors for PTLD are the type, length and intensity of immunosuppressive drug therapies. There is an increased risk of PTLD in patients who received potent T-cell depleting antibodies (like OTK3 or anti-thymocyte globulin ATG) for induction therapy or for treatment of rejection. There would be a twofold higher risk for development of PTLD in patients receiving tacrolimus in comparison to cyclosporine. A special category of patients at particular risk for PTLD development are seronegative patients at the time of transplantation, receiving an organ from an EBV-seropositive donor (inducing a primary EBV infection after transplantation). An age effect on the development of PTLD is present, with the incidence highest among children < 10 years of age and adults > 60 years of age (Opelz & Henderson, 1993; Opelz & Döhler, 2003).

	Early disease (55%)	Polymorphic PTLD (30%)	Monomorphic PTLD (20%)
Clinical features	Infectious mononucleosis-like disease	Infectious mononucleosis-like disease, +/- weight loss, localizing symptoms	More gradual Fever, weight loss, localizing symptoms
Pathology	Preserved architecture, atypical cells infrequent	Signs of early malignant transformation	High-grade lymphoma with confluent transformed cells and marked atypia
Clonality	Polyclonal	Usually polyclonal	Monoclonal
Treatment	Reduce immunosuppression, acyclovir	Reduce immunosuppression, acyclovir, rituximab.	Reduce immunosuppression to low-dose steroids only, combination surgery, chemotherapy, radiotherapy, immunotherapy, rituximab
Prognosis	Good	Intermediate	Poor

Table 2. Summary of clinical and pathological features and management of the different types of post-transplant lymphoproliferative disorder (PTLD) (adapted from Magee CC, 2008).

In the prevention of PTLD, monitoring of EBV viral load in high-risk patients (who received large dose of immunosuppressive drugs for induction or allograft rejection) is recommended since reduction of immunosuppressive treatment can be considered if high viral loads are detected. Use of antiviral therapy as profylaxis for PTLD in high-risk patients is controversial.

Treatment of PTLD consists in the first place of reduction or discontinuation of the immunosuppressive therapy (especially cyclosporine CsA, tacrolimus and mycophenolate mofetil MMF) to reestablish host defense mechanisms. Concomitantly, prednisone can be increased to prevent allograft rejection. This can lead to complete and durable resolution of some lymphomas, especially of early and polymorphic PTLD (sometimes in combination with antiviral therapy such as acyclovir and ganciclovir). Evidence for the treatment of PTLD with antiviral therapy is lacking and it is not used in monomorphic PTLD. For monomorphic PTLD, besides reduction or discontinuation of immunosuppressive therapy, other therapeutic strategies must be considered. In localized disease, surgical resection can be an option, for example transplant nephrectomy when PTLD is restricted to the renal graft. The use of rituximab RTX as first-line therapy is increasing, because of its low toxicity and high specificity. RTX is a chimeric monoclonal antibody against the B-cell-specific CD 20 antigen (widely expressed on B lymphocytes). Treatment consists of doses of 375 mg/m^2 intravenously weekly for a total of 4 weeks. In case of diffuse lymphomas, lack of response to RTX or CD20 negative lymphoma, chemotherapy (e.g. CHOP cyclophosphamide, doxorubicin, vincristine and prednisone) can be considered (Andreone et al., 2003; Bakker et al., 2007).

5. Immunosuppressive drugs and the risk of malignancy after transplantation

The principal factor influencing the risk of posttransplant malignancy is the overall level of immunosuppressive treatment. Indeed, in a prospective, randomised trial comparing low-dose cyclosporine CsA (trough blood concentrations 75-125 ng/mL) versus high-dose CsA (trough blood concentrations 150-250 ng/mL) both in combination with azathioprine AZA, a clear correlation between high-dose regimen and more secondary malignant disorders was demonstrated (Dantal et al., 1998). This may also explain why the incidence of post-transplantation malignancy is more frequent in heart transplant recipients (which usually receive more intense immunosuppression) than in renal transplant recipients. In transplant patients with cancer, a significant reduction or even cessation of the immunosuppressive therapy is advised.

There is some evidence that also the type of immunosuppressive agent would matter. However, since in most cases combinations of several immunosuppressive drugs are used, clear data concerning individual therapies are lacking and sometimes conflicting. The purine analogue a**zathioprine AZA** has been associated with increased risk of skin cancer, possibly as a result of increased photosensitivity to ultraviolet A light (Perrett et al., 2008).

In 1999, one study suggested that the **calcineurin inhibitor cyclosporine CsA** could promote cancer progression *in vitro* and *in vivo* in an immunodeficient mouse model by a direct cellular effect, independent of any effect on the host immune system. This would be mediated by stimulation of transforming growth factor β TGF-β production, which may lead to development of morphological transformation of cells from a non-invasive phenotype to an invasive phenotype and which may promote tumor invasiveness and metastasic spread (Hojo et al., 1999). Similar results were seen with **tacrolimus**, with increase in the number of pulmonary metastases and TGF-β overexpression in mouse renal cell carcinoma receiving tacrolimus (Maluccio et al., 2003).

In contrast, there is growing data suggesting that **inhibitors of the mammalian target of rapamycin mTOR** (**sirolimus** and **everolimus**) have antioncogenic properties and are therefore associated with a reduced risk for some malignancies and longer times for malignancies to develop. This can be explained by the fact that mTOR inhibitors repress several enzymes along the intracellular signaling pathways that play a role in the development and progression of different cancers (like p70 S6K, IL-10, and cyclins), resulting in deceleration or inhibition of cell-cycle progression, increased sensitivity to apoptosis and reduced angiogenesis.

There are several clinical trials linking the use of mTOR inhibitors to reduced incidence of malignancies. In 2004, Mathew et al. reviewed 5 multicenter studies, comparing the cancer risk for different immunosuppressive regimens. Two studies containing 1295 patients randomized to receive CsA in combination with sirolimus, AZA or placebo. After 2 years, they saw a significant lower incidence of skin cancer in the sirolimus-group (2% in a low-

dose group, 2.8% in a high-dose group) compared to the placebo-group (6.9%). Compared to the AZA-group (4.3%), the difference was not statistically significant. Two other trials (161 patients) compared maintenance therapy based on sirolimus or CsA (both in combination with steroids and AZA or mycophenolate mofetil MMF). In the CsA based-group, 5% of patients had some form of malignancy after 2 years, compared to 0% in the sirolimus-based group. In the fifth trial (525 patients), CsA withdrawal 3 months after renal transplantation in combination with steroids and increased sirolimus trough levels (20 to 30 ng/ml during year 1, 15 to 25 ng/ml thereafter) was compared with a continuous regimen of CsA, steroids and sirolimus (trough levels 5 to 15 ng/ml). After 2 years, the incidence of overall malignancies was significant lower in the CsA-elimination group (4.2% compared to 9.8%) (Mathew et al., 2004). The long-term results of this last trial are incorporated in the Rapamune Maintenance Trial (430 patients). Similarly, after 5 years follow-up, patients in the CsA withdrawal group had a reduced incidence of both skin and nonskin malignancies. What's more, the median time to first skin carcinoma was significantly shorter in the CsA group (491 days) compared to the withdrawal group (1,126 days) (Campistol et al., 2006).
A large registry (United Network for Organ Sharing database) reporting 33,249 renal transplant patients whose maintenance immunosuppression contained an mTOR-inhibitor, an mTOR-inhibitor in combination with a calcineurin inhibitor CNI or a CNI alone, showed reduction in the overall incidence of *de novo* malignancy in patients receiving an mTOR-inhibitor. After a mean follow-up of 2.3 years, an incidence of 0.6% was seen in the mTOR-inhibitor alone or the mTOR-inhibitor plus CNI group versus 1.8% in the CNI alone group (Kauffman et al., 2005). Similar results turned up in the Sirolimus Convert Trial where 830 renal allograft recipients receiving CNI-based immunosuppression were randomly assigned to convert to sirolimus or to continue CNI. The overall malignancy rates after 24 months were significantly lower in the sirolimus group (3.8%) versus the CNI group (11%). However, the number of adverse effects in the sirolimus group was higher than in the CNI group (Schena et al., 2009).
There is some evidence that sirolimus does not only prevent the occurrence of cancer, as described above, but is also promising in treating existing tumors. There would be some benefit of basing immunosuppression in patients with new-onset malignancy after transplantation on these drugs (especially for Kaposi's sarcoma). In 15 renal transplant recipients with biopsy-proven cutaneous Kaposi's sarcoma, cyclosporine and mycophenolate mofetil were stopped and sirolimus was started. After six months, all patients had complete clinical and histological regression of Kaposi's sarcoma lesions (Stallone et al., 2005). Gutierrez-Dalmau et al. reported similar results in 7 renal transplant patients after conversion of CNI to sirolimus (Gutierrez-Dalmau, 2005).
In patients with established malignancy after transplantation, some therapeutic options should be considered. It is clear that reduction of the total amount of immunosuppressive medication is very important. This should however be balanced against the risk of graft rejection and the quality of life with and without a functioning graft. The most serious effect of a reduction or cessation of therapy can be expected from malignancies with a greater increase in incidence after renal transplantation (like non-melanoma skin cancer, PTLD and Kaposi's sarcoma). Whether CNI should be converted into an mTOR-inhibitor is somewhat questionable. It is certainly advised for Kaposi's sarcoma. However, when considering switching CNI to mTOR inhibitors for other malignancies, it should be balanced against its frequent side effects, including increase in serum lipids, myelotoxicity, proteinuria, pneumopathy (hypersensitivity-like interstitial pneumonitis), dermatological

manifestations, some degree of oedema and aphtae. Up to one-third of patients starting sirolimus will stop because of side effects. When patients still need surgical intervention for the malignancy, potential wound healing complications attributed to mTOR-inhibitors should also be taken into account (Campistol et al., 2007; Cravedi P et al., 2009; Kidney Disease: Improving Global Outcomes (KDIGO) Transplant Work Group, 2009).

6. General recommendations for cancer screening after renal transplantation

Cancer should be a major focus in the long-term follow-up of renal transplant recipients. First and foremost, preventive measures should be taken, i.e. avoiding excessive immunosuppression (especially depleting anti-lymphocyte antibodies), screening transplant donors and recipients for cancer and avoiding carcinogenic factors (such as nicotin abuse, high sun exposure, etc.). Secondly, in order to detect malignancies in transplant patients at an early stage, periodic screening examinations are recommended. It is questioned whether guidelines for cancer screening for the general population are also applicable for renal transplant recipients, because the life expectancy of these patients is mostly less. Because of this, an individual approach for each patient is recommended, taking into account the individual prognosis and risk of developing malignancy (Webster et al., 2008). Based on the American (KDIGO Transplant Work Group, 2009) and European (European Best Practice Guidelines EBPG, 2002) transplantation professional guidelines, we can however suggest the following practical screening plan:

1. Annual examination of the skin and lip by a dermatologist (more frequently in high-risk patients, such as patients with a history of skin cancer).
2. Abdominal surveillance ultrasonography at least every three years to detect early stage renal cell carcinoma. Especially in high-risk patients including patients with a history of renal cell carcinoma or the presence of acquired cystic disease, analgesic nephropathy or tuberous sclerosis.
3. Standard cancer surveillance (appropriate for age) for neoplasms commonly seen in the general population:

- Colorectal cancer: colonoscopy every 5 years from the age of 50
- Breast cancer: breast exam and screening mammography every year from the age of 50 to 69 (from the age of 40 if mother or sister has had breast cancer)
- Cervical cancer: pap smear and pelvic exam every year for women within 3 years of onset of sexual activity or from the age of 21 (whichever comes first)
- Prostate cancer: digital rectal exam and PSA testing every year from the age of 50
- Hepatocellular cancer: abdominal ultrasound and alpha-feto protein testing every 6-12 months only in high-risk patients (cirrhosis or chronic viral hepatitis, especially HBV).

7. Conclusion

As short-term patient and graft survival have improved over the past few decades, long-term complications of kidney transplantation are becoming more important. The incidence of malignancies is considerably higher in renal transplant recipients than in the general population. In fact, malignancy is the third most common cause of patient death after renal transplantation (after cardiovascular events and infection). With longer graft survival and older donors (as well as recipients) and with the introduction of more potent immunosuppressive medication, malignancy is becoming even more common. Both clinicians and patients should be aware of this risk, making primary prevention a major concern. In addition, they should consider a cancer screening plan adapted to the patient's individual risk profile and life expectancy.

8. References

Andreone P, Gramenzi A, Lorenzini S, Biselli M, Cursaro C, Pileri S & Bernardi M. (2003). Posttransplantation lymphoproliferative disorders. *Archives of Internal Medicine,* Vol. 163, No. 17, (September 2003), pp. (1997-2004).

Antman K, Chuang Y. (2000). Kaposi's sarcoma. *New England Journal of Medicine,* Vol. 342, No. 14, (April 2000), pp. (1027-1038).

Bakker NA, van Imhoff GW, Verschuuren EAM & van Son WJ. (2007). Presentation and early detection of post-transplant lymphoproliferative disorder after solid organ transplantation. *Transplantation International,* Vol. 20, No. 3, (March 2007), pp. (433-438).

Birkeland SA, Løkkegaard H & Storm HH. (2000). Cancer risk in patients on dialysis and after renal transplantation. *Lancet,* Vol. 355, No. 9218, (May 2000), pp. (1886-1887).

Briggs JD. (2001). Causes of death after renal transplantation. *Nephrology, Dialysis and Transplantation,* Vol. 16, No. 8, (August 2001), pp. (1545-1549).

Campistol JM, Eris J, Oberbauer R, Friend P, Hutchison B, Morales JM, Claesson K, Stallone G, Russ G, Rostaing L, Kreis H, Burke JT, Brault Y, Scarola JA & Neylan JF for the Rapamune Maintenance Regimen Study Group. (2006). Sirolimus therapy after early cyclosporine withdrawal reduces the risk for cancer in adult renal transplantation. *Journal of the American Society of Nephrology,* Vol. 17: No. 2, (February 2006), pp. (581-589).

Campistol JM, Albanell J, Arns W, Boletis I, Dantal J, de Fijter JW, Mortensen SA, Neumayer HH, Oyen O, Pascual J, Pohanka E, Schena FP, Seron D, Sparacino V & Chapman JR. (2007). Use of proliferation signal inhibitors in the management of post-transplant malignancies - clinical guidance. *Nephrology, Dialysis and Transplantation,* Vol. 22, Suppl. 1, (May 2007), pp. (i36-i41).

Campistol JM & Schena FP. (2007). Kaposi's sarcoma in renal transplant recipients - the impact of proliferation signal inhibitors. *Nephrology, Dialysis and Transplantation,* Vol. 22, Suppl. 1, (May 2007), pp. (i17-i22).

Chen K, Craig JC & Shumack S. (2005). Oral retinoids for the prevention of skin cancers in solid organ transplant recipients: a systemic review of randomized controlled trials. *British Journal of Dermatology,* Vol. 152, No. 3, (March 2005), pp. (518-23).

Cravedi P, Ruggenenti P & Remuzzi G. (2009). Sirolimus to replace calcineurin inhibitors? Too early yet. *Lancet,* Vol. 373, No. 9671, (April 2009), pp. (1235-1236).

Dantal J, Hourmant M, Cantarovich D, Giral M, Blancho G, Dreno B & Soulillou JP. (1998). Effect of long-term immunosuppression in kidney-graft recipients on cancer incidence: randomised comparison of two cyclosporin regimens. *Lancet,* Vol. 351, No. 9103, (February 1998), pp. (623-628).

Dantal J & Pohanka E. (2007) Malignancies in renal transplantation: an unmet medical need. *Nephrology, Dialysis and Transplantation,* Vol. 22, Suppl. 1, (May 2007), pp. (i4-i10).

European best practice guidelines for renal transplantation. (2002). Section IV: Long-term management of the transplant recipient. IV.6. Cancer risk after renal transplantation. *Nephrology, Dialysis and Transplantation,* Vol. 17, Suppl. 4, (April 2002), pp. (31-36).

Euvrard S, Kanitakis J, Claudy A. (2003). Skin cancers after organ transplantation. *New England Journal of Medicine,* Vol. 348, No. 17, (April 2003), pp. (1681-1691).

Gutierrez-Dalmau A, Sanchez-Fructuoso A, Sanz-Guajardo A, Mazuecos A, Franco A, Rial MC, Iranzo P, Torregrosa JV, Oppenheimer F & Campistol JM. (2004). Efficacy of conversion to sirolimus in posttransplantation Kaposi's sarcoma. *Transplantation Proceedings,* Vol. 37, No. 9, (November 2005), pp. (3836-3838).

Hojo M, Morimoto T, Maluccio M, Asano T, Morimoto K, Lagman M, Shimbo T & Suthanthiran M. (1999). Cyclosporine induces cancer progression by a cell-autonomous mechanism. *Nature,* Vol. 397, No. 6719, (February 1999), pp. (530-534).

Kasiske, BL, Snyder, JJ, Gilbertson DT & Wang C. (2004). Cancer after kidney transplantation in the United States. *American Journal of Transplantation,* Vol. 4, No. 6, (June 2004), pp. (905-913).

Kauffman HM, Cherikh WS, Cheng Y, Hanto DW & Kahan BD. (2005). Maintenance immunosuppression with target-of-rapamycin inhibitors is associated with a reduced incidence of de novo malignancies. *Transplantation,* Vol. 80, No. 7, (October 2005), pp. (883-889).

Kidney Disease: Improving Global Outcomes (KDIGO) Transplant Work Group. (2009) KDIGO clinical practice guideline for the care of kidney transplant recipients. *American Journal of Transplantation,* Vol. 9, Suppl. 3, (October 2009), pp. (S1–S157).

Kovach BT, Murphy G, Otley CC, Shumack S, Ulrich C & Stasko T. (2006). Oral retinoids for chemoprevention of skin cancers in organ transplant recipients: results of a survey. *Transplantation Proceedings,* Vol. 38, No. 5, (June 2006), pp. (1366-1368).

Kovach BT & Stasko T. (2009). Skin cancer after transplantation. *Transplantation Reviews,* Vol. 23, No. 3, (July 2009), pp. (178-189).

Maluccio M, Sharma V, Lagman M, Vyas S, Yang H, Li B & Suthanthiran M. (2003). Tacrolimus enhances transforming growth factor-β1 expression and promotes tumor progression. *Transplantation,* Vol. 76, No. 3, (August 2003), pp. (597-602).

Magee CC, Javeed Ansari M & Milford EL. (2008). Renal transplantation : clinical managemant. In: *Brenner & Rector's The Kidney,* Brenner BM, pp. (2138-2167), Saunders Elsevier, ISBN 978-1-4160-3105-5, Philadephia.

Mathew T, Kreis H, Friend P. (2004). Two-year incidence of malignancy in sirolimus-treated renal transplant recipients: results from five multicenter studies. *Clinical Transplant,* Vol. 18, No. 4, (Augustus 2004), pp. (446-449).

Matin RN, Mesher D, Proby CM, Mc Gregor JM, Bouwes Bavinck JN, der Marmol V, Euvrard S, Ferrandiz C, Geusau A, Hacketal M, Ho WL, Hofbauer GFL, Imko-Walczuk B, Kanitakis J, Lally A, Lear JT, Lebbe C, Murphy GM, Piaserico S, Seckin D, Stockfleth E, Ulrich C, Wojnarowska FT, Lin HY, Balch C & Harwood CA, on behalf of the Skin Care in Organ Transplant Patients Europe (SCOPE) group. (2008). Melanoma in organ transplant recipients: clinicopathological features and outcome in 100 cases. *American Journal of Transplantation,* Vol. 8, No. 9, (September 2008), pp. (1891-1900).

Morath C, Mueller M, Goldschmidt H, Schwenger V, Opelz G & Zeier M. (2004). Malignancy in renal transplantation. *Journal of the American Society of Nephrology,* Vol. 15, No. 6, (June 2004), pp. (1582-1588).

Opelz G & Henderson R. (1993). Incidence of non-Hodkin lymphoma in kindey and heart transplant recipients. *Lancet,* Vol. 342, No. 8886-8887, (December 1993), pp. (1514-1516).

Opelz G & Döhler B. (2003). Lymphomas after solid organ transplantation: a collaborative transplant study report. *American Journal of Transplantation,* Vol. 4, No. 2, (February 2003), pp. (222-230).

Otley CC, Stasko T, Tope WD & Lebwohl M. (2006). Chemoprevention of nonmelanoma skin cancer with systemic retinoids: practical dosing and management of adverse effects. *Dermatologic surgery,* Vol. 32, No. 4, (April 2006), pp. (562-568).

Perrett CM, Walker SL, O'Donovan P, Warwick J, Harwood CA, Karran P & Mc Gregor JM. (2008). Azathioprine treatment photosensitizes human skin to ultraviolet A radiation. *British Journal of Dermatology,* Vol. 159, No. 1, (July 2008), pp. (198-201).

Schena FP, Dascoe MD, Alberu J, del Carmen Rial M, Oberbauer R, Brennan DC, Campistol JM, Racusen L, Polinsky MS, Goldberg-Alberts R, Li H, Scarola J & Neylan JF for the Sirolimus CONVERT Trial Study Group. (2009) Conversion from calcineurin inhibitors to sirolimus maintenance therapy in renal allograft recipients: 24-month efficacy and safety results from the CONVERT trial. *Transplantation,* Vol. 87, No. 2, (January 2009), pp. (233-242).

Stallone G, Schena A, Infante B, Di Paolo S, Loverre A, Maggio G, Ranieri E, Gesualdo L, Schena FP, Grandaliano G. (2005). Sirolimus for Kaposi's sarcoma in renal-transplant recipients. *New England Journal of Medicine,* Vol. 352, No. 13, (March 2005), pp. (1317-23).

Vajdic CM, Mc Donald SP, McCredie MRE, van Leeuwen MT, Stewart JH, Law M, Chapman JR, Webster AC, Kaldor JM & Grulich AE. (2006). *Journal of the American Medical Association,* Vol. 296, No. 23, (December 2006), pp. 2823-2831.

Webster AC, Wong G, Craig JC & Chapman JR. (2008). Managing cancer risk and decision making after renal transplantation. *American Journal of Transplantation,* Vol. 8, No. 11, (November 2008), pp. (2185-91).

Zwald FO, Christenson LJ, Billingsley EM, Zeitouni NC, Ratner D, Bordeaux J, Patel MJ, Brown MD, Proby CM, Euvrard S, Otley CC & Stasko T for the Melanoma Working Group of The International Transplant Skin Cancer Collaborative (ITSCC) and Skin Care in Organ Transplant Patients, Europe (SCOPE).(2010). Melanoma in solid organ transplant recipients. *American Journal of Transplantation,* Vol. 10, No. 5, (May 2010), pp. (1297-1304).